WITHDRAWN
UTSA Libraries

RENEWALS 691-4574
DATE DUE

The Race Against Time

PSYCHOTHERAPY AND PSYCHOANALYSIS IN THE SECOND HALF OF LIFE

CRITICAL ISSUES IN PSYCHIATRY
An Educational Series for Residents and Clinicians

Series Editor: Sherwyn M. Woods, M.D., Ph.D.
University of Southern California School of Medicine
Los Angeles, California

Recent volumes in the series:

LAW IN THE PRACTICE OF PSYCHIATRY
Seymour L. Halleck, M.D.

NEUROPSYCHIATRIC FEATURES OF MEDICAL DISORDERS
James W. Jefferson, M.D., and John R. Marshall, M.D.

ADULT DEVELOPMENT: A New Dimension in Psychodynamic Theory
and Practice
Calvin A. Colarusso, M.D., and Robert A. Nemiroff, M.D.

SCHIZOPHRENIA
John S. Strauss, M.D., and William T. Carpenter, Jr., M.D.

EXTRAORDINARY DISORDERS OF HUMAN BEHAVIOR
Edited by Claude T. H. Friedmann, M.D., and Robert A. Faguet, M.D.

MARITAL THERAPY: A Combined Psychodynamic–Behavioral Approach
R. Taylor Segraves, M.D., Ph.D.

TREATMENT INTERVENTIONS IN HUMAN SEXUALITY
Edited by Carol C. Nadelson, M.D., and David B. Marcotte, M.D.

CLINICAL PERSPECTIVES ON THE SUPERVISION OF
PSYCHOANALYSIS AND PSYCHOTHERAPY
Edited by Leopold Caligor, Ph.D., Philip M. Bromberg, Ph.D.,
and James D. Meltzer, Ph.D.

MOOD DISORDERS: Toward a New Psychobiology
Peter C. Whybrow, M.D., Hagop S. Akiskal, M.D., and
William T. McKinney, Jr., M.D.

EMERGENCY PSYCHIATRY: Concepts, Methods, and Practices
Edited by Ellen L. Bassuk, M.D., and Ann W. Birk, Ph.D.

DRUG AND ALCOHOL ABUSE: A Clinical Guide to Diagnosis
and Treatment, Second Edition
Marc A. Schuckit, M.D.

THE RACE AGAINST TIME: Psychotherapy and Psychoanalysis
in the Second Half of Life
Robert A. Nemiroff, M.D., and Calvin A. Colarusso, M.D.

A Continuation Order Plan is available for this series. A continuation order will bring
delivery of each new volume immediately upon publication. Volumes are billed only
upon actual shipment. For further information please contact the publisher.

The Race Against Time

PSYCHOTHERAPY AND PSYCHOANALYSIS IN THE SECOND HALF OF LIFE

ROBERT A. NEMIROFF, M.D.
AND
CALVIN A. COLARUSSO, M.D.

University of California—San Diego
School of Medicine
La Jolla, California

PLENUM PRESS • NEW YORK AND LONDON

Library of Congress Cataloging in Publication Data

Main entry under title:

The Race against time.

(Critical issues in psychiatry)
Includes bibliographical references and index.
1. Aged—Mental health services. 2. Psychotherapy. 3. Psychoanalysis. I. Nemiroff,
Robert A. II. Colarusso, Calvin A. III. Series. [DNLM: 1. Psychoanalysis—in middle age. 2.
Psychoanalysis—in old age. 3. Psychotherapy—in middle age. 4. Psychotherapy—in old
age. WM 420 R118]
RC451.4.M54R33   1984   618.97′68914   84-17683
ISBN 0-306-41753-7

© 1985 Plenum Press, New York
A Division of Plenum Publishing Corporation
233 Spring Street, New York, N.Y. 10013

All rights reserved

No part of this book may be reproduced, stored in a retrieval system, or transmitted
in any form or by any means, electronic, mechanical, photocopying, microfilming,
recording, or otherwise, without written permission from the Publisher

Printed in the United States of America

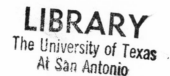

LIBRARY
The University of Texas
At San Antonio

Treasuring as we do the inspiration that their lives
provided for our own, we dedicate this book to Riva
Nemiroff, to the memory of George Nemiroff, and to
Sarah and Anthony Colarusso—our parents.

Robert A. Nemiroff, M.D.   Calvin A. Colarusso, M.D.

To everything there is a season, and a time to every purpose
  under heaven:
A time to be born, and a time to die;
A time to plant, and a time to pluck up that which is planted;
A time to kill, and a time to heal;
A time to break down, and a time to build up;
A time to weep, and a time to dance;
A time to cast away stones, and a time to gather stones
  together;
A time to embrace, and a time to lose;
A time to keep, and a time to cast away;
A time to rend, and a time to sew;
A time to keep silence, and a time to speak;
A time to love, and a time to hate;
A time for war, and a time for peace.

Ecclesiastes (Koheleth) 3: 1-8

Contributors

CLAIRE CATH, Department of Child Psychiatry, Tufts-New England Medical Center, Medford, Massachusetts

STANLEY H. CATH, Department of Psychiatry, Tufts University School of Medicine, Medford, Massachusetts

GENE D. COHEN, Department of Psychiatry, Georgetown University School of Medicine, Washington, D.C., and Program on Aging, National Institute of Mental Health, Bethesda, Maryland

JILL E. CRUSEY, Senior Medical Centers, San Diego, California

MARTIN GROTJAHN, Department of Psychiatry, University of Southern California, Los Angeles, California, and Southern California Psychoanalytic Society and Institute, Los Angeles, California

JOHN M. HASSLER, Department of Psychiatry, University of California at San Diego, La Jolla, California, and San Diego Psychoanalytic Institute, San Diego, California

H. P. HILDEBRAND, Department of Psychology, Brunel University, London, England, and Tavistock Clinic, London, England

RALPH J. KAHANA, Department of Psychiatry, Harvard Medical School, Cambridge, Massachusetts, and Beth Israel Hospital, Boston, Massachusetts

GARY A. LEVINSON, Department of Psychiatry, University of California at San Diego, La Jolla, California, and San Diego Psychoanalytic Institute, San Diego, California

ELI MILLER, Department of Psychiatry, University of California at San

Diego, La Jolla, California, and San Diego Psychoanalytic Institute, San Diego, California

MALKAH T. NOTMAN, Department of Psychiatry, Tufts University School of Medicine, Medford, Massachusetts

Foreword

This is the second book in the pioneering investigation of adult development by Robert A. Nemiroff and Calvin A. Colarusso. The first, *Adult Development: A New Dimension in Psychodynamic Theory and Practice*, arrived to critical acclaim in 1981. It presented a psychodynamic theory of development during the second half of life and a model of normal adult functioning. This book is the logical sequel, expanding and elaborating the original formulations and applying them to the clinical practice of psychotherapy and psychoanalysis. Nemiroff and Colarusso demonstrate that these are appropriate techniques for patients in the second half of life, regardless of age. They lay to rest many stereotypes and myths that have long interfered with the dynamic treatment of older patients, and they propose exciting new conceptualizations such as that of *adult developmental arrests*. The genetic approach reaches beyond childhood and adolescence and takes on important new meaning by incorporating an adult developmental past that influences both psychopathology and transference.

The relationship between theory and therapy is richly demonstrated in the clinical presentations, including ten detailed case histories of patients between the ages of 40 and 80. These and other clinical discussions provide ample evidence that a psychodynamic approach that is based on a sound adult developmental psychology can be extraordinarily effective. They also demonstrate both the similarities and differences in working with older versus younger patients.

This work is a major contribution in a long-neglected dimension of clinical psychiatry.

SHERWYN M. WOODS

Acknowledgments

The publication of any book is a collaborative effort, with contributions from many individuals. We feel particularly fortunate to have had the assistance of many highly knowledgeable, resourceful people, and we wish to acknowledge their significant contributions to *The Race Against Time*.

Sherwyn Woods, our editor, was immediately responsive to our wish to continue the exploration of the work begun in *Adult Development*. He has facilitated our efforts in every way and has made our work on *The Race Against Time* easy and enjoyable. The same may be said for our publisher, Plenum Press. We have had the very good fortune of working on both books with Hilary Evans, former senior editor at Plenum. Always, she cleared away any hurdles on the road from inception to finished product.

To establish the clinical focus of this book we needed detailed case histories, many more than we could provide from our own practices, so we approached our colleagues, some in San Diego, others elsewhere in the country, and one in England. We thank them, not only for their case histories but for their rich insights into development and patient care in the second half of life. We're sure the reader will share our appreciation of the contributions of Claire Cath, Stanley H. Cath, Gene D. Cohen, Jill E. Crusey, Martin Grotjahn, John M. Hassler, H. P. Hildebrand, Ralph J. Kahana, Gary A. Levinson, Eli Miller, and Malkah T. Notman. Special acknowledgment is given to Mary Jackuelyn Harris, who prepared an excellent survey of the literature for Chapter 2 while doing a psychiatric clerkship at the University of California, San Diego, School of Medicine.

We are fortunate to be associated with a university where our efforts are recognized and encouraged. We particularly wish to acknowledge the unfailing support and friendship of Lewis L. Judd, Professor and Chairman of the Department of Psychiatry at the University of California, San Diego.

Whenever our own writing efforts failed, our abilities in doubt, we turned for help to Barbara Wilkes Blomgren, a Senior Editor in the Department of Psychiatry at the University of California, San Diego; the cohesiveness of writing style is due to her efforts. We also acknowledge with gratitude the work of Maria Lofftus, Administrative Coordinator of the Residency Training Program, who graciously coordinated all aspects of manuscript preparation and myriad other tasks; Linda Greene and Yvonne Coleman who did a splendid typing job; and Julie Nemiroff who gave precious vacation time for library research.

Last but certainly not least, we thank our families, particularly our wives, Barbara Nemiroff and Jean Colarusso, for not begrudging the time spent in writing and for putting up with endless dirty cups and eraser crumbs on their dining room tables.

ROBERT A. NEMIROFF
CALVIN A. COLARUSSO

Contents

Introduction
AN OVERVIEW

ROBERT A. NEMIROFF AND CALVIN A. COLARUSSO

> Ay, note that Potter's wheel,
> That metaphor! and feel
> Why time spins fast, why passive lies our clay,—
> Thou, to whom fools propound,
> When the wine makes its round,
> "Since life fleets, all is change; the Past gone, seize to-day!"

> Robert Browning (1812–1889), *Rabbi Ben Ezra*

America is growing older. The latest census bureau information reveals that half of all Americans are now 30 or older. There are now 25.5 million people over 65 years old, 28% more than in 1970. Furthermore, the statistics portend a sharply rising median age over the next three decades. It is essential for the mental health profession to develop treatment strategies and respond to the needs of older patients. Ironically, there is probably no area in psychiatry and psychoanalysis in which there has been more misinformation, inconsistency, and stereotyping than in the treatment of the patient over 40.

In *Adult Development: A New Dimension in Psychodynamic Theory and Practice* (New York: Plenum Press, 1981), we presented a model of normal adult functioning and began to formulate a psychodynamic theory of development during the second half of life. Now in *The Race Against Time: Psychotherapy and Psychoanalysis in the Second Half of Life*, we expand on the model by presenting additional theoretical concepts, but our pri-

1

mary intent, aided by clinical contributions from 11 sensitive, experienced therapists, is to apply these ideas to the clinical situation. This is accomplished through the presentation of detailed case histories of psychotherapy and psychoanalysis of individuals from the ages of 40 through 80, followed by discussions by the primary authors (in Part II) and the therapists themselves (Parts II and III).

We hope this book will provide the therapist who is interested in working with older patients with a rich source of clinical data. We are not aware of another volume that collects as many detailed case histories and clinical approaches in one place. Throughout the book we and our collaborators have tried to define those specific therapeutic concepts and techniques that are relevant for work with older patients. The final chapter collects these major themes and ideas and relates them to the clinical material presented earlier. Whenever possible, technical concepts are enhanced by clinical illustration. As is always the case in clinical research, the clinical material itself becomes the raw data for further theory formation.

Based on current and past research, it is our conclusion that psychodynamically oriented psychotherapy and psychoanalyses are valid clinical techniques for selected patients in the second half of life, regardless of age.

To assist the reader in using this volume most effectively, what follows is a brief delineation of the organization of the book and some of the major ideas presented in each of the three main sections.

PART I

This book is a logical outgrowth of the ideas presented in *Adult Development*, and Chapter 1 is a review of that work. We encourage the reader who has the time and interest to read *Adult Development* before beginning *The Race Against Time*.

Chapter 2 is a selected review of heretofore largely neglected literature on psychotherapy and psychoanalysis with older patients. It begins with a consideration of the persistent stereotypes, barriers, and obstacles that interfere with effective work with older patients. Some of the avoidance of patients in this age group may be related to Freud's pessimism about the suitability for psychoanalysis of patients over 40—an attitude that is widely accepted today despite the later optimism of Abraham and Jung and the presence in more recent decades of proponents of both supportive and explorative approaches.

The reader may be particularly interested in the work of Butler and Lewis on the life review and adaptive value of reminiscence and Alvin Goldfarb's technique of working with dependency needs in very sick older patients. Also, Ralph J. Kahana, a contributor to this book, presents a very useful classification of patients into (a) those who are aging normally; (b) an intermediate group; and (c) those who are debilitated—primarily brain damaged. Most of the patients described in this book, primarily those who are suitable for dynamic work, fall into groups a and b.

A thorough diagnostic evaluation is the beginning of sound clinical intervention. In Chapter 3 we describe how the diagnostic process is altered by adult developmental concepts, particularly the taking of a developmental history of the life cycle, and we suggest that the therapist of older patients should have a working knowledge of adult developmental lines.

The concept of developmental arrest is well accepted in child analysis. Either through fixation and/or regression, a child's progression along a developmental line may be arrested. Because adult development consists of new phase-specific developmental tasks and intrapsychic conflict related to those developmental processes, we suggest that fixation and/or regression can also occur in adulthood, leading to adult developmental arrest, a new psychopathological concept proposed here for the first time and illustrated by clinical examples.

This idea suggests a new emphasis on the adult past. In an open-ended view of development, the genetic approach takes on a longitudinal perspective, incorporating experiences from adult developmental phases as well as from childhood. This has particularly important implications for transference, the subject of Chapter 4. There we suggest that, in addition to being elaborations of infantile experience, transference expressions in adults also reflect experiences and conflicts from developmental stages beyond childhood and the continuation of central developmental themes from childhood into adulthood. All three factors are represented by a psychic structure that is very different from that of childhood and that is continually undergoing refinement, regardless of the age of the patient. The clearest example of transference with roots in adulthood as well as childhood is multigenerational transference in which the patient treats the therapist as a son or daughter, bringing into the treatment unconscious attitudes and conflicts related to past experience as a parent. Particularly clear examples are found in Chapters 8 and 9.

Chapter 5, which deals with friendship in midlife, is a continuation of our efforts to formulate a psychodynamic theory of normal adult development. The literature on this perhaps most common human relationship is very sparse. We focus on two themes: (1) an exploration of the developmental forces that shape normal midlife friendships (which we feel are qualitatively different from earlier friendships), and (2) the effect of the therapist's work on his or her own friendships—particularly with colleagues and students.

PART II

Part II consists of five detailed case histories of patients between the ages of 40 and 80, described by five talented psychotherapists and psychoanalysts. Each is followed by our discussion. Our intent is a convincing demonstration of the following:

1. The nature of developmental processes in the second half of life
2. The vitality and resourcefulness of the human mind in regard to sexual and aggressive impulses and the capacity for introspection and self-analysis
3. The variety of diagnostic and therapeutic techniques usable with older patients, from psychoanalysis to a wide range of supportive techniques
4. The effect on therapists due to working with older patients. Creativity and flexibility are much in evidence in these case histories as is a striking degree of honesty about transference and countertransference reactions.

Each chapter contains myriad fascinating points, but it may be of interest to the reader to consider the following ideas. In "Turning Forty in Analysis" (Chapter 6), we are given the opportunity to study, through the high-powered microscope of psychoanalysis, the intrapsychic responses of a man and his analyst, John Hassler, to that critical demarcator of midlife, turning 40. The power of the universal midlife preoccupation with the developmental task of time limitation and personal death—and the strong defensive reactions against it—are presented in bold relief.

In Chapter 7, "The Development of Intimacy at Age Fifty," Eli Miller describes his psychoanalytic work with a man of 50 who had never achieved a meaningful relationship with a woman. The therapeutic results combat the notion that little can be done with long-standing, deeply entrenched inhibitions and character patterns. After reading this case report, therapists may be more inclined to consider doing dynamic therapy with patients whom they previously considered unsuitable.

Many younger therapists are intimidated by the prospect of treating individuals old enough to be their parents, particularly when such patients are of the opposite sex. Because of the honesty and forthrightness of therapists such as Jill E. Crusey, we are beginning to understand why. In Chapter 8, "Short-Term Psychodynamic Psychotherapy with a Sixty-Two-Year-Old Man," we see how quickly a powerful sexual transference can emerge, igniting equally forceful countertransference responses. For both patient and therapist, these feelings seem particularly inappropriate because the external reality mirrors the incestuous nature of the infantile wishes. We consider the exploration of the therapeutic processes involved in the treatment of older patients by considerably younger therapists to be an important frontier because the number of these interactions will undoubtedly increase in the future as the population ages and dynamic treatment for these age groups becomes commonplace.

One of the most intriguing chapters in this book is "New Beginnings at Seventy: A Decade of Psychotherapy in Late Adulthood" (Chapter 9) by Gary A. Levinson. On a weekly basis, using a combination of introspective and supportive approaches, Levinson dealt with extremely complex organic, psychological, and environmental factors that would have caused many therapists to throw up their hands in dismay. Levinson's work convincingly demonstrates a basic tenet of this book: When the therapist has an understanding of adult developmental processes and a deep respect for the developmental potential of his or her patient, regardless of age, remarkable therapeutic results can be achieved.

Gene D. Cohen certainly approached his patient with the deepest respect. In Chapter 10, "Psychotherapy with an Eighty-Year-Old Woman," he demonstrates how therapeutic acumen and openmindedness about developmental processes can lead to new and enriching work and interpersonal experience for a patient in late adulthood. We refer to Chapter 2 where it is demonstrated that there is avoidance of elderly patients by therapists because of fear that the patients may become debilitated or die. It is our thought that the therapist of the elderly should expect such an unfortunate eventuality and include as part of his therapeutic task helping the patient to adjust to the effects of a major illness or to prepare for death. In one of the most poignant vignettes in *The Race Against Time,* Cohen describes innovative interventions with his patient and the hospital staff after the patient suffered a stroke that left her demented.

PART III

Part III consists of a series of chapters by senior therapists who use clinical material to illustrate and underscore aspects of development in later life, particularly the loss of significant object ties. Then, Martin Grotjahn describes his own experience with illness and approaching death. In the final chapter, we summarize many of the ideas presented earlier with particular reference to treatment strategies.

In Chapter 11, "Object Loss and Development in the Second Half of Life," H. P. Hildebrand differentiates between patients who responded successfully to psychotherapy and to a second subgroup, identified for the first time, who did not (i.e., older patients who had the misfortune to lose an adult child through accident or illness). Hildebrand also presents the hypotheses that primal scene material in older patients may not only refer to parental intercourse but also to the problem that those in the second half of life have in facing their own death or the death of a spouse. This is illustrative of our thinking in *Adult Development* where we stressed that central developmental themes from childhood continue to play a critical intrapsychic role in the second half of life, which is often expressed through new phase-specific adult developmental issues and conflicts.

Loss of a spouse is considered in Chapters 11 and 12: "When a Husband Dies" by Malkah T. Notman and "When a Wife Dies" by Stanley H. and Claire Cath. Notman's patient came for treatment after a malignancy was discovered in her husband. She had been very dependent on him, and both she and her family feared the effect of his loss on her. Not only did the patient prepare for her spouse's demise, she also transformed their relationship prior to his death into one of rich emotional interaction and mutuality. Notman expresses surprise that so much change could be accomplished with so little therapeutic effort, pointing again to the exciting and rewarding experience awaiting the therapist of the elderly.

But such work is not always easy or without considerable emotional consequence for the therapist. Stanley H. Cath used the technique of conjoint therapeutic alliance to help him and his patient deal with the inevitable death of the patient's wife from a metastatic malignancy. The technique of involving Claire Cath in the treatment process was not only useful to the patient and his wife; it helped Cath deal with the overwhelmingly complex countertransference race against therapeutic time. His flexibility in devising this new technique is but one of many examples of therapeutic ingeniousness in this collection of contributions.

As he deals with aging in relation to work and gratification, Ralph J. Kahana (Chapter 14) compares his therapeutic experiences with two men and uses the clinical material as a springboard to discuss the psychopathology of work and play, the relationship between childhood experience and adult functioning, the aims and strategies of dynamic psychotherapy with older patients, transference and countertransference responses, and therapeutic outcome. In addition to this clinical and theoretical contribution, we are indebted to Kahana for his other writings on psychiatry and the elderly that we discuss in Chapters 2 and 16.

The final contribution (Chapter 15) differs from all the others in that the author is both therapist and "patient." In a moving, often painfully honest commentary on "Being Sick and Facing Eighty," Martin Grotjahn brings us face-to-face with a critical and universal developmental task of the second half of life—facing personal death. In commenting on his failing health, thoughts about death, and the demise of many friends, he shares the richness of his family relationships and dignifies life for us all. In discussing the role of time limitation and personal death as a stimulus to *forward* development in *Adult Development* we said: "Confronting this quintessential experience can lead to ego functioning and integration of the highest order and produce the profoundest awareness of what it means to be human" (p. 77). Here is an eloquent statement of such awareness.

In our summation for *The Race Against Time*, we try to integrate the existing literature with the rich clinical and theoretical contributions of our collaborators and our own work to delineate some of the central issues in doing effective work with middle-aged and elderly patients. These are subdivided into the following:

1. The importance of a developmental orientation
2. The role of bodily changes in the psychology of adults
3. Sexual myths about the elderly and their effect on therapy

4. The nature of transference and countertransference in the second half of life, similarities and differences from earlier versions
5. The significance of limited object ties, therapeutic termination, and thoughts about death

As the reader turns to subsequent chapters we hope that he or she will recognize the power and usefulness of the developmental orientation for day-to-day work with patients. In *Adult Development* we described the study of developmental processes in adulthood as a psychiatric frontier. In this second book, we have taken another step into the wilderness by focusing on the relationships between theory and clinical practice. Despite the best efforts of those of us interested in adult development, our vision is limited, and our tools are rudimentary. Much remains to be done if we are to deepen our understanding of our patients and ourselves to further enrich their lives and our own.

I

New Concepts in Adult Development

Midway in the journey of our life I found myself in a dark wood, for the straight way was lost. Ah, how hard it is to tell what the wood was, wild, rugged, harsh, the very thought of it renews the fear! It is so bitter that death is hardly more so. But, to treat of the good that I found in it, I will tell of the other things I saw there.

Dante (1265–1321), *The Divine Comedy*

1

A Review of
Adult Development

ROBERT A. NEMIROFF AND CALVIN A. COLARUSSO

A concise reprise of the themes from our earlier book, *Adult Development: A New Dimension in Psychodynamic Theory and Practice* (Colarusso & Nemiroff, 1981), will provide a context for the material contained in this volume.

There is little new under the sun when the subject is man himself, so it is not surprising that the myths, religions, and literatures of ancient civilizations contained thoughtful, rather sophisticated ideas about the life course. For example, in Greece in the sixth century B.C., Solon described six periods of adulthood and assigned to each appropriate developmental tasks like learning to use one's capacities to the fullest or becoming a husband and father. In the following century, Plato described the truly educated man, the philosopher, as using enlightened reason to contemplate the realities of human life and the reasons for his existence, that is, his place in life and death (Erikson, 1978). On the other side of the world, Confucius described how, at 15, he had set his heart upon learning; by 30, he had planted his feet firmly on the ground; by 40 he no longer suffered from perplexities; at 50 he knew the biddings of heaven; and at 60 he allowed himself to follow the dictates of his heart because he no longer wished to overstep the boundaries of right. Central to the Confucian concept of adulthood is the metaphor of "the way," a sense of inner direction that ever guides the individual toward increased self-awareness and realization. Concerns with time, age, and change pervaded ancient Japanese thought as well. There, adulthood

11

was construed as a time of life requiring effort and attention as the individual strives to become freer and freer of the "self," to gain eventually the highly respected wisdom of old age.

The relevant basic themes we found in ancient writings can be summarized as follows:

1. A comprehensive, chronological life cycle can be described.
2. Adulthood is not static; the adult is in a constant state of dynamic change and flux, always "becoming" or "finding the way."
3. Development in adulthood is contiguous with that in childhood and old age.
4. There is continual need to define the adult self, especially with regard to the integrity of the inner person versus his or her external environment.
5. Adults must come to terms with their limited span and individual mortality. A preoccupation with time is an expression of these concerns.
6. The development and maintenance of the adult body and its relationship to the mind is a universal preoccupation.
7. Narcissism, that is, love of self, versus responsibility to the society in which one lives and the individuals in that society toward whom one bears responsibility as an adult, is a central issue in all civilized cultures.

THE PIONEER ADULT DEVELOPMENTALISTS

The scientific study of adulthood is essentially a phenomenon of this century, stimulated by the writings of four men: Arnold Van Gennep, Sigmund Freud, Carl Gustav Jung, and Erik H. Erikson. Van Gennep originally published his landmark monograph *The Rites of Passage* in 1908. In it he described the importance and meaning of the rituals surrounding such events as pregnancy and childbirth, menarche, betrothal and marriage, and death. His ideas are implicitly developmental and speak to the universal character of the process. He wrote:

> The life of an individual in any society is a series of passages from one age to another.... A man's life comes to be made up of a succession of stages with similar ends and beginnings.... For every one of these events there are ceremonies whose essential purpose is to enable the individual to pass from one defined position to another which is equally well defined. (1908/1960, p. 203)

For Sigmund Freud, who formulated the first modern systematic theory for the child's development, development was seen as the result of the interaction between maturational (biological) emergence and environmental stimulation. Intrinsic to the predictable developmental progression were basic transformations, regressions and advances. Following Freud, Rene Spitz (1965, p. 5) defined development as "the emergence of forms, of function, and of behavior which are the outcome of exchanges between the organism on one hand, the inner and outer environment on the other." That is the definition we have adopted. The concept of interlocking stages in the life cycle, incorporating the numerous sketchy, still-controversial stages of adulthood follows directly upon Freud's familiar oral, anal, oedipal, latency, and adolescent stages of childhood.

The particularly *adult* developmentalist among the early psychoanalysts was Jung, whose interest in the second half of life is evident in most of his writings. He described a continuing process of physical and psychological separation from parents occurring in the 20s and 30s and viewed age 40 as a time of significant psychological change, growth, and transition. Presaging the work of cultural anthropologist David Guttman, Jung described how men in their 40s become more aware of the "feminine" side of themselves and women become more comfortable with the "masculine" aspects of their personalities. The archetypes *puer* (young) and *senex* (old) that Jung saw as fundamental polarities in each stage of life also find echoes among modern adult developmentalists (e.g., Levinson, Darrow, Klein, Levinson, & McKee, 1978).

The fourth major pioneer, Erik Erikson (1963), provided the first integrated psychosocial view of individual development through eight stages from birth to death. For us, as for him, development lies not in stability *per se* but in the changes necessary to transcend successive contradictions, conflicts, and states of disequilibrium. In a sense, all modern developmentalists are mining the claims staked out originally by Erikson.

Contemporary Adult Developmentalists

Much of the current interest in the nature of development in the second half of life was spurred by the almost simultaneous publication of three seminal books in the late 1970s: *The Seasons of a Man's Life* by Daniel Levinson and his associates at Yale (1978); *Adaptation to Life* by George

Vaillant of Harvard (1977); and *Transformations* by Roger Gould of the University of California at Los Angeles (1978). The three books share the same aim—exploration of the developmental process in the adult, but they differ in their approaches and methods.

Levinson and his associates studied 40 men between the ages of 35 and 40. From detailed interviews they constructed biographies from which they drew generalizations. Their psychosocial theory proposes a life cycle consisting of distinctive, identifiable eras of approximately 20 years, extending from birth to death and encompassing the evolution of a *life structure*, "the underlying design of the person's life at a given time...a patterning of self-in-world [which] requires us to take into account both self and world" (Newton & Levinson, 1979, p. 488). In systematic sequential *alternation*, stable periods of 6–7 years are followed by transition intervals of 4–5 years, each with its tasks to be met and mastered. We find the concept of stable periods followed by transitional phases very useful theoretically and clinically. Indeed, many of our patients, particularly the healthier ones, seem to alternate between such stable and transitional periods, and internal conflict during the transitional epochs was for many an impetus for seeking treatment.

The Harvard Grant Study has followed longitudinally the life courses of 268 undergraduate students from 1939 to the present. The current director, George Vaillant, has used these data to study adaptation in adulthood, particularly in terms of ego mechanisms of defense. His work illuminates the developmental nature of intrapsychic processes in the adult. The psychologically healthier members of the research sample used mature defenses much more frequently in midlife than they had in late adolescence and young adulthood. In agreement with all other major dynamic theories, Vaillant found conflict an integral, inescapable aspect of normal development.

In *Transformations: Growth and Change in Adult Life* (1978), Roger Gould explored the effects of childhood experience on adult development. He postulated four assumptions made by children that project the illusion of absolute safety (1978, p. 39): (1) "We'll always live with our parents and be their child"; (2) "They'll always be there to help when we can't do something on our own"; (3) "Their simplified version of our complicated inner reality is correct, as when they turn the light on in our bedroom to prove there are no ghosts"; and (4) "There is no real death or evil in the world." By the end of childhood these assumptions are abandoned intellectually, but they continue to have powerful influence emotionally. Gould concluded that adult consciousness emerges from challenging and mastering these false assumptions. If they are not abandoned emotionally, their protective nature impedes the risk taking necessary for emancipation, and the result is stagnation.

Part II of *Adult Development* contains a series of new concepts about various aspects of normal and pathological development in adulthood: hypotheses about the psychodynamic theory of adult development; narcissism in the adult development of the self; myths about the aging body; the father at midlife; and female midlife issues. We shall be referring frequently to those concepts as we try to integrate the ideas there with the focus on clinical theory and practice in *The Race Against Time*. For the reader who does not have available a copy of *Adult Development*, we will reiterate the concepts briefly.

BASIC HYPOTHESES

To lay a broad theoretical foundation for adult development, we postulated seven hypotheses. Hypothesis I asserts that the nature of the developmental processes is basically the same in the adult as in the child. Accepting Rene Spitz's definition of development mentioned earlier, we disputed the common idea that, compared to the child, the adult is relatively free from environmental influences. We suggested instead that for the achievement of new and phase-specific developmental tasks in adulthood, the individual is as dependent as is the child on the environment. In Hypothesis II, in contradistinction to the notion that the adult is a finished product, we suggested that development during the adult years is an ongoing, dynamic process. To differentiate child from adult development, we proposed in Hypothesis III that, whereas child development is focused primarily on the formation of psychic structure, adult development is concerned with the continuing evolution of existing psychic structure and with its use. Hypothesis IV deals with the relationship between childhood and adulthood, positing a continuous, vital interaction—the fundamental issues of childhood continuing in altered form as central aspects of adult life. In our opinion, attempts to explain all adult behavior and psychopathology in terms of childhood events is reductionistic. We proposed in Hypothesis V that developmental processes in adults are influenced by the adult past as well as childhood. Freud (1915a) emphasized the influence of the body on mental development in childhood and adolescence, but for some unaccountable reason he virtually ignored the body after that until dealing with the climacteric and old age. Our Hypothesis VI speaks to the effects of physical processes on psychological expression after adolescence and to the profound influences of the body and physical changes on development in adulthood. Finally, with Hypothesis VII, we addressed a paramount issue affecting the developmental process in the second half of life; namely, the growing awareness of death, suggesting that a central, phase-specific theme of adult development is a normative crisis precipitated by the recognition and acceptance of the finiteness of time and the inevitability of personal death. Physical signs of aging, the deaths of parents and friends, the maturing of children, and the growing understanding that not all one's life goals will be realized force upon the adult in middle age an unwanted awareness of temporal limitation that clashes with the "unmistakable tendency to put death to one side, to eliminate it from life" (Freud, 1915b, p. 289). We see this conflict as universal, containing within it the possibility of developmental progression or regression and arrest. As the clinical material throughout this book will attest, older patients—and therapists—almost inevitably become preoccupied with this central issue.

NARCISSISM AT MIDLIFE

A chapter of *Adult Development* is devoted to narcissistic features of normal and pathological development in adulthood. Under normal circumstances, people's interests are divided between concern for themselves (narcissism) and for the world of things and people around them (object love) (Moore & Fine, 1968, p. 62). We contended that it is not enough to resolve the narcissistic issues of early life because forces that modify the adult self are also fueled by narcissistic gratifications and disappointments. As the adult matures and engages life in all its ramifications, he or she develops *authenticity;* that is,

> a sense of intrapsychic recognition that one is singular (separated psychologically from parents, yet interdependent with important people in the present) and capable of making and accepting a realistic appraisal of living, including suffering, limitation, and personal death. Authenticity, therefore, includes the capacity to assess and accept what is real in both the external and internal worlds, regardless of the narcissistic injury involved. (Colarusso & Nemiroff, 1981, p. 86)

We proceeded to deal with narcissistic issues surrounding, in particular, the aging body, relationships, time and death, and work, creativity, and mentorship as they are manifested in the dynamic evolution of the self in adulthood.

For example, midlife brings conflict between wishes to deny physical aging and the need to accept loss of one's youthful body. Resolution of this normative conflict leads to reshaping of the body image and a more realistic appraisal of the middle-aged body, yielding heightened appreciation of the pleasures it can continue to provide if it is cared for appropriately. Similar conflict, narcissistic injury, and potential for developmental progression and further individuation versus stagnation and arrest are built into the constantly changing relationships with aging parents and grandparents, spouse, children, and mentees.

Time sense in childhood is mostly gratifying because the future seems unlimited. By midlife, time becomes a source of pain because of the growing realization that there is not enough of it left to allow the gratification of all wishes. This pain stimulates a reworking of attitudes toward time. The mature, authentic individual views his or her personal past with a minimum of denial and distortion; there is a strong sense of the present, a willingness to live life *now*, and ambivalence toward the future because it holds both the promise of additional pleasure and the inevitable end of all gratification through death.

THE AGING BODY

To understand better the influence of normal physical aging on psychological development in the second half of life, we undertook a computer-assisted survey of the medical and psychological literature on the normal functioning of the adult body and brain over time. The findings led to a chapter titled "Myths about the Aging Body" because many of the popular concepts about the brain and mental functioning in midlife and later life now appear to be erroneous. For example, many authors contest the notion that diminished estrogen and testosterone production is primarily responsible for decline in sexual functioning in the elderly, noting instead the importance of individual psychological factors, cultural attitudes, and availability of partners. Studies indicate that intelligence does not inevitably decline from the mid 20s on (Wechsler, 1941), but that in the presence of physical health and mental activity intelligence actually increases in most individuals into their 80s (Jarvik, 1973). Essentially, the adult brain is now seen as capable of structural modification resulting from psychological stimulation and activity; thus, modern research attests to the complexity of the body–mind interface and promises much potential for growth and change in the second half of life.

Most individuals do not experience a full-blown midlife "crisis." Rather, they engage in midlife transitions that are nevertheless often all encompassing and profound. In *Adult Development*, by comparing the myth and the reality of the life of the painter Paul Gauguin, we illustrated the tendency to simplify and romanticize midlife change and crisis in an attempt to avoid changes and the real adaptive work that must attend.

During the midlife transition an individual confronts versions of the following questions: Is this all there is in life? (I want more!) Have I accomplished anything significant? Will anyone remember me when I'm dead? Where has my time gone? Such questions express the normative conflict experienced by many healthy individuals who indeed are leading successful, responsible lives as they reassess and monitor the continuing changes taking place in their bodies, time perception, careers, relationships, and social and financial statuses. For most, the psychic pain involved in the midlife transition is suffered silently, in part because of the common idea that such thoughts and feelings are idiosyncratic and immature. Equally important, when internal resolution does lead to external change in such basic structures of life as marriage or career, the action is usually reasoned and considered. By contrast, a true midlife "crisis" is a major, revolutionary turning point that usually involves great emotional turmoil, significant symptomatology, and abrupt, pressured actions that disrupt long-standing patterns and relationships without a clear purpose.

SEXUAL INFLUENCES

In relation to the influence of gender on adult development, we described midlife (35–55 years) as a particularly formative time in the evolution of paternal identity for a man because of unique phase-specific interactions between issues of his own development and that of his adolescent children. Although everyone agrees that middle-aged parents react strongly to their adolescent children and that parental behavior is not simply a reaction to the adolescent but is also the result of equally or more salient developmental forces within the parent that are impinged upon by the adolescent, this is not widely appreciated. Adolescent children have youthful bodies, abundant futures, and many major life experiences ahead of them, all of which can produce awe and envy in a father who must, for instance, deal with his sexual responses to a maturing daughter, compete for her with boyfriends and suitors, and eventually watch her choose another and leave. With his son he must struggle against feelings of envy toward his youthful body, sexual wishes toward his girlfriends, and gradual abandonment of a position of dominance and control over another male. As his adolescent children mature, a father begins to contemplate grandfatherhood, anticipation of which can be a major stimulus to healthy psychic reorganization because it touches on many basic developmental themes: a kind of immortality through the narcissistically gratifying identification of one's genetic characteristics in children and grandchildren; the likelihood of recapturing the unqualified admiration and love of young children that are lost in the more realistic appraisals made by older ones; the reaffirmation of sexuality through the fertility of offspring; and the prospect of "spoiling" the grandchildren—the fantasized expression of impulses without restraint—that, through identification, applies to the self as well.

Many middle-aged women experience more painful, prolonged preoccupation with the physical signs of aging than do middle-aged men because prevailing sociocultural views equate female sexual desirability with a youthful body. Fears of being unsexed by age and losing love as a consequence are compensated for by success in roles as wife and mother. The menopausal experience used to be thought of as the dominant factor in the psychology of women and as an entirely negative experience representing the loss of procreativity. Within a broader conceptualization of midlife, the menopause becomes one of several important developmental experiences and not strictly a negative one. For many women, the sense of loss accompanying the cessation of menses is transcended by excitement about the future and a feeling of being "restored to themselves," free to pursue their own development rather than incessantly caring for the needs of others.

The middle-aged woman must reshape her relationships with parents, now older and dependent; a middle-aged husband, no longer idealized or exotic; and her children, who are establishing themselves as relatively independent individuals. Because of her deep involvement with them, she may experience increasing distance from her children as a loss akin to a death. The deaths of parents, particularly the mother, also emphasize the passage of time as well as the inevitability of personal death. A woman's sense of time is also influenced by what Neugarten (1973) calls the socially defined sense of time—the temporal appropriateness of major events of life—that is based on a male, not a female, life cycle, particularly in regard to career achievement. Work is a complex function that gives expression to erotic, narcissistic, and aggressive needs and impulses. Because society tends to relate achievement and success to paid employment, many women discount the value of their familial roles. Work outside the home is potentially more laden with conflict for women than for men because of their ambivalence about efforts to realize unfulfilled goals and values, to achieve increased status and self-esteem from a socioculturally valued role, and to adapt to and deal with age-related issues.

In response to the questions most commonly raised about development, we have made the following generalizations: Everyone must go through a life cycle based on such universal experiences as interactions between psyche and soma, maturational sequence, relationships to family and society, and aging and death. There is, however, a wide "normal" variation within these universals. *Normal* is a relative term encompassing mental activity and behavior that, based on current knowledge, fall within the broad range of predictable expectation, fulfill development potential, and are adaptive to the society in which they occur. Development is clearly a cross-cultural phenomenon and one that cuts across classes as well. In addition, it is strongly affected by changing social patterns, a fact indicating the need to study, conceptualize, and describe the effects upon the developmental process of such alternative life structures as the single state, divorce, widowhood, and homosexuality, in all of which one of the two major forces that shape development—the environment—is undergoing significant change. For those who choose to study the adult, these changes require new attitudes, an open-minded recognition of the limitations of our knowledge, and the evaluation of theories that take into account the actualities of how people live and behave.

CLINICAL APPLICATIONS

Part III of *Adult Development* in particular serves as an introduction to *The Race Against Time* because it deals with the application of theoretical concepts to the clinical situation. In it, we described the diagnostic procedures as elaborated by adult developmental concepts and suggested a comprehensive approach to the developmental history for the adult. Elaborations of those ideas and clinical applications are highlighted in

Chapters 3 and 6 through 9 of this volume. Recognition that the fundamental developmental issues of childhood continue as central aspects of adult life focuses the therapist's attention on three goals: (1) defining the relationships between infantile experience and adult symptoms; (2) elaborating the effects of the infantile experience on all subsequent developmental tasks, from childhood to adult; and (3) relating the insights to current, phase-specific arrests in development, leading to a reengagement of the adult developmental process.

The adult developmental orientation has implications also for other features of the treatment process such as free association, the working alliance, outside motivation and information, transference and countertransference, resistance, reconstruction, and termination.

It is assumed, often wrongly, that an adult patient can free associate readily. Actually, the process must be *learned* as treatment progresses, and when both patient and therapist understand that, neither is likely to become frustrated. A similar line of thought applies to the *working alliance*. It is not reasonable to expect that adult or child comes to treatment able to enter immediately into a smooth, effective therapeutic relationship. The speed with which a working alliance develops is related to the attainment of maturity along the developmental line of caring for the self. Usually, with neurotic patients, most aspects of the alliance are understood and integrated during the opening phase of treatment. However, with narcissistic and borderline patients, because of their severe problems with trust and other aspects of object relations, such integration may never be achieved.

Morton Shane (1977) suggests that the therapist pay attention to the effect of treatment on other developmental themes and relationships. For example, if marriage is understood as a process leading to increased capacity for intimacy, it is easier to empathize with a spouse who views therapy as a threat rather than an advantage. If the developmental aspects of the marriage are kept in mind, the therapist will be better able to assess the effect on the therapeutic process of outside motivation and outside information if he or she should meet the patient's spouse.

Transference is so important that we devote Chapter 4 to it in *The Race Against Time*, and several of the ideas elaborated there were first suggested in *Adult Development*, among them the effects of the adult past, influence of current relationships with parents, and use of the therapist as a transference object in ways that are not possible for young patients. In a similar way, *countertransference* reactions are seen as complex and multilayered and thus difficult to eradicate by single acts of self-analysis.

Through continual self-assessment, the therapist can understand better the developmental processes at work in both the patient and himself or herself and the interactions between the two. George Vaillant's (1977) construction of a developmental line for the *mechanisms of defense* can be of great help to the therapist in deciding what to interpret and when. In essence, phase-appropriate defenses are interpreted less often than are more primitive and maladaptive ones. Likewise, knowledge of adult development helps distinguish between *resistance* emanating from the therapeutic process and *avoidance* that is related to normative and timely developmental conflict.

The nature of the *reconstructions* that the therapist presents depends to a degree on the depth of his or her understanding of normal developmental processes. Once a reconstruction has been presented, its effect should reverberate throughout the patient's understanding of himself or herself as the new insight is applied to all phases of his or her life, providing a sense of continuity between past and present.

Among the criteria commonly used to determine readiness for *termination* are symptom relief, structural change, transference resolution, and improvement in self-esteem. Agreeing with the Report of the Conference on Psychoanalytic Education and Research (COPER), Commission IX (1974), we suggest that the resumption of normal development is a broader notion underlying and incorporating those criteria. Because the resumption of normal development is the overriding goal of therapy and normative crises and because transitions are to be expected in the future, both therapist and patient know that termination is flexible and open ended; it is the door to the consulting room left ajar. Neither patient nor therapist expects a perfect result from their collaboration but an increased ability to explore the external and internal worlds—in other words, to continue to grow.

Midlife developmental pressures can influence the onset and course of symptoms, and we discussed in *Adult Development* an approach to hysterical psychopathology in particular. During the middle years, individuals experience a need to act when confronted with the finiteness of their existence. The style of one's cognition dictates whether that experience occurs consciously or unconsciously. By definition, hysterical character defenses push ego-dystonic thoughts out of consciousness. For some, midlife provides a new freedom, another chance. Aspirations once postponed can now be pursued. Often, however, rationalizations for inactivity that have protected the ego from loss of self-esteem are dissolved by reality, and midlife development itself results in new stress that upsets established defenses and elicits more neurotic defensive operations.

The final chapter of *Adult Development* considered the implications of this orientation for the educational process, and we commented on the objectives in teaching developmental theory to mental health students, the developmental experiences of those students, the relationship between the student-therapist and supervisor, and two sample courses.

The objectives in teaching developmental theory are (1) to present the theory of the normal life cycle; (2) to relate developmental concepts to psychopathology, diagnosis, and treatment; (3) to use developmental concepts in curriculum planning and teaching; (4) to encourage research and writing about developmental concepts; and (5) to further the development of each student to its fullest.

In candidate selection, particular attention should be paid to those developmental lines that lead to the emergence of object relatedness and empathy, which are prerequisites for a psychotherapist. By tracing the developmental line of work identity, career choices can be validated or not in light of current objectives. It will be recognized that professional progress occurs at highly individual rates and is subject to regression and fixation. Further graduate and postgraduate education has a significant influence, which is not always positive, on other young adult developmental tasks such as intimacy and parenthood.

The teacher is emerging as the student is learning, and the transition to the role of teacher is an essential part of training. Becoming a therapist requires that the individual use himself or herself as the instrument of observation and treatment. This stresses the intrapsychic equilibrium but also serves as a vehicle for further development. The supervisory relationship is the crucible in which this new experience is integrated and understood, and both supervisor and supervisee are changed by its effects on their respective growth. The relationship is complicated by the involvement of a third party, the patient. The triangle is unique in each instance because the ages, developmental levels, and life circumstances of the individuals are always different and in flux.

Adult Development ends with outlines of two demonstration courses taught by us at the San Diego Psychoanalytic Institute and the University of California at San Diego. The goals of the courses were to integrate data on normal adulthood from biological, sociological, and psychological spheres with existing theory and clinical experience and to provide the students with a theoretical and practical grasp of the existing material and a desire to expand the frontier by research and study of their own.

REFERENCES

Colarusso, C. A., & Nemiroff, R. A. *Adult development: A new dimension in psychodynamic theory and practice.* New York: Plenum Press, 1981.

Conference on Psychoanalytic Education and Research, Commission IX. *Child analysis.* New York: American Psychoanalytic Association, 1974.

Erikson, E. H. *Childhood and society* (2nd ed.). New York: W. W. Norton, 1963.

Erikson, E. H. (Ed.). *Adulthood.* New York: W. W. Norton, 1978.

Freud, S. Instincts and their vicissitudes. In J. Strachey (Ed. and Trans.), *Standard edition* (14:109). London: Hogarth Press, 1915. (a)

Freud, S. Thoughts for the times on war and death. In J. Strachey (Ed. and Trans.), *Standard edition* (14:273). London: Hogarth Press, 1915. (b)

Gould, R. L. *Transformations: Growth and change in adult life.* New York: Simon & Schuster, 1978.

Jarvik, L. F. Intellectual function in later years. In L. F. Jarvik, C. Eisdorfer, & J. E. E. Blum (Eds.), *Intellectual functioning in adults.* New York: Springer, 1973.

Levinson, D. J., Darrow, C. N., Klein, E. B., Levinson, M. H., & McKee, B. *The seasons of a man's life.* New York: Knopf, 1978.

Moore, B., & Fine, B. *A glossary of psychoanalytic terms and concepts.* New York: American Psychoanalytic Association, 1968.

Neugarten, B. L. In I. Steinschein (Reporter), The experience of separation-individuation...through the course of life: Maturity, senescence, and sociological implications (panel report). *Journal of the American Psychoanalytic Association,* 1973, *21*, 633–645.

Newton, P. M., & Levinson, D. J. Crisis in adult development. In A. Lazare (Ed.), *Outpatient psychiatry: Diagnosis and treatment.* Baltimore: Williams & Wilkins, 1979.

Shane, M. A rationale for teaching analytic technique based on a developmental orientation and approach. *International Journal of Psycho-Analysis,* 1977, *58*, 95–108.

Spitz, R. *The first year of life.* New York: International Universities Press, 1965.

Vaillant, G. E. *Adaptation to life.* Boston: Little, Brown, 1977.

Van Gennep, A. *The rites of passage.* (M. B. Vizedom & G. L. Cafee, Trans). Chicago: University of Chicago Press, 1960. (Originally published, 1908)

Wechsler, D. Intellectual changes with age. *Mental Health in Later Maturity* (Suppl. 168). Federal Security Agency, United States Public Health Service, 1941.

2

The Literature on Psychotherapy and Psychoanalysis in the Second Half of Life

ROBERT A. NEMIROFF AND CALVIN A. COLARUSSO

OBSTACLES, BARRIERS, AND STEREOTYPES IN WORK WITH OLDER PATIENTS

Clinicians describing psychotherapeutic work with older patients almost invariably reflect the sense of resistance they experienced at the outset, citing a variety of obstacles to starting the work, barriers to performing the psychotherapeutic tasks, and societal and cultural stereotypes that inhibited them in their interactions with older patients. Butler and Lewis (1977) discuss the mental health profession's nihilism and negativism regarding the older patient. They consider them manifestations of "professional ageism" and therapist countertransference and list the following six issues:

1. The aged's stimulation of therapists' fears regarding their own eventual old age (*and, we would add, anxiety regarding death*)
2. Therapists' conflicts about their own parental relations
3. Felt impotence stemming from a belief in the ubiquity of untreatable organic states in the elderly
4. Desire to avoid "wasting" their skills on persons nearing death

5. Fears that an aged patient may die during treatment
6. Desire to avoid colleagues' negative evaluation of efforts directed
   toward the aged

The therapist's own anxieties in treating older patients must first be confronted and understood, particularly in their expression as counter-transference in the therapeutic process. In a comprehensive review, Rechtschaffen (1959) stated:

> The anxiety aroused by hostility toward a parent figure may lead to a water-ing down of the therapeutic process and to an exaggerated emphasis on sup-portive and covering-over procedures. Defending against his own anxiety, a therapist may propose only the most benign interpretations, and may assume an attitude of reverence toward an older patient that is out of keeping with the patient's actual readiness to examine himself. (p. 82)

THE MYTH OF RIGIDITY

Kahana (1978) has thoroughly discussed the problem of the older person's so-called rigidity as a significant attitudinal barrier on the part of the therapist. He describes how Guntrip (1975) had a second analy-sis relatively late in life and was able to recover, when he was in his 70s, valid and therapeutically significant childhood memories that were help-ful to a further understanding of his life. Grotjahn (1955) has found in a number of cases that resistance against unpleasant insights is frequently lessened in old age. Lifelong struggles and the demands of reality often characterize defenses. In much the same fashion, Wheelwright (1959) finds aging patients to be surprisingly flexible. He compares his older pa-tients to his younger ones and finds that patients in the second half of life may be less competitive and possessive because they have met a number of their life goals. He describes them as becoming more subjec-tively oriented and more concerned with who they are. Kahana describes the work of Fozard and Thomas (1975) who reviewed the results of psychological testing with physically healthy people over 50. In all the psychological functions measured, only one could be interpreted as dis-playing rigidity. That was a tendency toward slower reactions to stimuli due to the increase in time required for central information processing. Kahana (1978) summarizes the clinical evidence against the imputation of rigidity of thought process to patients over 50 in the following way:

> Thus, the evidence against a general imputation to patients over 50 includes reports of psychological improvement based on earlier psychoanalysis, reports

> based on later analysis and self-analysis, and observations of increased receptivity to insight and readiness for changes in values and life style in middle and later life. Many psychotherapists would agree with Berezin (1972) that rigidity and flexibility are not functions of age but rather of personality structure throughout life: a young person with rigid character structure will be rigid in old age, while those who are flexible when young will also be flexible when old. (p. 41)

Finally, Weisman (1978, p. 52) makes the interesting interpretation that the stereotyping of older people as being too rigid in their thought processes or unsuitable for explorative psychotherapy "is a fallacy based on the metaphor that increasing stubbornness or fixed ideas in the aged is a precursor to rigor mortis."

AN EXAMPLE OF ONE THERAPIST'S INITIAL RELUCTANCE TO TREAT THE OLDER PATIENT

In a personal account, psychiatrist Richard Rubin (1977) describes his own initial counterproductive attitudes including pessimistic theoretical opinions, countertransference, educational differences, and cultural biases in the therapeutic approach to the older patient. He describes his first attempt at psychotherapy with an elderly patient in the second year of his residency at the University of New Mexico. Rotating through a community satellite clinic that included consultation to a small service center for the elderly, Rubin was asked by an outreach nurse specializing in geriatric care to evaluate a 69-year-old man in distress. On taking a history, he found that the patient was intensely preoccupied with memories of his wife who had died 5 years before. The preoccupation took the form of frequently imagining her presence and repeating familiar conversations from their 26 years of marriage. The patient experienced frequent crying spells, considerable anxiety, insomnia, withdrawal from people, and somatic preoccupation. Having lost his job and moved 2,000 miles from his home, he spent a great deal of time trying to be admitted to the medical wards of various VA hospitals. Otherwise, he spent his time in bars. Habitual excessive drinking and nutritional neglect had produced a polyneuropathy that impeded his walking. A mental status exam showed signs of mild organic cerebral impairment manifested by short-term memory difficulties, some concreteness, and a tendency to ramble. Rubin's main diagnosis was unresolved grief reaction, and his plan of treatment was psychotherapy, beginning with encouraging the patient to review the events around his losses. The patient entered psychotherapy with enthusiasm and was able to talk about his life and feelings rather freely. However, despite a good beginning and an initially positive therapeutic alliance, Rubin found himself with doubts and reluctance to pursue the psychotherapy with the patient. Because of the openness and authenticity of Rubin's report, we quote it in detail (1977):

> I had never before attempted ongoing dynamic psychotherapy with an elderly patient, and I wondered if, despite significant motivating distress, his psychological mechanisms were inflexibly hardened by age. I was unfamiliar at that time with the literature on psychotherapy with the elderly and questioned the applicability of the methods I knew. My only previous experience with elderly patients had been with the severely ill in medical wards, psychiatric inpatient units, and nursing homes. I worried that the complexity and seriousness of this man's problems might make draining dependency demands on me. Behind this concern lay my own fears of possibly losing independence through social isolation and disability in the future. I thought about my rash optimism in minimizing the influence of his organic cerebral deficits. Would he be emotionally too labile or ramble about with little direction and coherence, preventing psychotherapeutic progress? In light of these weaknesses, would his attachment to alcohol be a stronger, more immediate source of gratification than dynamically more important issues?... In addition to professional concerns, I felt deficient in personal understanding of the elderly in my own family. Like many of my generation, I grew up in a suburb. My grandparents lived in a distant city, and visits were hectic affairs on holidays, involving many other relatives. Little time was spent at pursuing individual acquaintance, and they died before I was old enough to learn about their lives. I do not remember being offered understanding of what the recent generations still held in memory; life's purpose seemed more with the future and hopes for change than review of the past. (p. 219)

Rubin's statement of his conflicts and concerns in treating the patient with psychotherapy mirrors many similar statements by other clinicians and testifies to the accuracy of Butler and Lewis's (1977) list of issues (see p. 41). Rubin was able to overcome his reluctance and encouraged his patient to describe his feelings during the long months of his wife's dying from cancer. Much unresolved grief work was accomplished, and the patient was able to extend the work beyond the feelings and events surrounding his wife's death to important issues and conflicts in his current life. Transference developed and intensified during the treatment, and those feelings were interpreted to the patient with beneficial results. Dr. Rubin relied heavily on the "life review" technique first described by Butler (1963) as

> a naturally occurring universal mental process characterized by the progressive return to consciousness of past experiences and, particularly, the resurgence of unresolved conflicts; simultaneously, and normally, these reviewed experiences and conflicts can be surveyed and reintegrated. (p. 65)

Emphasis on reminiscence was an important vehicle for the psychotherapy; through it, and especially in the change in form and content of the patient's stories, transference feelings evolved, grief work was accomplished, and the patient's self-esteem and current life situation improved significantly.

Summarizing psychotherapy with the 69-year-old Mr. A., Rubin (1977) states:

> Direct experience with a patient can provide the learning therapist with an opportunity to overcome stereotyped bias, prejudices, and countertransference feelings. An evocative relationship facilitates awareness of these often unconscious influences on behavior...further, a successful therapy case can symbolically provide an exercise in mastery, allowing the therapist to accept his fears of disability and death, instead of reacting defensively. Hearing Mr. A.'s pains, hardships, and grief helped me to objectify, understand and deal with these human phenomena in my therapeutic work. (p. 223)

In applying the life review therapy model, Rubin derived important personal benefits; in this connection, he quotes Lewis and Butler (1974):

> One of the interesting fringe benefits for therapists and listeners is in obtaining a rich supply of information and models for their own eventual old age. (p. 165)

STANDARD PSYCHOANALYTIC TREATMENT OF OLDER PATIENTS

Early literature regarding psychoanalytic treatment of older individuals was influenced by Freud's pessimism. In a comprehensive review, Rechtschaffen (1959) outlines Freud's reasons for the inadvisability of treating older patients psychoanalytically. Freud (1905/1924, p. 264) wrote, "Near or above the fifties the elasticity of the mental process, on which the treatment depends, is as a rule lacking—old people are no longer educable." In addition, Freud felt that older people had too much life history behind them for successful analysis. He wrote that "the mass of material to be dealt with would prolong the duration of the treatment indefinitely" (1905/1924, p. 264). Implicit in that objection was the assumption that a successful analysis involves a complete reconstruction of the life history and a resolution of all the major conflicts experienced during a lifetime. Finally, Freud (1906/1942) was concerned about the relatively limited future of older patients. Even if the analysis was successful, the patient would have only a short interval in which to enjoy his or her newfound mental health. Freud seemed to be raising a cost-effectiveness argument, implying that in younger persons the investment of time, money, and effort was worthwhile, but that in older patients it was not. Kahana (1978) offers the following perspectives about Freud's own life and work:

> As his biographers have noted (Jones, 1953, 1955, 1957; Schur, 1972), Freud was unusually concerned with his own mortality and had an utter and life-long dislike of aging, especially if it entailed any decline in his creativity. In retrospect, *these attitudes contrast ironically with his eventual longevity, his remarkable scientific and literary achievements in later life, and his courage in facing prolonged illness and death* [italics added]. Although he characteristically tended to re-examine, update and elaborate, or discard and replace his scientific conclusions, he never revised his opinion on the age limit for patients in analysis. This was despite his own later discoveries, especially in the areas of narcissism and the structural point of view, which increased the scope and effectiveness of treatment. (p. 39)

Fifteen years later, Abraham (1949) struck a considerably more optimistic note in his descriptions of psychoanalytic work with patients in their 50s who had chronic neuroses. In fact, he went as far as to say that "to my surprise a considerable number of them reacted very favorably to the treatment. I might add that I count some of those cures as my most successful results" (p. 316). Jelliffee (1925) had similar results from remarkably successful classical analysis of older patients. He too felt that "chronological, physiological, and psychological age do not go hand in hand" (p. 9).

Those early reports were followed by two divergent schools of thought. Alexander and French (1946), Fenichel (1945), Hollender (1952), and Wayne (1953), writing in the 1940s, again expressed caution about working with older patients and argued for a primarily supportive approach that emphasized education, environmental modification, indeterminate termination, and a gentle handling of resistance. In contrast, others such as Kaufman (1937), King (1980), Jacques (1965), Sandler (1978), and Segal (1958) held firmly to the conviction that in many cases classical psychoanalytic technique need not be modified.

Special mention should be made of the pioneering work in gerontological psychiatry done over the years by the members of the Boston Society for Gerontologic Psychiatry. The leadership of Martin A. Berezin, Stanley H. Cath, Ralph J. Kahana, Sidney Levin, Norman E. Zinberg, and other Boston analysts has fostered many creative studies in the area of psychotherapy and psychoanalysis with the older patient. As only one example, we call attention to the symposium of the society entitled "Psychoanalysis in Later Life: Problems in the Psychoanalysis of an Aging Narcissistic Patient'' in which Sandler (1978) presented the case of an architect who was in analysis from ages 58 to 66. While driving with his wife, the patient had suddenly experienced chest pain and was racked with intense sobbing. Medical examination revealed no organic pathology, and the patient came for analytic consultation and eventual treatment because of panic over his sudden loss of emotional control. The case was perceptively discussed by Kahana (1978), Myerson (1978), and Weisman (1978). Sandler's case illustrates brilliantly how a standard psychoanalysis can be extremely useful to a man in late middle age who is approaching old age and suffering from neurotic symptoms embedded in a narcissistic matrix. The case is a landmark study because of Sandler's presentation of extensive and exquisite clinical detail and process. The transference developed fully over the course of the analysis, and Sandler sensitively interprets transference feelings and her own reactions to the patient. In his insightful discussion, Kahana (1978) delineates the three phases of the analysis:

> The patient began with intense feelings of shame and an attitude of idealizing the analyst. During the initial one and one-half year period, he experienced, through the transference, an awakening of libidinal and narcissistic elements, signalled by his preoccupation with the analyst. The second phase of three years featured the main work of clarifying and interpreting the patient's motivations and defenses, as they became apparent in the transference and his efforts to redirect his life. The analyst could show Mr. X. how he defended against his fears of sexual, aggressive and exhibitionistic urges by efforts to be loved and admired as ''good,'' by projecting his aggression and by hiding his achievements. As he recognized his competitive envy and compulsive traits he became more aware of his anger, and his academic work improved. With the reluctant realization that his wife did not want him, he entered into a relationship with a more receptive woman and began to analyze his fears of women. Interpretation of his defensive projection of aggression onto women led to the memory of his temper tantrums as a child. Then, after an actual achievement in his studies he was able to acknowledge his wish for success. This, in turn, led to the rediscovery of his mother's grandiosity and snobbishness, and to consciousness of his own hidden grandiose fantasies. The final two and a half years of analysis were marked by relinquishment of these grandiose wishes. His communications became more direct and genuine, and his plans more realistic. As termination approached, he was able to express hitherto repressed anger at his siblings, and finally to recall pleasant childhood experiences. His idealization of objects and excessive demands on himself had moderated. (pp. 43–44)

Kahana (1978) went on to describe how therapeutic movement in this case included the following:

> Awakening of feelings, loosening of defenses, mobilization of conflicts at phal-
> lic and prephallic developmental levels, representation in dreams of uncon-
> scious wishes and fears, response to skillful interpretations, recovery of mem-
> ories, increasing insight, better resolution of conflicts and reorientation of his
> life. (pp. 44–45)

Sandler (1978) was acutely sensitive to the developmental issues of aging and death anxiety in her patient.

> I gradually became aware of how Mr. X. had from his early years always felt
> intensely in conflict about assertiveness and success. To grow up, to compete,
> and to succeed were all seen as attacks on the outside world, and he always
> feared and expected revenge or retaliation. As he became older and weaker,
> having to face illness and death constantly reminded him of these increas-
> ing dangers, and reinforced his defensive retreat into the narcissistic position
> of having to please and placate. He desperately needed to attach himself to
> his highly idealized and narcissistically invested objects. (p. 14)

In summary interpretation, Sandler (1978) says:

> It was then possible to connect all of this with his feelings of despair at the
> prospect of death and of leaving things unfinished, and with the feeling that
> he had never been able to clear things properly with his father. Gradually,
> his bitterness, anger, and guilt toward his father diminished and he was able
> to express sadness and a sense of loss at having been estranged from him.
> *I felt acutely that the completion of an additional piece of mourning for his father helped
> him to prepare for his own old age and to mourn for his own postself* [italics added].
> (p. 33)

Currently, there is a renewal of interest in the psychoanalysis of older
patients. King (1980) has succinctly summarized some of the pressures
that bring older people to psychoanalysis.

> 1. The fear of the diminution or loss of sexual potency and the impact
> this would have on relationships.
> 2. The threat of redundancy, or displacement in work roles by younger
> people, and awareness of the possible failure of the effectiveness of their
> professional skills, linked with the fear that they would not be able to cope
> with retirement, and would lose their sense of identity and worth when they
> lost their professional or work role.
> 3. Anxieties arising in marital relationships after children have left home
> and parents can no longer use their children to mask problems arising in their
> relationship with each other.
> 4. The awareness of their own aging, possible illness, and consequent de-
> pendence on others, and the anxiety this arouses in them.
> 5. The inevitability of their own death and the realization that they may
> not now be able to achieve the goals they set for themselves, and what they
> can achieve and enjoy in life may be limited, with consequent feelings of
> depression or deprivation. (p. 154)

King states that by understanding of transference and countertransference phenomena in the context of the previously mentioned life cycle pressures, important conflicts of the older patient can be better brought into focus and made accessible for psychoanalytic work.

In extending King's work, Cohen (1982) has described how psychoanalysts increasingly find themselves confronted with middle-aged and elderly patients who come to psychoanalysis for the first time because of exacerbation of their narcissistic problems. These individuals have made lifelong attempts at "self-cure," building a precarious equilibrium around an omnipotent and idealized self that has hidden excessive envious and destructive feelings. With the onset of aging, including the decline of psychological and physical capacities, the emergence of death anxiety, and the loss of loved ones, there is an upsurge of underlying envy, destructiveness, and loneliness. Cohen (1982), agreeing with studies of Rosenfeld (1978) and Kernberg (1980), emphasizes the intense fears of dependency in these patients. Specifically, he states that it is important "in aging to retain the capacity to recognize and seek environmental help that often becomes a necessity and means recognizing one's sense of dependency" (p. 154). It is possible for analysis to mitigate excessive envy and rivalry, thus diminishing the sense of loneliness involved in growing older.

And recently, in a number of ground-breaking studies, George Pollock (1981a) has described successful psychoanalytic work with individuals in their 50s, 60s, 70s, and 80s, advancing the concept of "the mourning–liberation process," a universal transformation that allows for adaptation to change, loss, transition, and disequilibrium. The process goes on throughout life and has the potential of stimulating development at all ages. Pollock has found that middle-aged and older adults retain a considerable capacity for insight, therapeutically induced transference, dream analysis, self-observation, motivation for change, mobilization of libidinal and constrictive aggressive energies, and the institution of a mourning–liberation process.

SPECIALIZED TECHNIQUES IN THE PSYCHOTHERAPY OF THE OLDER PATIENT

In the preceding section we reviewed selected literature regarding the standard psychoanalytic treatments of the older patient. In this section we consider the work of clinicians who have suggested a variety of modifications and specialized techniques in the treatment of patients in middle and late life. Kahana (1980) has offered a very useful scheme for organizing the therapeutic approach to the older patient, suggesting that older patients who come for treatment be divided into three groups (1) aging, (2) an intermediate group, and (3) the debilitated aged. He describes those in the first group as experiencing

> physical changes in appearance, attractiveness, strength, agility and reaction time; physical illnesses that are manageable rather than critical; some fluctuation and recession of instinctual drives; conflict over and reassessment of the balance between ideal aspirations and actual achievement, whether in personal development, social relationships, community activities, work or creative efforts; the prospect of retirement from work; awareness of limitation of time and of the eventual reality of dying; the deaths of people who are significant to them; and changes in their relationships with spouses, children, friends and co-workers. (p. 318)

In the intermediate group are those patients who experience states of crisis stemming from severe physical and mental illness, losses by death, divorce or radical change in personal relationships, or failures in their work" (p. 318). The last group, the debilitated aged

> show in varying combinations and degrees: the limiting and burdening effects of chronic, multiple or dangerous illness, with diminished functional reserves of organ systems; manifestations of brain damage; constriction of activities; inability to maintain themselves without considerable assistance from their families, community resources or institutional facilities; a dominance of pregenital drives; and the depletion of stimulation, affectation and satisfaction, the recurrence of grief reactions, and the strengthening of defenses against painful affects resulting from repeated, cumulative losses of significant people. (p. 318)

In reviewing his clinical experience with these three groups Kahana found that almost all the patients in all three groups suffered from some form of depression. In the aging group the depression ranged from neurotic (reactive) to psychotic; in the intermediate group the depression tended to the more severe (psychotic); and the debilitated group had anaclitic depressions associated with depletion of functions and satisfactions and agitated depressions and depression associated with senile brain disease.

This typology of patients into three groups provides a systematic approach to treatment strategies. Thus, psychotherapy with the aging group is aimed at structural or intrapsychic change as well as restitution of personality functioning or basic support. For the intermediate group treatment strategies are centered around crisis intervention with the goal being the restitution of optimum functioning. The illnesses here are of crisis proportions in reaction to physical disease or personal losses. Therefore, prevention of future recurrences is important. With the debilitated aged groups, Kahana finds that therapeutic strategies are centered around measures of basic support for the treatment of anaclitic depressions set off by brain damage, physical aging, or multiple personal losses. In this group, oral dependency issues predominate, and the therapist must be prepared to work, possibly intensively, with the patient's family.

NEW TECHNIQUES

Adaptive Value of Reminiscence

A significant number of patients in the aging group can be treated with the standard methods of psychoanalytic psychotherapy and psychoanalysis. The goals involve attempting to bring about intrapsychic structural change, including better integration of drive derivatives, further development of ego and superego functions, and improved cohesion of the self. Emotional insight is the chief vehicle for therapeutic change. Bibring (1954) has described insight as occurring at two levels: (1) clarification via the giving of understanding of what is preconscious, that is, that which is just outside immediate attention, and (2) the bringing to consciousness via interpretation rather well-defended unconscious mental contents. Recent work has shown that the utilization of reminiscence in patients in the second half of life can add considerably to the therapist's armamentarium by facilitating the process of exploration and the attainment of emotional insight (Barns, Sach, & Shore, 1973; Berezin & Cath, 1965; Busse & Pfeiffer, 1965; Lewis, 1973; Lewis & Butler, 1974).

Pollock (1981b) has described the many ways in which reminiscence is important in work with adult patients, particularly the elderly. These include adaptational attempts, relational communicative attempts, and self-therapeutic attempts. Pollock writes:

> The recollections or fantasies of the past expressed in reminiscences help the elderly maintain a sense of continuity between past and present and between inside and outside. The events, relationships, and feelings recalled also maintain a sense of "me-ness." These recollection—reminiscences bridge time and maintain the sense of individual personality, especially when there is an in-

ner awareness of diminishing ego intactness and competency. In some individuals, the frequently repeated tales of the past are similar to the repeti-
tions, remembering, and working-through sequences observed in the
psychoanalytic treatment situation. In some, the obsessive reiteration—and—
recounting is similar to mourning work where recalling-and-expressing is part
of the self-healing process. In some elderly, the recounting allows the inves-
tigator to observe the consistencies of the accounts as they are restated. . . .
I have found that reminiscence is a way of returning to the past, especially
to periods of life when satisfactions and mastering took place. In some, the
return is to past traumatic situations where attempts to "work through" these
past, but still present, intense mental and emotional disturbances seem clear.
The insight of the psychoanalytic observer allows for understanding the meaning of what is otherwise considered "the ramblings of old men and women."
(p. 280)

The most systematic approach to the utilization of reminiscence in
insight-oriented psychotherapy with the older patient has been by Butler and co-workers. Butler (1963) had early postulated the *life review* as
a prominent developmental process of late life. After years of research,
Lewis and Butler (1974) defined it as

a universal mental process brought about by the realization of approaching
dissolution and death. It marks the lives of all older persons in some manner as their myths of invulnerability or immortality give way and death begins to be viewed as an imminent personal reality. (p. 165)

For many older people, this process seems to serve a positive psychotherapeutic function, helping them to reflect on their lives "in order to resolve, reorganize, and reintegrate what is troubling or preoccupying"
(1974, p. 165). In patients in early old age, the life review can take on
surprising intensity; some individuals are amazed at their own ability to
recall earlier life events with sudden and remarkable clarity. Lewis and
Butler quote their patients as saying "It's as though it happened only
yesterday"; "I felt as though I was there." The clarity of these reminiscences extends to striking memories of smell, taste, and touch as well
as sight and sound. In many of their patients, the capacity for free association is enhanced by reminiscing, and memories that were deeply
buried in the unconscious are recovered. There is, of course, some variation in the intensity of individual experience, ranging from mild nostalgia and storytelling to a feverish preoccupation with documenting their
experience.

As part of the psychotherapeutic process, Lewis and Butler (1974)
have devised several methods of evoking memory in older persons that
they find both useful and enjoyable.

1. *Written or taped autobiographies.* In these the therapist searches for clues, noting omissions as well as inclusions. A particularly poignant example given by Butler and Lewis is that of a man who provided an intricate history of his professional and social life with newspaper clippings, letters from important persons, and pictures of himself and his wife but nothing about his two children except a few news items. The therapist noticed this paucity of data, questioned the patient, and learned that the son, then 45 years old, had not spoken to his parents in 20 years and that their daughter had minimal contact as well.

2. *Pilgrimages* (in person or through correspondence). Lewis and Butler (1974) encourage older patients to go to the locations of birth, childhood, youth, and young adult life. During these pilgrimages the patient is encouraged to rediscover the past by recalling and talking over old times with family, neighbors, and friends. In one such case, a 69-year-old man, who after talking with persons who had known him in his childhood town recalled that as a little boy he had tried to make himself into a "noble image."

> I was orphaned at nine years of age. I was so scared that I decided to be the best boy there was. To avoid the orphan home secluded behind high brick walls, I vowed to go to church and Sunday school and never to swear, smoke, drink, steal, cheat, or hurt persons or animals. I would work hard to buy presents for everyone, scrub the floors, shovel snow, and split wood. The formula seemed to work, and the philosophy gained a strong hold on me. People tell me I never grieved openly or got angry. Now I'm understanding why I'm still such a damn nice guy all the time! (Lewis & Butler, 1974, p. 167)

3. *Reunions.* Patients are encouraged to attend reunions including high school, college classes, church, and family meetings. These offer a unique opportunity for the intensification of the life review. Lewis and Butler (1974) state that "an individual can look at himself in the context of other meaningful people and take a measure of where he stands in the course of the life cycle." (p. 167)

4. *Genealogy.* Many older people develop a keen interest in their family roots, sometimes for the first time in their lives. It is useful for the therapist to participate in these studies of their parents, grandparents, and distant ancestors, as the patients strive to find themselves in history and to take comfort in the fact that they are part of a line. Lewis and Butler (1974) feel that "one of the ways the old seem to resolve fears of death is to gain a sense of other family members having died before them" (p. 167).

5. *Scrapbooks, photo albums, old letters, and other memorabilia.* Lewis and Butler frequently ask older persons to bring such items to therapy sessions where therapist and patient go through them together. They find this an especially pleasant form of interviewing for the older patient as it quickly establishes positive rapport.

6. *Summation of life work.* For those who have had little in the way of family, that is, no spouse or little contact with grown children, a particularly useful technique is a specific focus on their life's work. For many people work has been their most meaningful participation in the world. Lewis and Butler ask people for a verbal or written summation of their work that will reflect what they regard as their contribution and also the history of their particular craft. They report that some of these summations have grown into full-scale books or published poetry and music.

7. *Preserving ethnic identity.* Lewis and Butler pay special attention to their patient's ethnic heritage. Because many first-generation Americans have been busy in establishing themselves, they have repressed important and meaningful aspects of their backgrounds. The authors have found that a resurrection and reconstruction of their ethnic identity can have positive personal and social value.

The life review process has many therapeutic possibilities. It affords opportunities to reexamine the whole of one's life and to put it in reasonable perspective. By doing this, there is the chance to solve old problems, to make amends, and to restore harmony with friends and relatives. Lewis and Butler report that family members have been known to decide to talk to one another after 30 or 40 years of angry silence. Further, the process seems to revive dreams of youth and some regret for what was not accomplished, along with appreciation for one's achievements. There is the opportunity to understand and accept personal foibles and to take full responsibility for acts that cause true harm but also to differentiate between real and neurotic guilt. Fears of death and dissolution may be confronted, and some of the anxiety associated with invulnerability may be mitigated. Lewis and Butler describe how pride in one's life and feelings of serenity often center around having done one's best, which includes giving oneself the benefit of the doubt in difficult or extenuating circumstances. Practically, as a result of the life review, individuals may revise their wills, give away unnecessary possessions, and generally simplify their lives. It is found that creativity may be restimulated or emerge for the first time in an individual's life in the form of memoirs, art, music, handicrafts, or teaching. Basically, the life review techniques can serve as a stimulus for the older patient deciding "how I want to live the rest of my life." Finally Lewis and Butler (1974) sum up their methods by saying,

> The success of the life review depends on the outcome of the struggle to resolve old issues of resentment, guilt, bitterness, mistrust, dependence, and nihilism. All the really significant emotional options remain available until the moment of death—love, hate, reconciliation, self-assertion, and self-esteem. (p. 169)

Utilization of Dependency Feelings

In contrast to working with the intact and integrated older patients, in Kahana's "aging group" special techniques have been evolved to work with severely impaired older patients. Foremost in this endeavor has been the work of Goldfarb, who has applied psychoanalytic thinking in a particularly creative way for the very old, specifically the brain damaged, residents of a home for the aged, patients who suffer from major somatic changes, intellectual impairment, and socioeconomic and personal losses. Basically, Goldfarb (1955, 1967) uses to the utmost the dependency inherent in the patient–physician relationship. Goldfarb and Sheps (1954) base their psychotherapy technique on the following data:

1. In their cases, they observed fear and rage arising in a context of increasing helplessness due to loss of physical, social, and economic resources.
2. The helplessness of these aged sick caused them, invariably, to press parental powers onto the therapist. They identified the therapist with a son or a daughter, marriage partner, relative, or friend upon whom they had leaned in the past.
3. The behavior the patients demonstrated in response to feeling helpless seemed to be motivated by their desire to obtain some pleasure through mastery by dominating or controlling others.

Goldfarb and Sheps saw that the role of the powerful parent that these increasingly helpless patients thrust on the therapist gave an opportunity to foster the illusion that the therapist was indeed such a powerful figure. In the role of omnipotent parental surrogate, the therapist can provide gratification of emotional needs for punishment, affection, respect, and protection. Goldfarb and Sheps (1954) describe the treatment as follows:

> By utilizing the role that the security-seeking aged sick force on him, guilt, fear, rage and depression can be ameliorated or their social manifestations altered. The patient's sense of helplessness is then decreased. Some successes in performance which follow tend to further increase the patient's sense of worth and strength. Therapy consists of brief (five to fifteen minutes) sessions which are as widely spaced as the status and progress of the patient permits. Each of the interviews is "structured" so that the patient leaves with a sense of triumph, of victory derived from having won an ally or from having dominated the therapist. The therapist attempts to have the patient leave not with the feeling of guilt but of conquest (triumph). (p. 183)

Thus, the aim of this technique is to increase *the self-esteem* of the patient in a transaction with a parent–surrogate therapist. The patient experiences the transaction as a struggle with a powerful figure from which he emerges a deserving victor, and the victory is viewed by the patient as proof of his strength and worth. Actually, Goldfarb and Sheps (1954) see the "struggle" as purely an illusion of the patient, that is, a product of his distortion of reality. In essence, the therapist accepts the role of the feared and resented parent and permits himself or herself to be persuaded to the patient's point of view or expectations. The authors (1954) conclude that

> the promotion of the illusion that the therapist was mastered and his power was available to them was a source of pleasure for those patients in whom healthy affectionate attitudes were poorly developed or had been lost; whose sense of worthlessness and disbelief that they could be loved was so great that the only bond between people they could envision was one of power. (p. 190)

Kahana (1980) describes Goldfarb's utilization of the dependency technique in the following example of a married woman in her mid-70s who was in the throes of an agitated depression, including both hypochondriasis and a significant degree of loss of recent memory:

> She came to the psychiatrist's office accompanied by family members, usually by her husband and one or more children. Initially fearful of the interviews and urgently requesting relief, she cast her younger therapist in the role of a savior or at least a superior court judge. He demurred and cautioned her overvaluation but could not entirely escape this omnipotent role. In a later session, when she felt better, she clasped him in her arms, said that she loved him—teasing that he mustn't tell his wife—and at the end of the session gave him a kiss. He was, of course, pleased with her improvement and he accepted her positive expression as he might from any affectionate older relative. (p. 319)

We have described some of the obstacles, barriers, and stereotypes that clinicians face in the treatment of older patients, including stimulation of therapists' fears regarding their own eventual old age and death and unresolved conflicts about their own parents, feelings of futility about treating organic states in the elderly, and time "wasted" on persons near death as well as patients' fears of actually dying and concerns about lowered status in the eyes of colleagues from treating a geriatric population. The mythical imputation to older people of automatic mental "rigidity" was examined and described, noting that the experience of many investigators suggests instead that patients who are flexible when young will also be flexible when old. Although Freud's early pessimism has set a negative tone, the literature abounds with examples of very creative psychoanalytic work with patients between the ages of 40 and 80. Currently, more middle-aged and older patients seem to be presenting for psychoanalytic psychotherapy and psychoanalysis proper, for the first time in their lives, with a variety of neurotic symptoms, including depression that is enmeshed in a narcissistic matrix. Finally, two specialized techniques for treating older patients—the use of reminiscence, specifically the life review therapy of Butler and co-workers, and utilization of the dependency technique in the aged sick by Goldfarb and co-workers—were described in some detail.

REFERENCES

Abraham, K. The applicability of psycho-analytic treatment to patients at an advanced age. In *Selected papers of psychoanalysis*. London: Hogarth Press, 1949.

Alexander, F. G., & French, T. M. *Psychoanalytic therapy: Principles and applications.* New York: Ronald Press, 1946.

Barns, E. K., Sach, A. A., & Shore, H. Guidelines to treatment approaches, modalities and methods for use with the aged. *Gerontologist*, 1973, *13*(4), 313–327.

Berezin, M. A., & Cath, S. H. (Eds.). *Geriatric psychiatry: Grief, loss and emotional disorders in the aging process.* New York: International Universities Press, 1965.

Berezin, M. A. Psychodynamic considerations of aging and the aged. *American Journal of Psychiatry*, 1972, *128*, 1485–1491.

Bibring, E. Psychoanalysis and the dynamic psychotherapies. *Journal of the American Psychoanalytic Association*, 1954, *2*, 745–770.

Busse, E. W., & Pfeiffer, E. Introduction. In E. W. Busse & E. Pfeiffer (Eds.), *Behavior and adaptation in late life.* Boston: Little, Brown, 1969.

Butler, R. N. The life review: An interpretation of reminiscence in the aged. *Psychiatry*, 1963, *26*, 65–75.

Butler R. N., & Lewis, M. I. *Aging and mental health: Positive psychosocial approaches.* St. Louis: Mosby, 1977.

Cohen, N. A. On loneliness and the aging process. *International Journal of Psycho-Analysis*, 1982, *63*, 149–155.

Fenichel, O. *The psychoanalytic theory of neurosis.* New York: Norton, 1945.

Fozard, J. L., & Thomas, J. C., Jr. Psychology of aging. Basic factors and some psychiatric applications. In J. G. Howells (Ed.), *Modern perspectives in the psychiatry of old age*. New York: Brunner/Mazel, 1975.

Freud, S. On psychotherapy. In *Collected papers* (Vol. 1). London: Hogarth Press, 1924. (Originally published, 1905.)

Freud, S. Sexuality in the aetiology of the neuroses. In *Collected papers* (Vol 1). London: Hogarth Press, 1942. (Originally published, 1906.)

Goldfarb, A. L. One aspect of the psychodynamics of the therapeutic situation with aged patients. *Psychoanalytic Review*, 1955, 42, 180–187.

Goldfarb, A. L. *Psychiatry in geriatrics, medical clinics of North America*. Philadelphia: W. B. Saunders Co., 1967.

Goldfarb, A. L., & Sheps, J. Psychotherapy of the aged. *Psychosomatic Medicine*, 1954, 15(3).

Grotjahn, M. Analytic psychotherapy with the elderly. *Psychoanalytic Review*, 1955, 42, 419–427.

Guntrip, H. My experience of analysis with Fairbairn and Winnicott. *International Review of Psychoanalysis*, 1975, 2, 145–156.

Hollender, M. H. Individualizing the aged. *Social Casework*, 1952, 33, 337–342.

Jacques, E. Death and the mid-life crisis. *International Journal of Psychoanalysis*, 1965, 46, 502–514.

Jelliffe, S. E. The old age factor in psycho-analytic therapy. *Medical Journal Records*, 1925, 121, 7–12.

Jones, E. *The life and work of Sigmund Freud* (Vol. 1). New York: Basic Books, 1953.

Jones, E. *The life and work of Sigmund Freud* (Vol. 2). New York: Basic Books, 1955.

Jones, E. *The life and work of Sigmund Freud* (Vol. 3). New York: Basic Books, 1957.

Kahana, R. Psychoanalysis in later life. Discussion. *Journal of Geriatric Psychiatry*, 1978, 11, 37–49.

Kaufman, M. R. Psychoanalysis in late-life depressions. *Psychoanalytic Quarterly*, 1937, 6, 308–335.

Kahana, R. J. Psychotherapy with the elderly. In T. B. Karasu & L. Bellak (Eds.), *Specialized techniques in individual psychotherapy*. New York: Brunner/Mazel, 1980.

Kernberg, O. *Internal world and external reality*. New York: Jason Aronson, 1980.

King, P. H. The life cycle as indicated by the nature of the transference in the psychoanalysis of the middle-aged and elderly. *International Journal of Psychoanalysis*, 1980, 61, 153–160.

Lewis, C. N. The adaptive value of reminiscence in old age. *Journal of Geriatric Psychiatry*, 1973, 5, 117–121.

Lewis, M., & Butler, R. N. Life review therapy. *Geriatrics*, 1974, 29, 165–173.

Myerson, P. G. Psychoanalysis in later life. Discussion. *Journal of Geriatric Psychiatry*, 1978, 11(37), 57–66.

Pollock, G. H. Aging or aged: development or pathology. In S. I. Greenspan & G. H. Pollock (Eds.), *The course of life: Psychoanalytic contributions toward understanding personality development* (Vol. 3). Washington, D.C.: U.S. Government Printing Office, 1981. (a)

Pollock, G. H. Reminiscence and insight. *Psychoanalytic Study of the Child*, 1981, 36, 278–287. (b)

Rechtschaffen, A. Psychotherapy with geriatric patients: A review of the literature. *Journal of Gerontology*, 1959, 14, 73–84.

Rosenfeld, H. A. Notes on the psychopathology and psychoanalytic treatment of some borderline patients. *International Journal of Psychoanalysis*, 1978, 59, 215–221.

Rubin, R. Learning to overcome reluctance for psychotherapy with the elderly. *Journal of Geriatric Psychiatry*, 1977, 10, 215–227.

Sandler, A. Psychoanalysis in later life: Problems in the psychoanalysis of an aging narcissistic patient. *Journal of Geriatric Psychiatry*, 1978, 11(37), 5–36.

Segal, H. Fear of death: Notes on the analysis of an old man. *International Journal of Psychoanalysis*, 1958, *34*, 178–181.

Schur, M. *Freud: Living and dying*. New York: International Universities Press, 1972.

Weisman, A. Psychoanalysis in later life. Discussion. *Journal of Geriatric Psychiatry*, 1978, *11*(37), 51–55.

Wheelwright, J. B. Some comments on the aging process. *Psychiatry*, 1959, *22*, 407–411.

Wayne, G. J. Modified psychoanalytic therapy in senescence. *Psychoanalytic Review*, 1953, *40*, 99–116.

3

Adult Development
and Psychoanalytic Diagnosis
and Treatment

ROBERT A. NEMIROFF AND CALVIN A. COLARUSSO

Although Erikson's (1963) concepts of the life cycle have been accepted generally among social scientists, psychoanalysts have only lately begun to attend to issues of development beyond adolescence. As we noted, Gould (1978) and Levinson, Darrow, Klein, & Levinson (1978) present empirical data describing specific stages of complex adult growth and transition; Vaillant (1977) demonstrates an evolution and change in the ego mechanisms of defense in a 40-year longitudinal study of normal men; Pribram (1971) and others offer evidence that, structurally, the brain progresses *and* regresses in adulthood; and Jarvik, Eisdofer, & Blum (1973) reverse earlier notions of an inevitable decline in intellectual acuity with age, showing that with continued mental activity, intelligence can expand even into old age.

A few psychoanalytic authors have begun to write about the life cycle. Pollock (1971) has shown the importance and pervasiveness of mourning processes for adaptation and growth throughout life. King (1980) has described continual identity formation in her psychoanalytic

The material in this chapter is adapted from a paper presented at the 1981 winter meeting of the American Psychoanalytic Association in New York City.

work with patients in the second half of life. Panels at the American Psychoanalytic Association (Marcus, 1973; Steinschein, 1973; Winestine, 1973) have focused on the separation–individuation process throughout the life cycle. More recently, Greenspan and Pollock (1981) edited a three-volume work entitled *The Course of Life* in which a number of psychoanalytic authors addressed developmental continuity throughout the life course.

In 1974, organized psychoanalysis did begin to lay a foundation for a theory of normal lifelong development. In a report on child analysis at the Conference on Psychoanalytic Education and Research (COPER IX, 1974), it was suggested that the developmental orientation has important implications for clinical work because it provides a new framework in which to view the adult. If a patient *of any age* were understood to be in the midst of dynamic change, to be still developing, diagnosis and treatment could focus on current, phase-specific adult developmental tasks as well as on earlier experiences and conflicts. Attending primarily to the potential for healthy development, the analyst would have a better opportunity to pursue an interest in the whole person. Psychopathology is redefined primarily as deviation from normal development, an outgrowth of inadequate developmental achievement. Conflict remains an inescapable part of all development, and either healthy progress or impairment and arrest can be its outcome. Thus, the goal of treatment in adults as well as in children is not simply the removal of symptoms but the elimination of blocks to the continued evolution of the personality.

In this chapter, we will discuss further implications of adult developmental theory for clinical work, elaborating the developmental dimension to complement well-established frameworks of psychoanalytic formulation (e.g., genetic, dynamic, structural) and organizing our ideas around a few key concepts: (1) the adult developmental diagnosis as an organizing approach to the assessment of analytic patients and a constant reference point during transference evolution, interpretation, working through, and termination; (2) adult developmental lines, an expansion of the concept of childhood developmental lines; (3) adult developmental arrest, another elaboration of an established concept from child analysis, to demonstrate the importance and salience of events from the adult past; and (4) developmental resonance, the awareness of developmental issues affecting both analyst and analysand.

THE ADULT DEVELOPMENTAL DIAGNOSIS

Detailed developmental histories are routine in the evaluation of children but often neglected in the assessment of adult patients. The omission persists because of the too widely held notion that developmental processes play a minor role in the adult, and, indeed, there has not been a comprehensive adult developmental theory to provide appropriate diagnostic tools. We find that a developmental history describing the entire life experience—from conception to the present—is invaluable in working with an adult patient. On the basis of our theoretical constructs about development and our work with patients, we have formulated an outline for such a history (Colarusso & Nemiroff, 1981).

As an illustration, consider one crucial area of adult developmental history—the ongoing relationships between middle-aged patients and their parents. The idea is to trace the adult course of the relationships between the grown child and the parents because those interactions continue to have a very significant effect upon development. For example, during the initial interview for analysis, a 43-year-old man was very surprised by the intensity of emotion that welled up in him when he was asked about the death of his mother when he was 39. The analyst's questions about the circumstances of her death, the funeral, its effect on the patient's life, and so forth led to a series of associations from both his childhood and his adult years that greatly impressed upon him the power of the diagnostic/therapeutic process and increased his desire for treatment.

Feelings about parents remain dynamically charged in older patients and, if not dismissed by the therapist as irrelevant reminiscences, their expression can lead to considerable insight and therapeutic progress. Even patients who are in their 50s, 60s, and 70s will focus readily on their parents, who are usually dead by that time. Feelings about adult interactions with siblings, alive or dead, are of a similar order of importance and should be explored in the same way. Underlying this approach to the continuous family history is the conviction that familial interactions, real and/or intrapsychic, continue to have a significant impact on development through the second half of life.

Treatment recommendations should follow from the diagnostic conclusions reached after a thorough evaluation, and the adult developmental framework allows flexibility and latitude in planning treatment because older patients are recognized as suitable for dynamic forms of treatment, including intensive psychotherapy and psychoanalysis. Their current developmental problems, understood as far more than recapitulations of a distant past or preludes to death, take on new importance for the analyst, and that enriches the working relationship.

In practice, while taking a developmental history from an adult patient, the diagnostician can be conceptualizing the material simultaneously in two ways that we will describe in detail: chronologically in terms of developmental stages that provide continuity with the stages of childhood, and in terms of developmental lines, singling out and following major themes.

Some recent authors, including Levinson *et al.* (1978) and Gould (1978), have elucidated much complexity in developmental stages. For the purposes of this discussion, we will use Erikson's (1963) division of adulthood into three major phases: early, middle, and late. The assignment of chronological ages to these phases is approximate and is meant to be descriptive rather than definitive. Likewise, the list of tasks we include within each phase is not exhaustive.

Stages and Developmental Tasks of Adulthood

Early adulthood (ages 20 to 40)
  Separating psychologically from parents
  Accepting responsibility for one's own body
  Becoming aware of one's personal history and time limitation
  Integrating sexual experience (homosexual, heterosexual)
  Developing capacity for intimacy with a partner
  Deciding whether to have children
  Relating to children
  Establishing adult relationships with parents
  Acquiring marketable skills
  Choosing a career
  Becoming a ''mentee''
  Using money to further development
  Assuming a social role
  Adopting ethical and spiritual values

Middle adulthood (ages 40 to 60)
  Dealing with bodily changes or illness and altered body image
  Adjusting to midlife changes in sexuality

Accepting the limitation of personal time

Adjusting to aging, illnesses, and deaths of parents and contemporaries

Dealing with the realities of death

Deepening relationships with grown children, grandchildren

Maintaining long-standing and creating new friendships

Developing resonance with people of all ages

Refining work identity

Transmitting skills and values to the young (mentor relationships)

Allocating financial resources, generatively

Accepting social responsibility and change

Late adulthood (age 60 and above)

Maintaining physical health

Adapting to physical infirmities or permanent impairment

Using remaining time in gratifying ways (integrity versus despair)

Adapting to loss of partner, friends

Remaining oriented to present and future, not unduly preoccupied with the past

Forming new emotional ties, seeking and maintaining social contacts

Reversing roles with children, grandchildren

Attending to sexual needs and expression

Continuing meaningful work and play

Using financial resources wisely, for self and others

ADULT DEVELOPMENTAL LINES

In assessing any particular aspect of an adult's development, the concept of developmental lines is very useful. Anna Freud (1963) originally described the manner and sequence in which various aspects of a child's personality unfold as a result of interactions between biological and environmental factors, thus breaking development into manageable components for clarity and study. Well-known childhood developmental lines include those from sucking to rational eating, from wetting and soiling to bladder and bowel control, and lines from the body to the toy and from play to work.

Similar lines of development can be constructed for the adult to help the diagnostician organize his or her thoughts and provide a framework in which to phrase appropriate questions and formulate diagnoses and treatment. We have begun to formulate adult developmental lines for the following issues: (1) intimacy, love, and sex,(2) the adult body, (3) time and death, (4) relationships to children, (5) relationships to parents, (6) mentor relationships, (7) relationships with society, (8) work, (9) play, and (10) financial behavior.

An example of the developmental line of adult intimacy, love, and sex is as follows.

Late teens, early 20s
  Finding appropriate heterosexual partners
  Desire for sexual and nonsexual closeness
  Emergence of capacity for heterosexual caring, tenderness
  Ability to use the body comfortably as a sexual instrument
  Continued resolution of homosexual trends

20s and 30s
  Capacity to invest in one person, based on ability to trust enough,
    to expose and tolerate imperfections in the self and the partner
  Continued broadening of sexual exploration and activity
  Wish for children as an expression of love, union, and sexuality
  Ability to share children with partner

40s and 50s
  Increased recognition of the value of long-standing relationships
  Redefinition of relationship to partner as children grow and leave
  Ability to care for partner in face of illness, aging, and physical
    retrogression
  Capacity to share new activities, interests, and people
  Continuation of active sex life
  Acceptance of diminished intensity of sexual drive
  Acceptance of loss of procreative ability in women

60s and 70s
  Capacity to tolerate loss, deaths of partner and friends
  Ability to form new sustaining ties with friends, children, grand-
    children
  Continuation of active sex life, including masturbation in absence of
    a partner
  Ability to live alone

Each person in the course of normal development in young adult-hood strives for (or reacts against) meaningful heterosexual love and intimacy just as surely as every child encounters the oedipal struggle or the separation–individuation issues. Intimacy is not the same as the ability to have sexual intercourse; it builds on the sexual experience gained in adolescence by incorporating dimensions of genuine caring, tenderness, and mutuality. Subsequent adult experience adds new dimensions, as outlined previously in the developmental line. The analyst locates his or her patient on this developmental continuum, determines the degree of normality or pathology present, and plans his or her diagnostic and therapeutic interventions accordingly. An example of an adult developmental history is included in the following section.

ADULT DEVELOPMENTAL ARREST

The concept of developmental arrest has also proved to be useful to child analysts (Nagera, 1964; Weil, 1953). Through fixation or regression or a combination of the two, a child's progress along a developmental line may be arrested. Likewise, phase-specific stimuli to development occur in adulthood, and development may be arrested in the face of those developmental tasks. Important to this concept is a new emphasis on the adult past (Colarusso & Nemiroff, 1979, 1981; Shane, 1977). In an open-ended view of development, the genetic approach takes on a longitudinal dimension, incorporating experiences that occur in all phases of life. Thus, in addition to the patient's childhood and adolescence, the therapist must consider young adult, and perhaps middle-age, experience as well. What follows is an example of a detailed developmental history including child *and* adult developmental information in which adult developmental arrest is illustrated.

The patient, a successful 31-year-old attorney, was analyzed because of feeling unhappy in his relationships with women. He described a repetitive pattern of disrupting those relationships when he felt too involved and "trapped." Married in his mid-20s, Mr. B. continued to be sexually involved with other women. After several months of marriage, the patient abruptly divorced his wife without external provocation. The memory of that sudden, inexplicable action continued to pain him 6 years later. At the start of his analysis, Mr. B. was seriously involved with another woman but found himself wanting to leave her. While lying with his head in her lap, he had the idea of "wanting to stab her in the vagina with a knife." He became frightened about this thought and sought analysis.

Developmental History

The patient is the eldest son of an intact family that includes father, mother, younger sister, and younger brothers. Mr. B. was a planned, full-term baby. There were no particular problems with the pregnancy, although he was told that his mother suffered from mild depression both before and after his birth. She was involved in his care on a full-time basis. For unknown reasons, breast feeding was begun and then interrupted soon thereafter. This was told to the analyst when the patient was describing his lifelong fascination with breasts. Physical milestones of development such as sitting, standing, and walking occurred within normal limits. Mr. B. was told that he was completely toilet trained before the age of 2 and, according to family lore, there were never any regressions from "this perfect toilet training." The patient reacted strongly to the birth of his sister when he was 2, and he remembers many battles with her during childhood. When Mr. B. was 3, his mother, who had been a constant figure in his life, was badly hurt in an automobile accident and remained hospitalized for almost a year. Mr. B. has no memory for this interval, during which the family lived with the maternal grandmother.

The oedipal years were characterized by frequent paternal absences of 2 to 3 weeks. Mr. B. remembers missing his father during that time and wishing that he could accompany him. When his father was away, his mother often invited Mr. B. to sleep with her. The patient recalled vivid memories of lying in bed with his mother, aware of her negligee, thinking about touching or sucking on her breasts. But his mother could also be punitive. One day when B. was 6 or 7, his mother discovered him involved in sex play with another boy. She overreacted and told him over and over again that he was "bad" for such activity.

Although Mr. B. was able to separate easily from his mother to attend school, he was described by several of his teachers as a mildly hyperactive child who had difficulty sitting still and concentrating. The patient had some initial problems with reading, likely on a neurotic basis, but soon he became a good student. Mr. B. had many friends and was well accepted by the peer group. During latency, his relationship with his father remained difficult because his father continued to travel and considered Mr. B. to be a "destructive, selfish child, only interested in himself and never taking the time to think."

Puberty occurred at 13. Masturbatory fantasies were centered on girls' breasts. In school, where B. was becoming a fine student, he had vivid memories of continually trying to look down girls' blouses. He started to date on a regular basis toward the end of high school. His father's business travel continued, but Mr. B. no longer slept in mother's bed; instead, the two of them would watch television late into the night. He remembered feeling overwhelming sexual desire for her that often culminated in masturbation, accompanied by conscious sexual thoughts about her. During those years his father developed a serious problem with alcohol. In addition to intensifying the tension between father and son, the drinking created a new bond between mother and son as they worked closely together to control the father's behavior.

Initial young adult development was quite positive. Mr. B. was accepted at the college of his choice, which was at a considerable distance from home; he greatly enjoyed himself, doing well scholastically, athletically, and socially. Eventually, he decided upon law as a career and was accepted at an outstanding school. There he met his future wife. Mr. B. was very attracted to her, particularly because of her ample breasts. After a brief courtship, they married impulsively.

However, almost immediately after marriage, Mr. B. found himself obsessed with other female law students, particularly the wife of a close friend. He was hardly married a month when he started a torrid affair with the woman. Against his wife's pleadings, in a callous and cavalier fashion, he abruptly divorced her, to the dismay of family and friends. After finishing law school successfully, Mr. B. entered a prominent law firm. He saw many women in "Don Juan" one-night stands but eventually became seriously involved with an attractive female lawyer. Mr. B. felt that she was "perfect," but he was troubled by feelings of being trapped. He was drawn to her but struggled with his wish to run. The recurrent and insistent idea of wanting to stab her in the vagina with a knife tortured him. He also found himself suffering remorse over the memory of his behavior toward his divorced wife; he felt he still loved her and could not make sense out of his irrational behavior toward her.

Mr. B.'s analysis revealed considerable preoedipal and oedipal rage that interfered with the achievement of intimacy and a loving relationship with a woman. In the transference, he relived early narcissistic injuries relating to both his mother and father as is demonstrated by the following dream and associations.

In a dream Mr. B. is called by a colleague and asked to recommend a good attorney. Mr. B. gives a name, the person is dissatisfied, so Mr. B. gives his own name and then feels agonized that he has to sell himself. He cries out in the dream, "Why do I have to be so defensive and always justify myself?"

His associations are to feelings of inferiority. Things are going well in his law practice, but it will collapse—that is why he has to give his own name inappropriately and oversell himself. He associates to the injuries in his life: his mother's depression, the births of sister and brothers, and his father's alcoholism and unavailability. Mr. B. feels the analyst always evades his questions, as his father did. His father must have held back from him because the patient was inferior. Really, he wants to go home with the analyst and be there all the time. "What I really want is to wrap my legs around you and get inside of you. I want to have you all to myself, that there be no end to our sessions, no weekends, no vacations. But I can't stand talking to you like this." The analyst asks what frightens him so about these feelings. "It would give you so much control over me. It's what I wanted from my mother, but she would completely take me over. I can't trust her. Now I see, with your help, how I have my girlfriend, you, and my mother all mixed up. You and my girlfriend are not my mother."

The patient also feared his rage, which he experienced as murderous. Closeness with the analyst and his girlfriend had to be avoided; he had to protect them from being destroyed. Mr. B. reexperienced feelings of wanting to crush his sister's head with a hammer. His mother was hospitalized, and his father went away on business trips because he was such a destructive child. He was a killer, and his parents were fragile. He had better keep his distance from people.

This patient had both significant childhood traumas and a developmental arrest in young adulthood when he began to struggle seriously with conflicts over intimacy and love. The adult developmental arrest was precipitated by the sudden divorce that was experienced as a significant adult trauma as was the continued inability to make a commitment to one woman. Although the analysis considered all aspects of Mr. B.'s life, it was decidedly helpful to both patient and analyst to *focus* on the adult developmental arrest and the barriers to intimacy and loving relationships with women because the emphasis on both childhood events *and* adult experiences increased the analyst's armamentarium and the patient's understanding. The developmental perspective played a major role in helping to orient and organize the analysis. Although the patient dealt with many aspects of his childhood, current reality, and transference during the 5-year treatment, his central problem was the inability to achieve intimacy with a woman during his young adult years. Eventually, he gained considerable emotional perspective about the origins and ramifications of this barrier and was able to make a commitment to an appropriate woman and continue to progress along the adult developmental line of intimacy, love, and sex.

DEVELOPMENTAL RESONANCE

We introduce the term *developmental resonance* to describe the therapist's awareness of developmental themes in both the patient and himself or herself. Empathy is understood to be an essential ingredient in the therapeutic process. The therapist cannot fully appreciate or understand transferences without feeling what his patients feel, envisioning himself or herself in their places. The developmental framework adds a new dimension to the meaning of empathy and a new facet to transference by demonstrating that patient and analyst share the same developmental continuum. As individuals, they must deal with the same themes in childhood (infantile sexuality, separation from parents, learning, etc.) and adulthood (adult sexuality, work, aging, etc.), although each has unique experiences and, in most instances, they are not at the same point on the continuum. Developmental resonance, then, is the therapist's capacity to share, respect, understand, and value the thoughts and feelings of patients of all ages because of the explicit awareness that he or she had, or likely will have, similar experiences. The following example illustrates the concept.

> A woman in her early 50s came for psychoanalytic psychotherapy because of pain as she watched her 23-year-old son struggle to leave home. The analyst's explanation of the son's continued search for identity—a task she felt he should have finished in his teens—relieved her fears that he was severely disturbed and stimulated her transference relationship to the analyst. The son's verbal abuse and rudeness, a defense against dependency, contrasted sharply with the analyst's kindness, understanding, and empathy and led to the emergence of a transference in which the therapist was seen as a good and caring son. This idealization facilitated the exploration of the mother's role in her son's conflict and her ambivalence about giving him up. At that point, the analyst became the equivalent of a transitional object facilitating the mother's separation from her child. As the son individuated, the patient regressively tried to reestablish the relationship in the transference through attempts to control the analyst and seduce him around issues of medication and a mutual interest in literature. "Let's read Chaucer. Why talk about such depressing stuff," she said. The resolution of the transference allowed the patient to focus on other phase-specific developmental issues such as the "empty nest syndrome"—what to do with life now that her children were raised—and her changing relationship with her husband. In the process, the analyst went from being "my good son" to being "my good friend."

In this instance, the analyst was able to empathize with the age-related experiences of the son, the patient, and himself and to make those three sets of feelings understandable to the patient. The analyst's appreciation of the mutual dynamic conflict—a mother and son at different points in their life cycles locked in the same intense struggle against separation—was the basis for the therapeutic interaction.

SUMMARY

The adult developmental framework is a new frontier for psychoanalytic diagnosis and treatment. In this chapter we have introduced four concepts: (1) the adult developmental diagnosis as an organizing approach to the assessment of patients; (2) adult developmental lines, an expansion of the concept of developmental lines beyond childhood to the entire life cycle; (3) adult developmental arrest, demonstrating the importance of the past from both childhood and adulthood; and (4) developmental resonance, the interaction of the developmental issues in the relationship between analyst and patient.

REFERENCES

Colarusso, C. A., & Nemiroff, R. A. Some observations and hypotheses about the psychoanalytic theory of adult development. *International Journal of Psycho-Analysis*, 1979, *60*, 59–71.

Colarusso, C. A., & Nemiroff, R. A. *Adult development: A new dimension in psychodynamic theory and practice*. New York: Plenum Press, 1981.

Conference on Psychoanalytic Education and Research. Commission IX. *Child Analysis*. New York: American Psychoanalytic Association, 1974.

Erikson, E. H. *Childhood and society* (2nd ed.). New York: W. W. Norton, 1963.

Freud, A. The concept of developmental lines. *Psychoanalytic Study of the Child*, 1963, *18*, 245–265.

Greenspan, S. I., & Pollack, G. H. *The course of life: Psychoanalytic contributions toward understanding personality development. Infancy and early childhood* (Vol. I); *Latency, adolescence and youth* (Vol. II); and *Adulthood and aging* (Vol. III). Washington D.C.: U.S. Government Printing Office, 1981.

Gould, R. L. *Transformations: Growth and change in adult life*. New York: Simon & Schuster, 1978.

Jarvik, L. J., Eisdofer, C., & Blum, J. E. *Intellectual functioning in adults*. New York: Springer, 1973.

King, P. The life cycle as indicated by the nature of the transference in the psychoanalysis of the middle-aged and elderly. *International Journal of Psycho-Analysis*, 1980, *61*, 153–160.

Levinson, D. J., Darrow, C. N., Klein, E. B., Levinson, M. H., & McKee, B. *The seasons of a man's life*. New York: Knopf, 1978.

Marcus, J. (Reporter). The experience of separation–individuation...through the course of life: Adolescence and maturity (Panel report). *Journal of the American Psychoanalytic Association*, 1973, *21*, 155–167.

Nagera, H. On arrest in development, fixation, and regression. *Psychoanalytic Study of the Child*, 1964, *19*, 222–239.

Pollock, G. H. Mourning and adaptation. *International Journal of Psycho-Analysis*, 1971, *42*, 341–361.

Pribram, K. *Languages of the brain: Experimental paradoxes and principles in neuropsychology*. Englewood Cliffs, N.J.: Prentice-Hall, 1971.

Shane, M. A rationale for teaching analytic technique based on a developmental orientation and approach. *International Journal of Psycho-Analysis*, 1977, *58*, 95–108.

Steinschein, I. (Reporter). The experience of separation–individuation. . .through the course of life: Maturity, senescence, and sociological implication (Panel report). *Journal of the American Psychoanalytic Association*. 1973, *21*, 633–645.

Vaillant, G. E. *Adaptation to life*. Boston: Little, Brown, 1977.

Weil, A. P. Certain severe disturbances of ego development in childhood. *Psychoanalytic Study of the Child*, 1953, *8*, 271–286.

Winestine, M. (Reporter). The experience of separation–individuation. . .through the course of life: Infancy and childhood (Panel report). *Journal of the American Psychoanalytic Association*, 1973, *21*, 135–154.

4

Adult Development and Transference

ROBERT A. NEMIROFF AND CALVIN A. COLARUSSO

Transference has been defined as the displacement of patterns of feelings and behavior that were originally experienced with significant figures of one's childhood to individuals in one's current relationships (Moore & Fine, 1968, p. 92). Transference has always been understood to have its roots in the infantile past. Freud focused on the events of the oedipal phase and the infantile neurosis as the source of neurotic transference (Freud, 1905, 1912, 1913, 1915–1917). Gradually, other analysts (Kernberg, 1975; Klein, 1948, Kohut, 1971, 1977; Kramer, 1979) explored the relationships between preoedipal development and transference.

As we have pointed out, the most prevalent psychoanalytic conception today does not hold that adults undergo dynamic development. Indeed, such distinguished developmentalists as Anna Freud, Humberto Nagera, and W. Ernst Freud (1965) wrote in their work on the adult profile:

> In this instance assessment is concerned not with an ongoing process but with a finished product in which, by implication, the ultimate developmental stages should have been reached. The developmental point of view may be upheld only insofar as success or failure to reach this level or to maintain it determines the so-called maturity or immaturity of the adult personality. (p. 10)

The paper on which this chapter is based was presented by Dr. Colarusso at the spring 1981 meeting of the American Psychoanalytic Association in San Juan as part of a panel entitled "The Changing Vistas of Transference: The Effect of Developmental Concepts on the Understanding of Transference."

Their statement may not be limited so much by a failure to see the adult as dynamic and changing as by what they choose to call *development*. For them, as for the majority of analysts, the term refers primarily to the formation of psychic structure, a process that is confined to childhood and adolescence.

The view of adulthood that we and some others hold agrees with the following statement by Morton Shane (1977):

> The use of the developmental approach implies that the analytic patient, regardless of age, is considered to be still in the process of ongoing development as opposed to merely being in possession of a past that influences his present conscious and unconscious life. (pp. 95–96)

Likewise, we remind the reader that the definition of development to which we adhere is that of Rene Spitz (1965, p. 5): "The emergence of exchanges between the organism on one hand, and the inner and outer environment on the other."

Whereas most analysts readily acknowledge the developmental role of organic maturation and physical progression in childhood and adolescence, few acknowledge that the forces of physical aging and retrogression may be equally important factors in developmental processes in the second half of life. With respect to the effects of bodily changes on adult development, we maintain that the organism *continues* as a dominant influence in the developmental processes and is expressed psychologically through the normative increasing awareness of physical aging and a growing preoccupation with time limitation and the inevitability of personal death. As at all points throughout life, depending on individual experience, the phase-specific developmental tasks that must be engaged can serve as stimuli to developmental progression, that is, significant intrapsychic growth or as niduses for arrest and fixation.

And what of the other pole of development—the inner and outer environment? It is a psychoanalytic truism that the outer environment as characterized, for instance, by the mother of infancy or the oedipal father has a powerful effect on childhood development. But, as with the body, the environment is usually afforded an inconsequential role in adult development. Witness the following statement by Eissler (1975):

> In early life periods, biology and the primary demands of reality furnish the guidelines of a necessary development. The guidelines of latency, puberty and adolescence are increasingly defined by the demands of culture and sexual maturation. The adult, though, should be more or less free, even though limited by the general biological framework. In the ideal case internal processes

are autonomous and are not primarily determined by immediate biological or sociocultural factors, as occurs in the preceding phases of development. (p. 139)

In contradistinction, we have suggested that in the achievement of new and phase-specific developmental tasks the adult is as dependent as the child on the environment. Parents and play are replaced by spouse, children, and work. Mature sexual activity and the gradual emergence of the capacity for intimacy are impossible to achieve without a loved and loving partner. Creativity and work, even of the most introspective kind such as music or literature, are influenced by existing forms and styles and are intended to be communicated to others.

DIFFERENCES BETWEEN THE DEVELOPMENTAL PROCESSES IN CHILDHOOD AND ADULTHOOD

It is important for our consideration of the effect of developmental concepts on the understanding of transference that we address the *differences* between the developmental processes in the child and the adult. One aspect of difference is reflected in our hypothesis that whereas childhood development is focused primarily on the formation of psychic structure, adult development is concerned with the continuing evolution of existing psychic structure and with its use (Colarusso & Nemiroff, 1981).

Part of the reason the adult has been conceptualized as static may be a failure to recognize the scope of psychic change in adulthood. The appearance in childhood of basic ego functions, the superego and ego ideal, has been designated as development but not so the sometimes sweeping changes that occur in those basic structures in adulthood. Settlage (1973) uses the word *rearrangements* to describe this evolution in adulthood, whereas Benedek (1975) uses the term *psychological reorganization* for the same processes. Both terms may be inadequate to describe the great degree of change in psychic structure that occurs in adulthood. Take, for example, the experience of parenthood. We have described the change in the internal representation of the concept *father* as that role changes over time (Colarusso & Nemiroff, 1982). The experiences of being the 25-year-old father of a 3-year-old child, relating to a living father of 55 and to a young wife deeply involved in child care, and those of being a 45-year-old father of late adolescents and young adults, relating to an aging or dead father and preoccupied with the aging process in oneself and one's wife, can be so different and result in such altered intra-psychic representations that perhaps the only thing in common is the name given to the experience. The changes in psychic structure that oc-cur in adults are analogous to gutting the inside of a building and retain-ing the facade for historical purposes; the interior becomes very differ-ent, but the same face is presented to the external world. We construe such changes as developmental because they result from exchanges be-tween the organism and environment, and they are as significant for the normal adult as the formation of psychic structure is for the normal child.

The attitude of an analyst toward the evolving transference presented by his or her patient is very likely to be influenced by his or her mental set about what constitutes development. Without a sense of the adult as immersed in an ongoing developmental process, he or she may minimize the effect of adult experience on transference phenomena, and his or her interpretations would represent the transference phenomena as repeti-tions of childhood experience alone rather than elaborations from a lifetime.

Although transference has been seen as an "amalgam of past and present, infantile and adult" (Curtis, 1979, p. 178), few analytic theore-ticians have seen the adult years as a potential *source* of transference. It is our contention that in addition to being new elaborations of infantile experience, transference phenomena in adults are also expressions of new experiences and conflicts from developmental stages beyond child-hood. Both factors and the continuation of central developmental themes from childhood into adulthood are represented in the present by psy-chic structure that is very different from that which existed in childhood and which is undergoing continuous change and refinement.

According to Coltrera (1979), although Freud clearly understood childhood experience to be the source of transference phenomena in the adult, he wrestled until his death with the question of the effect of more recent events on psychopathology and transference:

> In their strict sense, genetic interpretation and reconstruction may be said to be concerned with genetically significant, usually childhood, intrapsychic events. While this is strictly true in the reconstructions of the infantile neu-roses of Little Hans and the Wolf Man, it was not so in the cases of the Rat Man or the eighteen-year-old Katharine—the girl Freud met while on vacation—whose reconstructions concerned more recent events. As the Kris Study Group (Fine *et al.*, 1971) pointed out, Freud's (1909) saying of the Rat Man, "He must have known," was implicitly an interpretation of psychically significant *recent* events. This continuous and seemingly ambiguous shifting between an earlier past and a more recent past in the focus of genetic interpre-

tation existed in Freud's mind right up to his last paper on reconstruction in 1937 and must be looked upon as an early and critical declension of the genetic view to include not only the past's determinacy in the present, but an appreciation of how the present can influence the recollection of the past. (p. 291)

Shane (1977) has formulated the following developmental conceptualization of transference:

> With a developmental approach, however, transference, and particularly the transference neurosis, while involving crucial pathogenic elements from the past displaced onto the present, does not involve the past *exclusively*. In fact, the potency of primary objects to elicit powerful developmental conflicts in the present (albeit with strong reverberations to the repressed past) is seen throughout adolescence and indeed into adult life. (p. 102)

THE ADULT PAST AS A SOURCE OF TRANSFERENCE

The advent of a developmentally dynamic psychology of adulthood now allows reconsideration of the effect of events in adulthood on the nature of transference and expansion of the use of the genetic approach (reference to the past) to place greater emphasis on adult experience in which psychogenesis takes on a longitudinal dimension, incorporating new developmental conflicts and experiences occurring at each phase throughout the life course. In such a conceptual framework, the adult past can be an important source of transference.

It is well recognized that the events of the oedipal past express themselves in the neurotic process and in the transference neurosis in adults. Increasingly, through the work of Peter Blos (1980) and others, the effect of the adolescent past on transference is being recognized in adults, demonstrating that a developmental phase beyond the oedipal phase is indeed a source of transference. But how are the young adult past and the middle-age past represented in the transference? These later developmental experiences certainly relate to and are influenced by the events of childhood, but they cannot be fully explained by them, hence the need to broaden the concept. The following clinical example serves well to illustrate our point.

> Mr. L. was 38 when he entered treatment because of an absence of feeling and sexual impotence. Highly successful and creative in his business, he was unable to sustain any degree of sexual or emotional closeness with his wife of many years. Numerous infantile experiences obviously contributed to his behavior, such as a seductive mother, a sexually inhibited,

distant father who preached the evils of sex, and surgery on the genitals during the oedipal phase. Sexual development was hampered throughout adolescence, but in his twenties the patient was able to marry, father a child, and achieve academically. Sexual performance gradually improved during the early years of marriage, indicating some mastery of infantile sexual conflicts through adult sexual experience. Suddenly at age 30, the patient developed a testicular cancer which was treated with surgery and irradiation, leading to sterilization.

This patient's cancer experience was understood by the analyst in two ways: as a significant trauma in its own right and as a major interference with young adult development, particularly the tasks related to the achievement of intimacy and parenthood. The patient's idiosyncratic psychological response to the physical trauma was considerable intrapsychic conflict resulting in inhibition of aggression and in sexual and emotional withdrawal. The opening phase of the analysis, begun 5 years after the surgery, was characterized by a pleasant cooperative attitude and deference toward the analyst. Initially, the cancer experience was studiously avoided, but eventually the patient described it with great emotion. Recognition by the analyst of the effect of the cancer on L.'s adult aspirations—his wish to father a second child and hope for the growth of sexual intimacy with his wife, which had been developing spontaneously at the time—was the key to establishing a therapeutic alliance. To this patient, particularly at the beginning of his analysis, the adult past was more important than the infantile past. If the analyst had minimized or ignored the patient's focus on the recent experience or interpreted prematurely the transparent infantile transference determinants, the therapeutic alliance might not have developed as smoothly as it did. Valuing the adult past as meaningful in its own right helped the analyst engage the patient with sensitivity and empathy, thus creating an environment in which transference could emerge and be elaborated.

When associations about the surgery itself began to emerge, the patient's attitude toward the analyst changed. He became quarrelsome, hostile, suspicious, even embittered. These responses were understood to be primarily feelings about the cancer surgery, that is, transference emanating from an adult experience despite the fact that feelings from the oedipal genital surgery were also involved. Attempts to analyze these transference responses were met with verbal abuse and threats to end the analysis. The patient, accustomed to his pattern of deference toward physicians—understood by the analyst to be an inhibition against his rage at them for both surgical assaults—was chagrined and puzzled by these uncharacteristic feelings and behavior. Gradually, it became apparent that he had recreated in the transference first his fear of and later his rage at the physicians who had sterilized him. His growing emotional dependence on the analyst and his inability to control those feelings stimulated recall of the profound helplessness he has experienced in relation to the physicians who "dominated me, treated me like a guinea pig, and ruined my life. I hated them and was terrified of them. I can see now that I've been feeling the same way about you."

The analysis of this adult experience and the transference it generated was, of course, only one aspect of the analysis. It is emphasized here to demonstrate our point. Considerable work was done in terms of the transference on feelings about the oedipal surgical experience as well. Nevertheless, this patient's transference could not have been understood simply as a new edition or elaboration of an infantile event and conflict because different developmental tasks and processes had been compromised by the adult trauma. The surgery during the oedipal period compromised that phase of development and contributed to the failure to "resolve" the infantile neurosis; the later cancer surgery seriously compromised the adult developmental tasks of intimacy and parenthood.

In this man, or in any patient, the analysis of infantile derivatives is undiminished in importance by the incorporation of the adult past as a potential source of transference. The adult developmental framework complements earlier analytic theory and may be particularly helpful in elucidating the interrelationships between transference phenomena rooted in childhood and in adulthood. This is a matter of considerable technical interest that will be discussed later in this chapter.

THE ADULT OEDIPAL COMPLEX

Another theme that affects the evolution and expression of transference in the adult is contained in our hypothesis that the fundamental developmental issues of childhood continue as central aspects of adult life but in altered form (Colarusso & Nemiroff, 1981, p. 67). If we look at major developmental issues in terms of the life cycle rather than as isolated events limited to only certain stages of development, they become integral parts of normal adult experience. We shall use the oedipal complex—the core of the transference neurosis—as the example of a childhood theme that continues as a central aspect of adult life. The continuation of the oedipal complex into adulthood is not a new idea. Freud (1924) spoke of it in *The Dissolution of the Oedipal Complex*, and Pearson (1958), Benedek (1975), and others have touched on it. With the exception of Leo Rangell (1953), however, few have dealt with oedipal phenomena as central, continuing factors in normal adult development. We have described the following evidence of oedipal phenomena in the normal adult (Colarusso & Nemiroff, 1981):

> Each parent reacts to the budding sexuality of adolescent children with at least occasional over-restriction or seductiveness. Aware of the muting of sexual prowess in midlife and unconsciously jealous of the adolescent's abundant future, the parent retaliates against his offspring (Pearson, 1958). Competitiveness and envy of girlfriends or boyfriends, fiances, and eventually husbands and wives of grown children provide ample evidence of the triangular relationships that exist among parents, children, and children's spouses. Fathers' protectiveness of their daughters' virtue and encouragement of their sons' lack of it, and mothers-in-law's almost universal tendency to compete for their children are all too obvious evidence of the nature of adult oedipal experience. (p. 68)

These oedipal phenomena are responded to by the normal adult with capabilities that make the experience qualitatively different from that of the child. The analyst must distinguish between and interrelate the oedipal productions from his or her patient that are generated by infantile and adult experience, respectively.

THE NEGATIVE OEDIPAL COMPLEX

The negative oedipal complex has also been expanded beyond the confines of the oedipal period. Peter Blos (1980) recently made the following statement:

> The negative oedipal complex is resolved normally toward the end of adolescence. Thus, the totality of the oedipal complex comes to its final and inclusive settlement.... The resolution of the negative oedipus complex is one—if not *the* major task of adolescence. (p. 147)

The elaboration of the influence of negative oedipal themes on adolescent development, particularly in regard to the formation of the ego ideal and adult character, is an important insight that expands our knowledge of the formation of psychic structure. We do not agree, however, that either the oedipal or the negative oedipal complex comes to its final and inclusive settlement in adolescence. Both continue to influence psychic life throughout the adult years. For an illustration of this, we return to the developmental phenomenology of fatherhood and our postulation of negative oedipal currents in the middle-aged father who is traversing a particularly formative time in the evolution of paternal identity. Reengagement and further resolution of negative oedipal themes, which were not possible before this period, and their manifestation in the transference can occur in the following manner. A father must gradually relinquish active control of his adolescent son as the boy insists on increasing autonomy. This necessitates a shift in the balance of power between them as the younger male moves toward self-mastery. In the face of this normal conflict, the father may experience rage and helplessness and a sense of weakness, even passivity, in relation to his son because he must leave behind his role as parent of a young child. Because many gratifications of that role were related to the direct expression and sublimation of feelings of aggression through domination and control, the transition can be a painful one. Overreactions may take the form of attempts to maintain dominance or, through reversal, the opposite may occur when the father neglects the paternal limit-setting role and tries to imitate his son instead. Both types of behavior can emerge in the transference phenomena.

> It is our impression that the capacity for paternal generativity (Erikson, 1963) is determined in part by the resolution of this conflict. Through adult reworking, generativity is linked to masculinity as the passive, loving trends within a father's character are expressed by his care, unintrusive support, and facilitation of the emergent sexuality, independence, and separateness of late adolescent and young-adult sons and daughters. (Colarusso & Nemiroff, 1981, p. 132)

Case Study

A 44-year-old man was deeply troubled by the emergence of wishes to see the analyst's penis. Gradually, these thoughts were related to wishes from childhood to see his father's penis and wishes in the present to see that of his teenaged son. Through the analysis of transference fantasies about sexual activity between himself and the analyst, it gradually became clear that the patient envied the sexual prowess of both his father of childhood and his son of the present and recent past and unconsciously coveted their penises in fantasies of homosexual activity and castration. The wishes toward his father and his son, which first appeared in the transference, had to be analyzed and interpreted, relating the infantile past with the adult present.

As these feelings and wishes became conscious, the patient reacted by attempting to control the analyst and restrict his son's dating activities. Only gradually, as he analyzed his positive and negative oedipal wishes—in the transference toward the analyst and in his role as a father toward his son—was he able to assume a less intrusive, more supportive attitude toward his son's emerging autonomy and sexual development.

A conceptualization of this middle-age man's transference as expressing both current midlife developmental conflict and *at the same time* the recapitulation of oedipal and adolescent themes from his childhood past increases the complexity of the analytic work, but it provides a framework in which transference variables from all phases of development, including the present, may be considered.

THE INFANTILE AND ADULT NEUROSIS: INTERRELATIONS AND EFFECT ON TRANSFERENCE

If the individual is in the midst of dynamic change in adulthood and transference stems from the adult past and the continuation of childhood developmental themes into adulthood, what is the relationship between childhood and adult experience in the formation of the adult neurosis and how is this relationship manifested in the transference?

The continued study of both infantile and adult neuroses has led prominent analytic theoreticians to the conclusion that the relationship is a complex one. As demonstrated by Blos (1972), Ritvo (1974), Loewald (1979), and others, there is not always a direct, traceable relationship between the infantile and adult neurosis. Yet the events of the oedipal phase are clearly linked to the adult psychopathology. We believe that the adult developmental framework may shed some light on the relationship between the infantile neurosis and subsequent experience.

Developmental experience during the preoedipal and oedipal phases *predisposes* an individual to the possibility of an adult neurosis. During the oedipal phase, for the first time, sexual and aggressive impulses are expressed primarily through the framework of triangular object relationships. Because of the combination of drive expression and ego development that occurs then, the psychic apparatus is capable of responding, for the first time, with neurotic symptom formation. A new mental response to conflict, namely, the infantile neurosis, occurs. Subsequent developmental phases, both in childhood and adulthood, participate in the following way. When the infantile neurosis is not "resolved," the neurotic pattern may continue unabated from the oedipal stage onward, traceable through each subsequent phase of development where it is elaborated by subsequent experience. On the other hand, the neurotic patterns may disappear, only to be precipitated later by events at some subsequent stage of development. The adult presentation of the neurosis is the result of the infantile predisposition, the subsequent elaboration, *and* current developmental experience. All of these factors are condensed into the symptom picture forged by the psychic apparatus of the present. In a sense, adult experience rewrites the experience from childhood, shaping its presentation in the adult transference. Thus, all three aspects (organization and predisposition, subsequent elaboration, and adult presentation) are important in understanding neurotic transference and in determining technique.

Coltrera (1979) has a developmental orientation similar to ours. He has stated:

> One becomes ever more impressed that the transference neurosis is very much developmentally determined, its character and focus changing throughout the life cycle according to phase-specific developmental and conflict resolutions and their subsequent internalizations. A growing body of literature on serial analysis done in the same patient...attest[s] to the transmutation of the transference neurosis throughout genetic series, different in character and form during different developmental times. (p. 305)

The following clinical example from a 47-year-old man, in his fourth year of analysis, illustrates these concepts.

> The patient, Mr. B., presented with marked anxiety, fear of heights, and a pronounced fear of premature death from a heart attack. Youngest of three children, B. was raised in an intact family. His preoedipal years were characterized by relatively stable development. Despite seductive interactions around toilet training, he entered the oedipal phase without significant symptoms. As reconstructed by analyst and patient in the analysis, the oedipal phase was characterized by seductive closeness to mother (parental nudity, enemas, and wiping the patient after bowel movements until he was 8), and a quiet, distant relationship with his father. Mr. B. had memories of nightmares and fears of the dark that diminished during latency. Thus, during the oedipal phase he had experienced an infantile neurosis and produced typical oedipal symptomatology that predisposed him to a later neurosis.
> But it was not until late latency, when he rather suddenly required major surgery shortly after his father had a heart attack, that a clinical neurosis appeared, which consisted of pronounced fears of the dark, exaggerated concerns about his own and his father's health, and a strong

obsessional inhibition against stepping on cracks. Mr. B.'s concern for his father's health intensified over the next few years as did his phobic and obsessional symptoms, until in his midadolescence his father died. The patient, so acutely preoccupied with the prospect of his father's death, was unable to mourn when the death actually occurred. The surgery and paternal illness and death precipitated and organized the neurosis.

As adolescence continued, the neurosis became increasingly focused on bodily concerns. By his late teens, Mr. B. was severely inhibiting his physical activity and sexuality and relying on medications to magically guard against his fears of death.

The adult years prior to the analysis were characterized by a steady, low-grade preoccupation with physical health, an increasing tendency toward self-medication, and marked sexual and work inhibitions. Analysis was precipitated by job-related concerns. The presenting complaints centered on anxiety about these events and a phobia that was becoming incapacitating.

Clearly, this man's neurosis was elaborated in each subsequent phase of development and upon presentation was also an expression of his adult developmental concerns with work achievement and aging. "I'm 47 years old; I don't expect to live beyond 50; my father died when he was 49."

The transference was the main vehicle for the expression of each facet of this man's neurosis. At various times the analyst was represented not only as a parent of childhood (the father who did not care, the seductive mother) but also as the dangerous physician from late latency. The analyst was also represented as the "cheap whore" from his young adult past who encouraged him to engage in new forms of sexual activity that would kill him—a heart attack while in bed—or turn him into a depraved sexual maniac. Another representation was the uncaring boss who would fire him (throw him out of analysis) if he knew of Mr. B.'s anger and criticism.

Thus, transference from *all* stages of development brought the neurosis to life in the analysis, demonstrating how each developmental phase participated in the clinical picture the patient presented.

Such a conceptualization of the adult neurosis suggests the following technical considerations. It would not have been enough to help the patient gradually see the relationship between the infantile and adult neurosis—in other words, the oedipal and preoedipal reconstructions. That was but one step in the therapeutic process. It remained for patient and analyst to detail the elaboration of the neurosis in adolescence and adulthood (relating it to such significant life events as the father's death and the patient's surgery) and to describe the neurotic interference with normal adolescent and adult developmental tasks. Then, as has been described by Shane (1979), the patient could apply the insights and freedom gained in the analysis to his present and future development and return to the mainstream of development as free as possible from the powerful skewing effect of his neurosis.

SUMMARY

The adult developmental framework, a psychoanalytic frontier, may add a new and complementary dimension to existing theory about transference. By shedding light on the developmental processes in the adult and relating these to childhood experience, the adult developmental framework influences the analyst's attitude toward his or her adult patient and increases his or her understanding of transference material from all phases of life. A more comprehensive understanding of the neurotic process and advances in technique may be other useful results of continued study in this field.

REFERENCES

Benedek, T. Depression during the life cycle. In E. J. Anthony & T. Benedek (Eds.), *Depression and human existence*. Boston: Little, Brown, 1975.

Blos, P. The epigenesis of the adult neurosis. *Psychoanalytic Study of the Child*, 1972, 27, 106–135.

Blos, P. The life cycle as indicated by the nature of the transference in the psychoanalysis of adolescents. *International Journal of Psychoanalysis*, 1980, 61, 145–152.

Colarusso, C. A., & Nemiroff, R. A. *Adult development: A new dimension in psychodynamic theory and practice*. New York: Plenum Press, 1981.

Colarusso, C. A., & Nemiroff, R. A. The father at midlife: Crisis and growth of paternal identity. In S. Cath, A. Gurwitz, & J. M. Ross (Eds.), *Father and child*. Boston: Little, Brown, 1982.

Coltrera, J. Truth from genetic illusion: The transference and the fate of the infantile neurosis. *Journal of the American Psychoanalytic Association*, 1979, 27(Supplement), 289–314.

Curtis, H. The concept of therapeutic alliance: Implications for the "widening scope." *Journal of the American Psychoanalytic Association*, 1979, 27(Supplement), 159–192.

Eissler, K. On possible effects of aging on the practice of psychoanalysis: An essay. *Journal of the Philadelphia Association of Psychoanalysis*, 1975, 11, 138–152.

Erikson, E. H. Eight ages of man. In *Childhood and society* (2nd ed.). New York: W. W. Norton, 1963.

Fine, B. D., Joseph, E. D., & Waldhorn, H. R. (Eds.). *Recollection and reconstruction. Reconstruction in psychoanalysis*. Kris Study Group Monograph, IV. New York: International Universities Press, 1971.

Freud, A., Nagera, H., & Freud, E. Metapsychological assessment of the adult personality. *Psychoanalytic Study of the Child*, 1965, 29, 9.

Freud, S. Fragment of an analysis of a case of hysteria. In J. Strachey (Ed. and trans.), *Standard edition* (7:3). London: Hogarth Press, 1905.

Freud, S. Notes upon a case of obsessional neurosis. In J. Strachey (Ed. and trans.), *Standard edition* (10:153). London: Hogarth Press, 1909.

Freud, S. The dynamics of transference. In J. Strachey (Ed. and trans.), *Standard edition* (12:97). London: Hogarth Press, 1912.

Freud, S. On beginning the treatment. In J. Strachey (Ed. and trans.), *Standard edition* (12:121). London: Hogarth Press, 1913.

Freud, S. Papers on metapsychology. In J. Strachey (Ed. and trans.), *Standard edition* (14:105). London: Hogarth Press, 1915-1917.

Freud, S. The dissolution of the oedipus complex. In J. Strachey (Ed. and trans.), *Standard edition* (19:173). London: Hogarth Press, 1924.

Kernberg, O. *Borderline conditions and pathological narcissism*. New York: Aronson, 1975.

Klein, M. The Oedipus complex in the light of early anxieties. In *Contributions to psychoanalysis, 1921-1945*. London: Hogarth Press, 1948.

Kohut, H. *The analysis of the self*. New York: International Universities Press, 1971.

Kohut, H. *The restoration of the self*. New York: International Universities Press, 1977.

Kramer, S. The technical significance and application of Mahler's separation-individuation theory. *Journal of the American Psychoanalytic Association*. 1979, 27(Supplement), 241-262.

Loewald, H. The waning of the oedipal complex. *Journal of the American Psychoanalytic Association*. 1979, 27, 751.

Moore, B., & Fine, B. *A glossary of psychoanalytic terms and concepts* (2nd ed.). New York: American Psychoanalytic Association, 1968.

Pearson, G. *Adolescence and the conflict of generations*. New York: W. W. Norton, 1958.

Rangell, L. The role of the parent in the oedipus complex. *Bulletin of the Menninger Clinic*, 1953, 19, 9-15.

Ritvo, S. Current status of the concept of infantile neurosis. *Psychoanalytic Study of the Child*, 1974, 29, 159-182.

Settlage, C. The experience of separation-individuation...through the course of life: Infancy and childhood (Panel report. M. Winestine, Reporter). *Journal of the American Psychoanalytic Association*, 1973, 21, 135-154.

Shane, M. A rationale for teaching analytic technique based on a developmental orientation and approach. *International Journal of Psychoanalysis*, 1977, 58, 95-108.

Shane, M. The developmental approach to "working through" in the analytic process. *International Journal of Psycho-analysis*, 1979, 60, 375-382.

Spitz, R. *The first year of life*. New York: International Universities Press, 1965.

5
Friendship in Midlife
WITH REFERENCE TO THE THERAPIST AND HIS WORK

ROBERT A. NEMIROFF AND CALVIN A. COLARUSSO

> It is astonishing how little has been written in the psychoanalytic literature on this perhaps most frequent of all human relations [friendship]. The references which do exist are generally glancing, scanty, and *en passant*. There is, to my knowledge, scarcely a psychoanalytic study centered on this subject in depth. (Rangell, 1963, p. 3)

That statement, made over two decades ago, is still essentially true. The reasons are undoubtedly many. Among them are the relative youth of psychoanalysis as a science, an early preoccupation with psychopathology, and a later focus on development in childhood. Increasingly, in recent years the scope of interest and research has broadened to include the study of normality in the adult. In this chapter, we explore the developmental forces that shape normal midlife friendships and consider the effect of the therapist's work on his or her own friendships, particularly those with colleagues and students.

REVIEW OF THE LITERATURE

Freud's references to friendship are few, and his thoughts on the topic are highly insightful, but they are essentially undeveloped. Friendship, said Freud (1921), is a form of love, an expression of libido, stemming from the same source as sexual love that has sexual union as its aim.

> We do not separate from this—what in any case has its share in the name "love"—on the one hand, self love, and on the other, love of parents and

children, friendship and love for humanity in general, and also devotion to
concrete objects and to abstract ideas. (p. 90)

In the relationship between the sexes, the impulses "force their way toward sexual union, but in other circumstances *they are diverted from this
aim or are prevented from reaching it* [italics added] though always preserving enough of their original nature to keep their identity recognizable"
(pp. 90–91).

So a critical distinction between love and friendship is the aim-
inhibited expression of the impulses in friendship. However, these inhibited instincts

always preserve some few of their original sexual aims; even an affectionate
devotee, even a friend or an admirer, desires the physical proximity and the
right to the person who is now loved only in the "Pauline" sense. (1921, pp.
138–139)

Thus, "the inhibited instincts are capable of any degree of admixture
with the uninhibited; they can be transformed back into them, just as
they arose out of them" (p. 139). It is our impression that the aim-
inhibited nature of the impulses—and the possibility of reversal to direct
expression—defines the nature of friendship more than any other characteristic.

But human relationships, including friendships, are not based on
"love" alone.

Men are not gentle creatures who want to be loved, and who at the most can
defend themselves if they are attacked; they are, on the contrary creatures
among whose instinctual endowments is to be reckoned a powerful share of
aggressiveness. As a result, their neighbor is for them not only a potential
helper or sexual object, but also someone who tempts them to satisfy their
aggressiveness on him, to exploit his capacity for work without compensation, to use him sexually without his consent, to seize his possessions, to hu-
miliate him, to cause him pain, to torture and to kill him. (Freud, 1930, p. 111)

As with all other human interactions, friendships are also based on aggression. The character of friendship is determined by the aim-inhibited
expression of the aggression, not by the absence of it.

Little has been done to elaborate Freud's seminal ideas. As previously mentioned, Rangell's article (1963) "On Friendship" looms as the
one significant exception. Using the developmental and ego psychological ideas available at the time, Rangell described what might be called
a developmental line (A. Freud, 1963) of friendship during the childhood
years. The gratified infant first experiences friendly feeling toward his

or her mother. Later, similar feelings are directed toward a transitional object (Winnicott, 1953).

During the preoedipal and oedipal years, friendly feelings begin to be concentrated on persons other than nuclear family members, but the relationships are "transient, mostly nonspecific, internally directed, and self oriented, of use primarily for the consolidation of *inner* psychic development" (Rangell, 1963, p. 116).

Rangell (1963) puts considerable import (correctly so, it seems to us) on the resolution of the oedipal complex and passage into latency. With the resolution of the complex, "love, which has now reached an intense developmental peak, can be diluted and mitigated, objects (again) displaced, and aims inhibited and less than directly sought" (p. 17). Latency friendships result from the "widespread and more general sublimatory activity occurring at this time" (p. 17).

In Rangell's opinion, however (as opposed to our own), adolescence is the phase in which "friendships, in the true and technical sense. . . take root, begin to flourish, and become a center of activity" (p. 18).

DEFINITION

> There can be no friendship where there is no freedom. Friendship loves a free air, and will not be fenced up in straight and narrow enclosures. (William Penn)

Defining friendship is not an easy matter. Neither Freud nor Rangell gives a complete definition, possibly because the subject is too broad to be encompassed by a single statement. What follows is our attempt to provide a psychoanalytic definition of friendship, integrating thoughts of Freud, Rangell, and us.

> Friendship is an extrafamilial object relationship based on mutuality, equality and freedom of choice, in which the expression of sexual and aggressive impulses is predominantly aim inhibited.

Like all other relationships, friendships are psychically determined, and they serve conscious and unconscious purposes of drive expression.

By limiting friendships to extrafamilial relationships, our definition rules out many significant interactions in which friendly feelings occur—such as those between lovers (heterosexual or homosexual), spouses, parents and children, and siblings. This exclusion was made because the essential nature of those interactions is determined by either the direct expression of sexual and aggressive impulses (lovers and spouses) or by inequality and the absence of choice (parents and children, and siblings).

Friendships are defined primarily by the aim-inhibited expression of impulses. However, because of the power of the drives, this is often a difficult condition to maintain. Consequently, friends can be transformed into lovers or enemies—and sometimes back again into friends. Because of the relatively limited capacity of the childhood ego vis-à-vis the drives, this tendency toward fluidity is common in childhood, whereas the maintenance of a stable state of friendship over an extended period of time is more characteristic of adulthood.

It should also be noted that his definition does not discriminate on the basis of sex. Rangell points out that, although he does not specifically say so, Freud seems to be limiting friendships to same-sex relationships. It is our impression that true friendships between members of the opposite sexes can occur throughout life but happen with greater frequency in adulthood for reasons to be examined later.

Finally, our definition allows for friendships between individuals of different ages and developmental phases. The ability to form friendships across the barriers imposed by age and developmental differences is again most characteristic of mature individuals in the second half of life. True equality may be difficult to achieve and maintain in these friendships.

THE EMERGENCE IN LATENCY OF THE CAPACITY FOR FRIENDSHIP

In her definitive article on play in childhood, Lilli Peller (1954) described the effect of major developmental themes upon the nature and form of play. In essence, she described how play facilitated the engagement and mastery of phase-specific, normative tasks. For instance, play during the anal phase centered around the child's experience with the preoedipal mother, "the unfathomable source of comfort as well as of fear and terror" (p. 186). Through countless repetitions, the child deals with the mother's enormous power. "I can do to you what mother did to me" (p. 186). At this stage of development, the child plays alone or with the mother, sometimes using transitional objects as well.

During the oedipal phase, play changes dramatically. The variation in form and substance is in response to the emergence of new developmental tasks and the continued growth of the ego. Aware that he or she is small and left out of adult pleasures, the oedipal child creates compensatory fantasy play in which he or she is big and powerful—the center of attraction. Other children are increasingly involved, but the play usually revolves around the fantasy of a single child who, at least for the moment, dominates the others and assigns them roles in his or her idiosyncratic fantasy.

Can these children be considered friends? Certainly friendly feelings are often observed. But, according to our criteria, the oedipal-age child is not yet capable of genuine friendship. The relationship may be extrafamilial but is not characterized by equality, mutuality, or aim inhibition. The oedipal-age child's ego and forming superego are not yet integrated enough to consistently inhibit the direct expression of sexual and aggressive impulses.

A person's capacity for friendship, however, is partially determined by the "object lesson" he or she learned from the oedipal struggle and its resolution: That it *is* possible to have meaningful, need-fulfilling relationships with others without the property of exclusivity. To the extent that this lesson is imperfectly learned (and this is always the case), jealousy has a role in friendship. Thus, jealousy is a component of friendship even when the relationship is overtly aim inhibited (Braun, 1982).

During latency, dramatic changes in psychic structure occur with the continued growth of the ego and the internalization of the superego. The internalization of the superego is a critically important step in the development of the capacity for friendships because it propels the child away from the direct expression of impulses toward the original objects and toward the displaced, inhibited, sublimated expression of impulses toward others.

Play and friendships are intimately linked during latency. According to Peller, latency play, which is characterized by group activity with sharply defined rules (a reflection of the growth in the capacity for peer relationships and the internalization of the superego), deals with the following anxiety, "I have to face authority, threatening dangerous authority, all by myself" (1954, p. 191). The compensatory fantasy underlying the group activity may be paraphrased as follows: We are a group of brothers mutually and jealously guarding our perogatives. We are not alone; we are united; we follow rules to the letter. For example, each member of a latency-age soccer team (male, female, or mixed) plays a required, defined, interlocking role with all other members. Thus, the thrust of latency development facilitates a new form of object relationship with peers: It is interlocking and mutual; that is, it is interdependent.

In summary, all the components described in our definition are present in normal latency development. Extrafamilial relationships are self-initiated and freely chosen. Consistent inhibition of impulses is increasingly the norm rather than the exception. These and other basic characteristics of genuine friendship, namely mutality and interdependence, are readily observed when they have become part of the fabric of latency-age object relationships and play.

FRIENDSHIP AND OBJECT LOSS IN ADOLESCENCE AND EARLY ADULTHOOD

From the latency period onward, friendships are an integral part of human experience, a vital form of object relationships. *At each subsequent developmental phase, including adolescence and young adulthood, the character and substance of healthy friendships are determined in part by the mutual need to engage and resolve major, phase-specific developmental tasks.*

Sometimes developmental pressures may strain the capacity for friendship to the limit. In early adolescence, in particular, the strength of the drives vis-à-vis the ego often lead to breakdowns in aim inhibition as observed in both homosexual and heterosexual experimentation between peers. But, generally speaking, at no other time in life do friendships play such prominent roles in the developmental process. At this time, they facilitate the engagement and resolution of such developmental tasks of the phase as separation from parents and beginning integration of adult sexual and work identities.

In late adolescence and young adulthood, prior to the establishment of a committed heterosexual relationship and parenthood, friendships are often the primary source of emotional sustenance. Between the family of origin and the family of procreation, the late adolescent finds himself or herself in a state of relative object loss, with little opportunity for the direct expression of impulses in committed relationships. Friendships may become the major form of object relationship at this time of transition between childhood and adulthood.

A central developmental task of young adulthood is finding (a spouse) and creating (children) new objects to replace infantile ones, forming relationships that provide a new center of gravity for the adult years, that organize adulthood the way the relationship to parents organized childhood. Once these new, more permanent, less aim-inhibited relationships are established, friendships assume different and less central roles in the developmental process. Increasingly, friendships become vehicles for the expression of sexual and aggressive impulses related to marriage, parenthood, and work. However, when attempts at intimacy fail and children and spouse are lost through divorce, friendships may again become the most important form of object relationship.

In midlife, another major change in family structure occurs, again centering on object loss. In childhood, the child leaves the parent—and relies increasingly on friends. In midlife, the adult loses his or her children—and may rely increasingly on friends. It becomes more evident that a major purpose of friendships in both childhood and adulthood is to serve as a repository for impulses that cannot be directly expressed through the family.

DEVELOPMENTAL TASKS OF YOUNG ADULTHOOD AND MIDLIFE: THEIR EFFECT ON FRIENDSHIPS

It is our hypothesis that friendships in adulthood are qualitatively different from those at earlier stages of development. Because developmental processes are interlocking and sequential, one stage builds upon the other. More specifically, the engagement and resolution of the central developmental tasks of young adulthood change the nature of midlife friendships.

For example, middle-age friendships take place after the normal individual (in the 20s and 30s) establishes heterosexual intimacy. All friendships prior to this time occur before or during the formation of this basic aspect of the adult personality. The emergence of the capacity for intimacy is usually associated with late adolescent development, in keeping with the belief that significant development change ceases at the end of childhood, that is, at adolescence when (within such a framework) the primary purpose of development, the formation of psychic structure, has been completed.

Under ideal conditions, sexual development in adolescence and young adulthood procedes along the following lines. The profound biological upheaval of puberty requires major structural changes in the ego and superego and the formation of the ego ideal (Blos, 1968), leading to the integration of a new body image, the beginning establishment of an adult sexual identity, and the ability to engage in sexual intercourse. What is gradually added in young adulthood is a refinement of these structures and a change in aim, namely, engagement in sexual activity to achieve a new, more complete form of object love, which we call intimacy. *Intimacy* is the capacity to care for the sexual partner genuinely in his or her own right, with tenderness, love, and commitment. The early adolescent learns how his or her (and sometimes, others') body works. The late adolescent applies this knowledge to the opposite sex through heterosexual experimentation. The sexual object is more often than not used in the service of drive expression and establishment of a sexual identity. Building on this knowledge and experience, the young adult gradually adds the capacity for intimacy.

Clinical Example

Because the developmental process rarely occurs under ideal circumstances and may be encumbered by unresolved infantile issues, the engagement of the young adult developmental tasks of intimacy and marriage may severely test the sexual equilibrium achieved during adolescence, lead to the onset of symptomatic behavior, and effect longstanding, stable friendships.

The analysis of a 30-year-old neurotic man demonstrated such conflict.

> Married since his early 20s, the patient entered analysis because of major inhibitions in his chosen field of endeavor and vague feelings of "discomfort" about his marriage. During the opening phase of the analysis, it was discovered that the patient was unable to enjoy sexual relations with his wife, partly due to the occurrence of homosexual fantasies during intercourse. On occasion, during the 3-year period preceding the analysis, these wishes had been gratified, without conscious awareness, through a ménage à trois among the patient, his wife, and his best friend. The friendship had never been overtly homosexual prior to the ménage à trois. Under the guise of sexual openness and sophistication, the patient unconsciously used his friend to avoid the demands for intimacy within the marriage and to gratify his unrecognized homosexual wishes. As the behavior and underlying impulses were analyzed and understood, the patient terminated the ménage à trois, maintained both the marriage and the friendship, and developed an increased capacity for both.

MIDLIFE FRIENDSHIPS

We are suggesting that because of the establishment of an adult sexual identity in the young adult years and because of the gratification gained from adult sexual intimacy, mature midlife friendships (35–55) can be (but are not necessarily) relatively desexualized compared to those that occur earlier in life. Pressure to sexualize the friendship or share sexual anxieties (as in late adolescence and young adulthood) may be markedly diminished due to the adult developmental mastery of sexuality and intimacy. In addition, it is now easier to establish friendships with the opposite sex because direct gratification of sexual impulses in a separate heterosexual intimate relationship facilitates the maintenance of aim inhibition in the friendship.

Unlike friendships in latency and adolescence, and, to some extent in young adulthood, midlife friendships do not usually have the sense of urgency or the need for frequent or nearly constant physical presence of the friend. The midlife individual has neither the need to build new psychic structure (as do the latency-age child and adolescent) nor the pressing need to find new objects (as does the young adult). He or she may have many sources of gratification available to him or her through relationships with spouse, children, and colleagues.

Because of his or her unique position in the life cycle, he or she is easily able to initiate and sustain friendships with individuals of different ages as well as with chronological peers. It need not be assumed that the unconscious motivation underlying these relationships is different from any other. However, the capacity for sublimation, particularly of aggressive impulses, may be considerable. A friendship with an adolescent may be based in part on an identification with his or her youth and an envy of his or her abundant future in an attempt to bolster a sagging sexuality and painful feelings about aging. Friendship with young adults may serve the same psychic aims as well as provide an outlet for sexual and aggressive impulses related to parenthood and work. Friendships with older individuals may have multiple determinants, including longing for preoedipal parenting, oedipal sexual and aggressive gratification, or the passive gratifications of a "mentee" relating to an older mentor.

However, as at all other points in the life cycle, Freud's recognition that friends can rapidly become lovers or enemies remains completely valid. In the face of a disruption in marriage or intimacy and/or because of the pressure of other midlife developmental themes, (to be described later) friendships may quickly become vehicles for the direct expression of impulses.

In summary, then, midlife friendships have a definite character of their own because of previous engagement and "resolution" of the developmental tasks of childhood and young adulthood. In particular, we describe them as (1) capable of being relatively desexualized, compared to those in childhood and young adulthood because of the capacity for and experience with adult intimacy; (2) less urgent in their expression because they are not involved in the formation of psychic structure and because many avenues for direct impression of impulses are available; and (3) occurring with greater frequency with individuals of both sexes and from other developmental phases throughout the life cycle.

In some respects, the therapist, because of his or her attentiveness to the nature of his or her relationships with others, is especially well equipped to achieve the kind of mature, midlife friendships just described. But, because of the nature of his or her work, particularly the constant role as passive recipient of powerful sexual and aggressive transference feelings, his or her friendships may be subjected to special pressures.

The relationship between friends and between therapist and patient are alike in that both are primarily aim inhibited. Neither friend nor therapist is expected to use the relationship as an avenue for sexual or aggressive actions. Sometimes, the aim-inhibited nature of the relationship breaks down, and therapist and patient become lovers or enemies. But much more frequently, we suggest, the feelings generated in the therapist by his or her work are displaced onto nontherapeutic relationships such as those with spouse and children or friends.

Although the family is a constant repository of such displacement, friendships may be unconsciously singled out even more because they do not have the central importance of relationships within the family and therefore can be disrupted with less realistic consequences. In many instances, the disruption of a friendship may also cause less intrapsychic pain because it can be more easily rationalized and more easily replaced than a relationship with either a family member or a patient.

In addition, like all other human beings in the second half of life, the therapist is subject to the normative conflicts engendered by the incessant pressures of the adult developmental process. Should these conflicts be particularly severe or should he or she be subject to an unusual number of traumatic acts of fate such as severe personal illness or the premature loss of loved ones through death, both his work and his friendships may suffer even more.

MIDLIFE DEVELOPMENTAL TASKS AND THEIR EFFECT ON FRIENDSHIP

We suggest that the nature of midlife friendships may be illuminated by a consideration of the phase-specific developmental tasks of midlife. Although current knowledge of the developmental processes in adulthood is scanty, several basic themes central to development in midlife have been identified (Colarusso & Nemiroff, 1981).

Among the major developmental tasks of midlife (ages 35–55) are

1. Separating from grown children
2. Dealing with the aging body and increased awareness of time limitation and personal death
3. Maintaining intimacy in the face of significant physical, psychological, and environmental change
4. Elaborating creativity and work-related goals and achievements

We suggest that individual experience with these basic, universal themes determines the form, expression, and aim of midlife experience in general and midlife friendships in particular and provides a framework from which to describe and explore the latter.

PARENTHOOD IN MIDLIFE: ITS INFLUENCE ON FRIENDSHIPS

As described in Chapter 8 of *Adult Development* and in Chapter 4 of this book, parenthood is a complex developmental task that continues to occupy a central intrapsychic position in midlife as well as in young adulthood. In midlife, each parent struggles with the need to give up power and dominance over his or her child. Feelings of impotence, loss, dissolution, resignation, and rage inevitably follow and must be engaged and managed in some way.

If the parent happens to be a therapist, he or she may displace these disturbing feelings of weakness and rage into the therapeutic situation where his or her role is unchanged and his or her power is secure. Because of ethical prohibitions, however, he or she is more likely to unconsciously select relationships in which his or her thoughts and actions are not so sharply circumscribed by the superego.

The relationships that exist between and among therapists in professional and academic institutes seem particularly well suited for such displacements. The relationships are significant, ongoing, and centered, at least in part, on themes and issues that engender strong positive and negative feelings. Through position and power within the structure of committees, control over others may be exercised and heightened at a time when it is being surrendered (ambivalently to be sure) within the family. Further, some of the work within the professional organizations relates directly or indirectly to the training and progression of students, younger individuals who may easily be identified with the therapist/parent's rebellious offspring. Both student and maturing child are younger, have abundant futures, and sooner or later will establish themselves as free of the older parents' guidance and control.

Clinical Example

The relationship between midlife parenthood and midlife friendship is often observed in patients. One patient-father chose the path of confrontation.

> When his 17-year-old son returned home at 2 A.M. from a date, the father was waiting at the door, insisting that his son would get up at 5 A.M., as planned, to work with him in a project requiring strenuous manual labor. Throughout the day, the father attempted silently to "break" his son by working him to the point of exhaustion. By noon, it was the father who broke and called off the work. Although not a word was spoken, both father and son knew that a "moment of truth" had arrived and their relationship was changed forever.
>
> The father went directly to a close male friend and poured out his rage and frustration, condemning his son with four-letter words and threats of retaliation. At first, he was shocked by seemingly mocking laughter and only gradually was he able to acknowledge the friend's admiration of his son's courage, determination, physical prowess, and imagined sexual adventure the night before. The friend reminded the father that he, too, was once "young, cocky, smart, and tough."

The relationship between the midlife friendship and the father's development is readily seen. By listening and responding as he did, the friend provided first an opportunity for ventilation and then perspective. Later, through reassurance, he encouraged moderation of parental response and eventually facilitation of separation from the son and mourning for the lost parent–young son relationship.

Adult Developmental Observation

In the past few decades, child observation has become an important, accepted technique for gathering data to use in formulating psychoanalytic developmental theory. We believe that adult observation can serve the same function in regard to adult developmental theory. If one accepts the notion that the developmental process is lifelong, then adult development, as child development, can be studied through observation as well as through the clinical interaction between therapist and patient. An example of an adult observation that illustrates the point of this section follows.

> As their firstborn sons progressed through high school, two women in their mid-40s became fast friends. In addition to raising money for the school activities in which their sons were involved, thus maintaining a close involvement with the boys, they spent many hours talking about the boys' activities, girlfriends, and plans for college. Their husbands, who liked each other, became acquaintances, not friends. They directed their own feelings about their sons into other relationships. After the boys left for college the intensity of the friendship diminished, tending to peak again during vacation periods.

In this instance, the friendship served the basic midlife purpose of helping the women master the experience of separating from their firstborn. The friendship began at this point to serve as a vehicle for the redirection of impulses formerly invested in the children.

In summary, then, friends may serve as a source of ventilation, solace, and comfort as parents struggle with powerful conflicted feelings about their children. These less intense, more manageable, less conflicted object ties provide a vehicle for working through this and other developmental conflicts in the parent. New friendships may arise, and old ones may intensify or disappear as many of the libidinal and aggressive feelings formerly directed toward children are partially displaced onto friends.

MAINTAINING INTIMACY

Whereas the adolescent learns to engage in sexual activity and the young adult develops the capacity for intimacy, the middle-aged person is confronted with the difficult task of maintaining intimacy in the face of profound physical, psychological, and environmental changes. In order for intimacy to continue and deepen, individuals of both sexes must accept the significant aging process in their own and their partners' bodies, confront a growing awareness of time limitation and personal death, and adjust to significant alterations in family structure, such as the leaving of children. These are just some of the factors that effect the task of maintaining intimacy. For example, if the aging of the partner's body is not accepted, sexual closeness may be avoided. If the increased awareness of personal time limitation is not integrated, desperate and inappropriate attempts at new intimacies may be made before time runs out. When children leave, the marriage relationship is exposed in bold relief, as if caught at low tide. A redefinition of the marital relationship must be attempted, bringing with it new anxieties about, and opportunities for, intimacy.

Friends may play important, often critical roles in the maintenance and redefinition of intimacy in midlife. Libidinally derived feelings may be expressed more easily within the bonds of a friendship. Closeness and a sense of nondemanding loyalty may provide a framework within which to ventilate concerns about the spouse and to gain support. Aggressive feelings about one's partner may be verbalized to the friend. They may be expressed in various forms of adult play among friends, that is, hunting, tennis, or attendance at sporting events, or they may be displaced into the friendship.

The friendship(s) may allow for enough ventilation and gratification of impulses to support the continuation of the intimate relationship through a difficult phase or facilitate its dissolution.

Clinical Example

In the face of his wife's aging, a man in his early 50s turned to a younger woman. In a spirit of locker room comradery, he spoke openly to his closest friends of the sexual details of the affair, bragging about sexual prowess and adventure. As it appeared to the analyst (and partly to the patient as well), the woman seemed more interested in the gifts and money that he lavished on her than his sexual prowess. He did not tell his friends of his occasional impotence either with the girlfriend or his wife.

At first, the friends listened to his war stories and vicariously enjoyed the affair. However, their feelings turned to concern when he expressed a desire to leave his wife and business and move away with his girlfriend. Concurrent therapeutic efforts to understand and temper the desire for abrupt action were stymied by the excitement of the affair and an urgent wish for a new life. Dynamically, the behavior was understood as a flight from fears of aging, loss of sexual prowess, impotence, and multiple difficulties in the marriage. These midlife conflicts also had many readily apparent infantile determinants that were being presented concurrently in the transference.

The analyst watched as the patient's best friend confronted the patient, telling him his behavior was stupid and inappropriate, that his girlfriend did not really love him and was taking him for a ride. He was told that he was acting like "an old fool" and had better stop before he threw away his life. After an initial reaction of embarrassment and rage, the patient analyzed his response and eventually came to admire his friend's courage and appreciate the depth of his concern. The confrontation produced a postponement of the move and greater willingness to use the therapeutic process. Eventually, after a miniscandal, the patient broke off the affair and began to approach the complicated and painful issues in the marriage and in himself.

As the therapist, male or female, struggles to maintain intimacy in the marital relationship in the face of aging, in personal time limitation and changes in the structure of the family, he or she may seek gratification *within* the therapeutic relationship. Few relationships are as intimate as that between therapist and patient, particularly when a transference neurosis has developed. The relationship need not become physical because the psychological intimacy of the transference/countertransference union is a compensation in itself and, in the face of increasing concerns about the body as a sexual instrument, it may actually be preferred. These aim-inhibited unions, which are altered by the therapist's exaggerated need for closeness, resemble friendships in their structure. They are not the same, however, because the relationship was not freely chosen as a friendship by either party and is not based on equality, due to the transference and financial aspects involved.

Mature, stable friendships are extremely valuable to the middle-aged therapist because of the support and sustenance they can provide in the face of developmental pressures and the demands of therapeutic work.

WORK AS AN ORGANIZER OF FRIENDSHIP

A comprehensive psychoanalytic psychology of work has yet to be written. But it is obvious that few adult experiences occupy more time, are more emotionally consuming, or effect the evolution and use of the adult psychic structure more than work.

By providing time together, a frequent meeting place, a mutual conceptual framework or goal, and an expectation of the subordination of direct instinctual gratification to the work task, the work environment becomes a fertile field in which adult friendships may grow and flourish. A strong syncretic mesh exists between adult work and adult friendships because the need for the aim inhibition of impulses is central to both. Work-related friendships are also facilitated by the mutuality of interests. As one's identity is increasingly related to work and professional activity, and the nature of the work activity becomes more complex, those with a similar frame of reference, those who can understand, are singled out to be friends.

Because of the complicated, esoteric nature of psychotherapy and analysis, few who have not functioned as therapists themselves can truly understand the nature of the work. Further, the work is solitary by nature, and the isolation is heightened by the need for confidentiality. Therapists are constantly in conflict between the need to share the pressures of their work, seek advice and council, and the demands of confidentiality. There are numerous formal channels available to deal with these pressures, such as case conferences, supervision, and further personal treatment, but the graduate therapist does not always easily avail himself or herself of them. He or she may resort instead to more informal contact and consultation with colleagues who are friends. We suspect that such interchanges among therapist/friends are frequent because hardly anyone else is in a position to be of assistance.

These communications can run the gamut from well-thought-out interchanges in which the privacy of the patient is maintained to open breeches of confidentiality. The therapist as friend who understands both the demands of the work and the nature of normative developmental conflicts of midlife is in a truly unique position to observe and monitor the interaction between these two powerful sets of forces, providing support, advice, and direction as they are needed.

The sublimated expression of aggression is a major affective component in all work. The expression of aggressive impulses in work activity is frequently shared with co-workers who, for example, work together toward a predetermined goal. The collective channeling of the aggressive drive toward the work-related goal is facilitated when the co-workers are friends and impeded when they are enemies. Aggression toward a superior or rival may be more easily managed and expressed when it is shared with a friend or sometimes sublimated within the friendship. But the aggression generated by the work situation may also be displaced into the work-related friendships.

Again, the demands of dynamic psychotherapeutic work may be highlighted by contrast because the therapist must passively encourage the expression of hostile feelings toward himself or herself; he or she has no co-worker to shoulder the burden; or he or she may not express his or her own negative feelings within the work situation. Because the therapist is essentially sedentary, not even motoric release is available. It is our impression that this penned-up aggression is often displaced into organizational activities and in friendships and relationships with other therapists. This may explain in part the tendency toward conflict, acrimony, and splits that are so common in our professional organizations. The maintenance of "aim-inhibited" friendly relationships among colleagues in institutes and societies is difficult at best under such circumstances.

Clinical Vignette

In a sense, work is a stimulus to, and organizer of, friendships in adulthood as play is in childhood. Childhood friendships grow out of similarities of interests and the need to engage developmental themes and conflicts that are expressed in play. In adulthood, work occupies the same central position and performs the same function in regard to friendships.

> Mr. R. began analysis at age 38. Although not a central theme in his 5-year analysis, his experience in forming and developing friendships was observed and analyzed. Because he was a shy man, struggling greatly with significant neurotic anxieties and phobias, he was not able to easily reach out to others.
>
> Although he worked independently, he had continual contact throughout the day with co-workers who were performing parallel tasks. His initial feelings about male co-workers prevented the development of friendships because he saw them as superior and judgmental, "looking for cracks

in my armor, looking for ways to put the new guy down." These feelings were so strong about his boss that he continually sought ways to avoid him.

As his tendency to project his repressed hostility onto others was interpreted and eventually acknowledged, he was able to respond more easily to the overtures from his co-workers, and friendships with two of them began to develop. In midphase, when the negative transference was at its peak, in addition to attacking the analyst, the patient became a petty tyrant at work, challenging his friends and confronting his boss. As the transference was interpreted and gradually resolved, he tempered his critical response to his colleagues and broadened his circle of friends.

When a single woman became a colleague, a friendship, largely initiated by the woman, quickly began. The patient responded because he found the woman sexually attractive and enjoyed their mutual interests and similar backgrounds. As the relationship developed, Mr. R. began to consider, for the first time in his 10 years of marriage, having an affair. He related his dilemma to the analysis and work. "If my god damn sex life hadn't improved so much, I wouldn't be thinking like this, and if I didn't spend so much time working with her, I wouldn't be thinking about her. I spend more time with her than I do with my wife." The analysis of his feelings about the woman included infantile and adolescent derivatives and attitudes about his adult development. "I'm getting old. She's young and has a great body but I better not fool around at work; it's too important." In a sense, by providing greater access to his sexual wishes that led to increased sexual gratification with his wife, the analysis allowed the patient to recognize the value of aim inhibition within the friendship and to opt for a friendship over an affair.

ILLNESS, TIME LIMITATION, AND THE PROSPECT OF DEATH: EFFECT ON FRIENDSHIPS

In the course of midlife development, each individual must deal with the aging process in the body. We suggest that as the signs of aging become more apparent, a *normative conflict* ensues between wishes to deny the aging process and acceptance of the loss of a youthful body. The resolution of this universally experienced conflict leads to a more realistic appraisal of the midlife body, a reshaping of the body image, and a heightened sense of appreciation of the pleasures the body can continue to provide if properly cared for through appropriate activities. These psychic processes about the body are related to a second developmental task of midlife, the normative crisis precipitated by the recognition and acceptance of the finiteness of time and the inevitability of personal death (Colarusso & Nemiroff, 1981).

The power of this realization and increased acceptance of one's mortality can be a positive stimulus to further development, including a redefinition of the body image, a clarification and reordering of goals and priorities, and—most relevant to our focus on friendship—increased attention to and recognition of the value of significant object ties. Friendships become a vehicle for the expression, engagement, and resolution of these enormously powerful midlife themes.

When illness intervenes, this entire complex of thoughts and feelings, already central to mental life, is intensified because illness disturbs the sense of mutuality and equality in a friendship because the sick person is no longer fully able to participate. This imbalance stimulates libidinal wishes, which are expressed through administering to and caring for the friend. Family members and others close to the sick person also become objects of libidinal expression as is demonstrated by the increased administering to others in this time of need. These interactions among friends provide a sense of continuity to relationships in a time of potential loss, thus defending against the fear of loss of the friend and personal death. So, in the service of both impulse and defense, illness disturbs existing friendships, stimulates the expression of friendly feelings toward the ill person and those close to him or her, and draws other friends closer together through the mutual task of caring for those involved.

But aggressive impulses are stimulated as well because the illness makes the friend unavailable and therefore results in deprivation and loss of the gratifications obtained from the relationship. Feelings of hostility, competition, and envy, including death wishes, may also be stimulated by the illness and incapacitation. A situation is created in which oedipal themes in particular may be reignited or intensified.

Because illness becomes more prominent and common in midlife, friendships are increasingly structured by and redefined by such occurrences. We are suggesting that the increased incidence of illness in midlife and the implications that such events have on thoughts about time limitation and personal death become increasingly central to the maintenance and expression of friendships and may become critical factors in determining the deepening or dissolution of them.

Clinical Vignette

When Mr. R., the analytic patient referred to in the section on work (p. 89), was 42 years old and in his 4th year of analysis, a friend and colleague, then age 50, had a severe heart attack. The friend's illness became a central focus in the analysis and produced the following series of themes over several weeks. Mr. R.'s initial reaction was concern about his own health and death—"It could have been me. When will it be my turn?" He felt guilt over his concern about himself rather than his friend. Further conflict evolved around how much time to spend visiting his friend. He wanted to see him, missed him, but was upset by the friend's condition and the hospital setting.

Frequent phone calls to the friend's wife began to stimulate distressing fantasies that were blatantly oedipal in nature. Surely his friend's sexual prowess was compromised. He might even die. In either event, his wife would be "horny" and looking for "a good fuck." Because R. was in the late middle phase and had developed an excellent capacity to free associate, these thoughts, which were extremely distasteful to him, could be tolerated and thoroughly explored.

Similar feelings were brought into the transference. Perhaps the analyst would become ill. Certainly, his wife would also desire another man. Gradually the patient launched a full-fledged attack on the analyst— commenting that he was about as old as the sick friend, noting his gray hair and wrinkles, asking if he had had a treadmill test lately. A dream followed in which "a middle-aged man died suddenly, before his time. Funny, they didn't lay him out; they propped him up on a chair, just like the one you're sitting in." Such material, which was simultaneously a reflection of both the infantile neurosis and the patient's midlife developmental course, is common in the analyses of patients in this age group and confronts the analyst with an awareness of his or her own mortality. If unrecognized, these feelings may be a significant source of countertransference, or, as previously mentioned, they may be displaced into other relationships.

However, the analysis of these feelings did not prevent R. from caring for his friend and his wife in a genuine and loving way. As his friend recovered, the friendship continued, and it was strengthened by Mr. R.'s evidence of genuine concern in a time of need and by his greater understanding of his motivations and impulses.

SUMMARY

The developmental orientation provides a most suitable theoretical framework from which to study friendship—a subject that is neglected in the psychoanalytic literature. The new field of adult developmental theory, particularly the description of developmental tasks for the adult years, sheds considerable light on the nature of adult friendships by describing the uniquely adult factors that shape, alter, and force change and continuing evolution in these relationships. The psychotherapeutic and analytic situations are excellent sources of data about the nature of the adult developmental processes in general and adult friendships in particular.

The therapist, himself or herself is not immune from adult developmental forces and conflicts, and because of the nature of his or her work, additional strain may be placed upon his own friendships, particularly those with colleagues and students, and especially within professional organizations.

REFERENCES

Blos, P. Character formation in adolescence. *Psychoanalytic Study of the Child*, 1968, *23*, 245–263.

Braun, J. Personal communication, 1982.

Colarusso, C. A., & Nemiroff, R. A. *Adult development, A new dimension in psychodynamic theory and practice*. New York: Plenum Press, 1981.

Freud, A. The concept of developmental lines. *Psychoanalytic Study of the Child*, 1963, *18*, 245–265.

Freud, S. Group psychology and the analysis of the ego. In J. Strachey (Ed. and trans.), *Standard edition* (18:67). London: Hogarth Press, 1921.

Freud, S. Civilization and its discontents. In J. Strachey (Ed. and trans.), *Standard edition* (21:59). London: Hogarth Press, 1930.

Peller, L. Libidinal phases, ego development, and play. *Psychoanalytic Study of the Child*, 1954, *9*, 178–198.

Rangell, L. On friendship. *Journal of the American Psychoanalytic Association*, 1963, *11*, 3.

Shane, M. A rationale for teaching analytic technique based on a developmental orientation and approach. *International Journal of Psychoanalysis*, 1977, *58*, 95–108.

Winnicott, D. W. Transitional objects and transitional phenomena. *International Journal of Psychoanalysis*, 1953, *34*, 89–97.

II

Clinical Presentations

PSYCHOTHERAPY AND PSYCHOANALYSIS
OVER THE DECADES

"You are old, Father William," the young man said,
    "And your hair has become very white;
And yet you incessantly stand on your head—
    Do you think, at your age, it is right?"

"In my youth," Father William replied to his son,
    "I feared it might injure the brain;
But now that I'm perfectly sure I have none,
    Why, I do it again and again."

"You are old," said the youth, "as I mentioned before,
    And have grown most uncommonly fat;
Yet you turned a back somersault in at the door—
    Pray, what is the reason of that?"

"In my youth," said the sage, as he shook his gray locks,
    "I kept all my limbs very supple
By the use of this ointment—one shilling the box—
    Allow me to sell you a couple."

"You are old," said the youth, "and your jaws are too weak
    For anything tougher than suet;
Yet you finished the goose, with the bones and the beak;
    Pray, how did you manage to do it?"

"In my youth," said his father, "I took to the law,
    And argued each case with my wife;
And the muscular strength which it gave to my jaw,
    Has lasted the rest of my life."

"You are old," said the youth; "one would hardly suppose
    That your eye was as steady as ever;

PART II

Yet you balanced an eel on the end of your nose—
What made you so awfully clever?''

''I've answered three questions, and that is enough,''
Said his father; ''don't give yourself airs!
Do you think I can listen all day to such stuff?
Be off, or I'll kick you down-stairs!''

Lewis Carroll (1832–1898), *Father William*

6

Turning Forty in Analysis

John M. Hassler

Birthdays have a special meaning for everyone. For the American middle-class child, birthdays are occasions for expanding the sense of personal worth through peer acceptance and family love. Gifts, cakes, and other expressions of love are offered and received as proof of worth. For happy children, the present joys and affirmations matter more than reflections on past or future anticipations.

However, for adults, birthdays are occasions for introspection. Beyond the celebrations of worth, adults use them to review achievements and frustrations of the past and define hopes for the future.

> Men and women compare themselves with their friends, siblings, work colleagues, or parents in deciding whether they have made good, but it is always with a time line in mind. It is not the fact that one reaches 40, 50, or 60 which is itself important, but rather, "How am I doing for my age?" (Neugarten, 1979, p. 888)

A 40th birthday often has very special significance as one reviews all that has happened in life and anticipates all that is to come. It was subjectively the halfway point—35, half the biblical threescore and 10—that was viewed in the same way prior to the extension of longevity by good nutrition and medical care in the last few decades. The lifting of the denial of death is the central and crucial feature of the midlife phase (Jacques, 1965). As noted by Soddy (1967) in his study of men at middle age, both Arthur Schopenhauer and Albert Camus vividly described the awareness that struck them in their late 30s—that they had already lived half their lives and that death was inevitable (Camus, 1942/1960; Schopenhauer, 1851/1970).

Each man faces this reality in his own way. Bach accepted his cantorship at Leipzig at 38 and began to compose. Albert Schweitzer chose midlife as the time to retire from his career as a concert organist in Europe and become a physician in Africa. Major shifts in self-image, love relationships, and career directions frequently are provoked or facilitated by the lifting of the denial of aging and the realization that the halfway point of life has been reached. Suddenly, it is clear that life is half over and that the "race against time" cannot be stopped.

In psychoanalysis, birthdays may be used as foci for displacement and elaboration of a variety of neurotic or developmental conflicts. Beyond the special meaning of specific time events, the passage of time itself is a major implicit or explicit theme. Review of past development, the examination of present realities, and the preview of future hopes are often a part of many individual sessions. It is as if there were a compression of time, a time warp, allowing the patient to look at his or her whole life course from one vantage point. As I will note later, this compression gradually brings adult aging realities into sharp focus as the transference contaminations are analyzed. Until then, even the awareness of this unique vantage point on time is partly encapsulated in denial.

I propose, through the presentation of detailed clinical material from the psychoanalysis of Mr. B., to highlight the importance of time and the conflicts of aging in midlife. Conflicts in aging helped shape both the presenting concerns and the contours of his adaptive resolutions. The material in this case also provokes a few thoughts as to the countertransference problems of the therapist who is aging each day along with the patient.

THE ANALYSIS OF MR. B.

Mr. B. entered analysis when he was 36 and turned 40 12 months before termination. On center stage, the analytic process focused on the exploration and resolution of neurotic conflict. After a look at the overall case material, a review of those hours during the few weeks on either side of his 40th birthday will reveal how time and aging perceptions colored his neurotic conflicts and his use of the 40th birthday to focus on and move beyond the problems faced in the analysis. The case of Mr. B. details his intrapsychic adaptation to aging, thus providing data for the understanding of this basic, universal, adult developmental task.

Presenting Symptoms and Background

Mr. B., an intelligent, articulate architect, sought help after a year of depression, self-doubt, and intermittent resentment toward his adolescent daughter. The onset of his depression coincided with her pubescence.

The patient was the oldest of two children, a sister had been born when he was 2 years old. His mother was loving but hot tempered and would occasionally "knock heads together." The father, a successful builder, was caring and available in early childhood. At 3, Mr. B. recalled, he happily helped his father build the house they lived in during his childhood. When he was 10 his parents divorced. From that point onward, he viewed both mother and father as angry, aloof, and emotionally unavailable.

Mr. B. was a wanted child, the product of an uncomplicated pregnancy. He was breast-fed and was reportedly within the norm of all early maturational and developmental guidelines. There were no childhood surgeries or major illnesses. He did not recall weaning or toilet-training experiences, or later problems with eating or bowel and bladder control. Harsh toilet training was unlikely, although the patient remembered conflicts over control issues: "My mother ran the place. . . we all had to act by the numbers. . . she was rigid on dinner manners and clean rooms."

Although he had no recall of the event, the birth of his sister when he was 2 years of age prompted (as reconstructed in the analysis) a precipitous separation from his mother. Unresolved feelings about this experience later caused difficulties in marriage, due to Mr. B.'s exaggerated dependency needs, and figured prominently in the transference.

In addition to "helping" build the family house, he also shared his father's interest in guns. "I remember that I once found Dad's shotgun. . .I could barely lift it." Although Mr. B. did not recall explicit oedipal fantasies or fears, aside from highly disguised wishes to interrupt his parents behind locked bedroom doors "to show mother the snake I caught," material evolved from the transference neurosis that allowed for reconstruction.

At 5, while roughhousing in a treehouse, his 3-year-old sister fell and was nearly killed. This event shaped the family destiny ("my mother always said that that's why father left") and was so elaborated by the patient that he forever after felt like "a rotten kid. . .a potential killer." Soon after the accident, the father began working some distance from home. At 6 his mother also went off to work and during many evenings the patient was left in the care of baby-sitters "who would leave us in the attic to discipline us." Despite these problems, the boy "did O.K. until my parents divorced...I got real depressed...all my friends still had fathers." He rarely saw his father after puberty.

The patient always did well in school, although from the second grade on he was in trouble for taunting teachers and provoking fights. After high school he joined the marines. "I believed the ads about making a man out of you."

Puberty occurred at 13. Mr. B. remembered frequent masturbation but could not recall fantasies. Early in the analysis, he described his adolescent sex life as intercourse with a series of girls—"love 'em and leave 'em." However, midway in the analysis, he admitted penetrating his sister's best friend at age 14. "We were just playing...but it has always bothered me...as if I screwed my sister."

After the marine service he returned home, entered college, married in his sophomore year, and was content for the next 3 years. "I made the dean's list and felt comfortable with her [his wife] and her family." Marital discord began when a daughter was born and when undesirable job changes occurred. However, basic compatibility persisted until a year or two before the analysis—until his daughter reached puberty.

The Opening Phase

As the analysis began, Mr. B. highlighted his successes as a jogger of great endurance and as a skilled hunter. Concurrent with this breezy counterphobic confidence was a relative compliance noted by the analyst in his hellos and goodbyes and agreeability as to hours and fees. Toward the end of the early sessions there were also expressions of anger—"I feel trapped...forced to look at myself." The analytic situation reminded him of a repetitive dream from late adolescence when he was "an enlisted man lost in the hull of a large navy ship with signs everywhere that I am in officer's country and subject to punishment."

A session in the second month illustrates how his dread of attack for phallic-narcissistic display led to a withholding, mildly passive-aggressive stance with the analyst, similar to ones taken with his wife and mother. In this and all subsequent clinical examples, much of the patient material has been deleted or condensed for reasons of space and clarity. The activity of the analyst thus appears falsely exaggerated.

MR. B.: I couldn't stand to be close to my wife this morning when she wanted to hug me...(*etc.*).

ANALYST: How long have you felt this need to pull away?

MR. B.: I remember the old lady trying to push the shit out of me once...on a biology paper...I failed it anyway (*laugh*)...(*etc.*). I do perceive my wife as acting domineering...(*silence*)...I'm uncomfortable coming today, I don't want to talk about anything...I feel picked at, probed.

ANALYST: Like having to show off before me as with the boss in last week's dream? [In the dream he had to attend a meeting nude with his boss at his grammar school playground and be observed while a black girl performed fellatio on him.]

MR. B.: (*silence*)...I had a dream last night where I was on stage with a towel around my middle...I was supposed to ad lib lines that I didn't know...being exposed, how do I seem less conspicuous...like here, not at ease expressing all of the things that I think.

A few days after this session, Mr. B. recalled that his mother once made him dress and undress before his grandmother "because I was so slow dressing."

As Mr. B. gained confidence in the analytic process and resistances to the transference were interpreted, he began to see the analyst as less belittling and controlling and more as a direct danger to his masculinity. Intermittent impotence followed as he limited his sexual life to the weekends, free from the need to be "a good boy" at work and with the analyst. With great tentativeness, he began to describe liaisons with women at work and his wife's (his own, displaced) uneasiness at X-rated movies. He wondered if he was oversexed and if "screwing will make me psychotic?" Ongoing dread of attack was part of this concern within the transference as well, as was demonstrated in this session toward the end of the first year.

MR. B.: I had a dream the night before last that I have been reluctant to talk about...I was in a dinner theater with my wife watching a play and a guy reached over and grabbed me by the balls...I've had dreams of being squeezed by the balls for the last 2 or 3 years...it's never happened in reality.

ANALYST: What do you make of it?

MR. B.: It has no rhyme or reason. (*silence*)

ANALYST: Who was the man?

MR. B.: I felt uneasy years ago when I slept in a truck with a friend of mine while duck hunting...(*etc.*).

ANALYST: I wonder if the dream relates to feelings about me?

MR. B.: No, I don't think so...I've had this situation dream before...very vulnerable position.

ANALYST: Yesterday you spoke of uneasiness in here and when close to males.
MR. B.: Ya...certain amount of uneasiness...someone knowing all about you, taking your shields away.

As his fears within the transference were confronted by similar interventions over many months, Mr. B. became more ambitious at work and less submissive in the analysis. He began to arrive in slacks rather than Levis—"my rebel outfit."

Midphase

In the 2nd year of analytic work, Mr. B. began an affair with a very young clerk at his job. The liaison served initially as a resistance to examining sexual feelings toward his adolescent daughter and sister in adolescence. As analytic consideration of the affair evolved with interpretations of his projection, displacement, and splitting, genetic issues developed more clearly. The following material is representative of this phase of analytic work.

MR. B.: I'm preparing to take my daughter hunting and I had a dream last night where I was camping with her and trying to find a shotgun that would fit her, a 4-10 or a 28 gauge?... Then my sister and I were horsing around and I got real horny, so she started doing oral sex...I woke up and jumped on my wife, kind of incestuous.
ANALYST: Incestuous?... Can you elaborate a bit.
MR. B.: Well, I haven't had my sister in dreams for years, kind of scary, I don't really like my sister...because she reminds me of my mother...dominating bitch!
ANALYST: Why turn on to your sister last night?
MR. B.: I don't know...I was put out that one of the other guys brought his girlfriend into a man's domain when we were hunting last month... (*sat up*) Do you have a Kleenex, my damn glasses.
ANALYST: You're looking forward to hunting with your daughter...but I wonder if the preparations don't evoke conflicts you felt as a boy and as an adolescent with your sister and mother.
MR. B.: Ya, but not much turn on...my daughter used to jump in the shower occasionally with me...if I ever did get a hard-on it would scare her off from men.

Over the next many months, as this material evolved with more dreams of guns and family females, Mr. B. wondered if he should not mention that he had penetrated his sister's best friend on several occasions in early adolescence. He always feared that this sexual play had hurt his sister because she was an observer. During the months in which he examined this material, the analyst wondered if his fear of sexual impulses were not also complicated by his dread as a 5-year-old that he had almost killed his sister when she fell from the tree. As Mr. B. gradually reedited his view of adolescent impulses, he was able to recall that the 2 years of early adolescence prior to his mother's remarriage "weren't all that bad...I was kind of king of the roost."

As repressed adolescent conflicts over libidinal impulses were explored and resolved, material surfaced that allowed for a reconstruction of the infantile neurosis, prefaced by concerns of how the analyst would react.

MR. B.: I dreamt the other night that you and I were discussing something back and forth, argumentative...you had a more critical, forceful tone than your comments or questions here.
ANALYST: What do you fear that I would be critical of?
MR. B.: ...The other day I decided not to be the leader of this [social] group that I'm in...it is more authority than I want to get associated with.

Mr. B. went on to describe over the next few weeks how difficult it was to get up in the mornings for analysis. He reported a dream in which he warned people to leave his house (like the one that he had grown up in) and then "I got a gun and started shooting at them...they were a little irate." He associated to feeling as a boy that his father was stealing from him when the house was sold after the divorce. "I guess I thought they were stealing my manhood...in reality I couldn't defend myself...all I could do was carve my initials on everything...my mother helped my confusion along by claiming that it was all my dad's fault...she set us against him." Mr. B. recalled how isolated and empty he had felt—"I used to stay in bed all Saturday...no reason to get up...I guess I'd lost hope." He agreed with the analyst's comment that he had felt deserted by his father at 5, but that his denial and magical thinking helped partially block this loss until 11.

As transference analysis and genetic reconstruction progressed, Mr. B. reported many oedipal and primal scene dreams. The following is a representative example.

MR. B. (session 219): My wife was upset because I wouldn't snuggle with her last night; sometimes I don't want her close...but I dreamt that I was with my girlfriend in a summer cottage like the kind we vacationed in when I was a little boy...we were making mashed potatoes and they were getting soupy...I kept looking out the window to see if her husband was coming home.

ANALYST: What in your life now evokes images of a vacation cottage as a little boy?

MR. B.: I never cook with my girlfriend, but I must have with my mother...I was always afraid to get close...I felt left out...I remember her getting upset once when I knocked on the bedroom door to show her a worm that I had caught...they probably were getting it on.

ANALYST: In fact you don't fear your girlfriend's husband. As a boy you feared your father because you wanted mother.

As in the preceding material, for many subsequent months Mr. B. reworked in the transference various aspects of the oedipal situation. This was followed by a gradual shift in the description of his mother of childhood ("sitting around the fire reading stories to me") and increasing expressions of warmth for his wife. During this phase, a further reconstruction of the infantile neurosis was possible.

MR. B. (session 388): It's been a pretty good week...but I had the strangest dream...watching a movie with my wife (*feeling sheepish*) while a catapult was hurling balls from the United States into Russia...it reminds me of a repetitive dream at 7 where I was pleading with the government not to have an atomic war.

ANALYST: I wonder if this wasn't your view of parental intercourse contaminated by the fighting in the marriage.

MR. B.: My mother cried a lot, maybe I felt he hurt her...when I was a teenager she told me that he'd once been drinking on a date and had accidentally run down a pedestrian...maybe the nuclear fallout fears was what I feared from sex...I must have been turned on as a little boy...my girl sure was with me (*laugh*).

As the 3rd year of the analysis continued with further work on the transference neurosis and a freeing up of inhibitions to adult prerogative, Mr. B. followed through on some long-frustrated desires. He bought a new car, built a swimming pool, and spoke more of shopping and going to lunch with his wife and daughter.

Termination Phase

Around the 400th hour, Mr. B. announced that he wanted to terminate soon and set a date 4 months hence. Although the analyst acknowledged this desire, he did not directly support it in hopes that Mr. B. would allow himself greater working through of the remaining moderate narcissistic, preoedipal, and characterologic conflicts. On prior occasions, when fearing the analyst as a controlling mother or as a castrating father, Mr. B. would announce the termination of the analysis only to change his mind as these areas of resistance were examined. However, during these final few months, he presented less of a wish to escape than a desire to validate further his new sense of self and ego integrity. The following material is typical of this effort at synthesis.

MR. B.: I had these dreams where I was chasing this adolescent who had raped this girl and was going to throw him off a building...but the girl was not hurt, and it was the boy's parents' problem not mine...then, in another, it was like here in the office, but a courtroom where an old black man was acquitted of pornographic charges.
ANALYST: How might the dreams relate to analysis?
MR. B.: It is like my sister...her problems are hers, I don't want to be her pawn any more...I didn't cause them...same with my wife and daughter...I'm free to be myself.
ANALYST: Could you have seen your home as a boy and the analytic office as courtrooms?
MR. B.: (laugh)... No more, I'm acquitted.

Along with a final reworking of derivative conflicts from his infantile neurosis, Mr. B. also described during the final few months some insomnia, irritability, and loneliness, which seemed related to saying goodbye to the analyst. In the last session, he reported a dream from the night before where "my wife had let me down, I think she left me...it must have been you as someone very important for me...I'll let you know how I do in the future." I have heard from other patients that are friends of his that he is happy and successful.

MR. B.'S FORTIETH BIRTHDAY

Mr. B. turned 40 after 2 years and 335 hours of analysis. At this point, he was developing a deepening awareness of his childhood distortions and examining the derivative reenactments with the analyst. With the overall contours of the analysis in mind, the specific challenge of turning 40 may now be highlighted.

Propositions

The following propositions are helpful in conceptualizing the clinical material about the birthday.

1. Turning 40 prompted a significant, although partial and temporary, lifting of denial of the aging process.

2. After hundreds of analytic hours of introspection and psychological reflection, Mr. B. could look with less contamination at the adaptive choices of a 40-year-old. He could move beyond the emptiness and anguish of a passive-aggressive child and accept the more adaptive and pleasant identities and pleasures available to him at midlife.

3. At this point in the analysis, Mr. B. was beginning to change his view of the analyst. Instead of seeing him as a hostile parent, denying him access to the adult world, he began to express feelings of warmth, equality, and friendship.

4. With the move toward resolution of the transference distortions, a shift in his sense of self was occurring. Mr. B. was developing a broader perspective on his inner and outer worlds, shifting his characteristic object relatedness from withholding to giving, from rage over deprivation to pride in achievement.

Clinical Data

Three Weeks Prior to the Birthday

Twenty days prior to his birthday, Mr. B. presented the following material, which was typical of the preceding few months. He came back from a vacation weekend and began to complain.

MR. B.: I drove back in a hurry, I wanted to see my wife...but I was in a bad mood as soon as I got home...all we did was argue, she makes me so mad...over trivia.

ANALYST: What feelings are beneath the anger? As you mentioned, you were angry over trivia.

MR. B.: I just don't enjoy being with her...I don't know if she even has to say anything...it's almost as if I am not supposed to be in love with anyone...I try and talk with my wife but get nowhere, constant arguing...I don't seem to be able to change...I wonder if I give my daughter enough.

In the second session of this week, he started by looking further at withholding, but now from himself.

MR. B.: My daughter was out so we got it on...but somehow there is much more emotional release with my girlfriend...I smile after orgasm...yet rationally, I don't want her...it is almost as if I'm not supposed to show satisfaction, pleasure with my wife...guess I don't trust...don't see her as my friend, afraid to share my wish for warmth.

And then in his first reference to aging, he mentioned the following:

MR. B.: I guess I can't be a kid screwing around with my wife; yet I can be a kid with my girlfriend.
ANALYST: Only kids are allowed to express warmth and passion with women, not men?
MR. B.: Men and women are so screwed up...my daughter used to masturbate until it was raw...I told her not to wear it out...and with my girlfriend she'll sit next to me in the car with her pants off, but only if it is kid stuff...I guess I never had a grown-up man to watch...no affection at home.

In the third session of the week, while talking about the marital separation of a friend, he mentioned that he was feeling more assertive as a man.

MR. B.: It pisses me off that I was such a milk toast in the old days...I am angry at a lot of things these days, but I don't think it is my wife.

In the last session, Mr. B. mentioned that his girlfriend was upset over his recent indifference, "the affair is coming to an end."

Two Weeks Prior to the Birthday

After describing his "dutiful" participation in Easter services with his family, Mr. B. started the week by reporting a dream.

MR. B. (*dream*): I was playing poker with one of the ladies at work...I had a full house but didn't bet as much as I should have. She laid down four aces...I was so mad I almost hit her.
MR. B. (*associations*): I could have killed her, but why...I only bet a quarter...she reminds me of how my mother had to have everything her way...or maybe I set the game up to lose...recently I've thought a lot about those repetitive dreams of failing the design course in college...why in hell do I have these failure mode situations...I graduated years ago.

What is new in this particular week is his resolution to get beyond his conflict of "years ago." He has finally, after 2 years of talk, begun to play his cards. As material evolved later in that week:

MR. B.: I was talking with an older architect in town and found out that he is human...he has good kids and works hard...my daughter is great, too.
ANALYST: What allowed you warmth with him now?
MR. B.: Everyone seems a little more human...in the past I felt hugging a woman was like molesting her and hugging a man was for queers...I saw everything in terms of sex as a kid...as an adolescent, it was all I had.

One Week Prior to the Birthday

In the first session of the week:

MR. B.: I don't want a divorce, I used to...I get a lot of joy out of marriage.

At the beginning of the following session, he started with the following:

MR. B.: Heck of a day yesterday...I talked with a new junior associate who began working for me...she's only 25...a lot younger than I thought...I am feeling older and older, oh well.

In the final session of the week, the last before his birthday, he mentions the following for the first time:

MR. B.: My birthday is coming up...I don't want a cake...(*later in the session he comments*) I think I want to take a vacation for a day or two...the senior partner has been out all week; I wish there were more sunny days...I wish it were September and I could ride a bike around with the sun in my face.

In retrospect, he might be wishing to deny the opportunities of manhood and the dreads of aging and preserve some of the childhood fantasies of basking in love, "the sun."

First Week after the Birthday

In the first session of the week:

MR. B.: I don't feel like letting people fawn over me as if I can't take care of myself...I can't depend on my partner or my wife...no one else will cover my ass.

He then went on to describe his indifference to a surprise 40th birthday party attended by six couples that his partner had organized for him.

MR. B.: Forty candles on a cake are too many...but they were a nice group of people...one of the ladies was crying.
ANALYST: Why do you feel she cried?
MR. B.: A sad affair, birthdays...(*after a long silence he added*)...I kind of think that the thing with my girlfriend is over; it is not a very satisfying relationship....(*later in the session*) I have been irritated with everyone...and myself since I have the feeling I don't do the things I want to with my life...I feel pushed at home, and in my love life I feel like saying "fuck off world"...I'm pissed at everything including coming here 4 days a week but I stick to it to make life better.

The following day he started by reviewing how sick and weak he felt. This was the only time in the analysis that he complained of a cold, although he had colds at other times. He then went on:

MR. B.: I'm frosted at my parents for putting me in school a year early...I was smart enough but I just wasn't ready emotionally...(*later*)...my partner has been a real disappointment in life...maybe I put him in a role he didn't fit....(*later still*) maybe I have confused my girlfriend in the same way...she is a burden...I find it difficult to remember that she is only 26...there is quite a disparity between 26 and 40...the needs are different...I don't want to start all over again....(*etc.*)...I don't seem to be getting anywhere...maybe tomorrow I'll feel better...(*silence*)...I'm also irritated at turning 40...it beats the alternatives, but I'm tired of all the problems; I spend my whole life learning how to grow up.

In the third session of the week following his birthday, after complaining about his cold, Mr. B. presented this dream.

MR. B. (*dream*): At the stadium, quarterbacking a professional football team, crowded stands...I was on the better team but couldn't pass to save my ass; it was halftime and I was talking with Ed...he had a lot of money bet on the point spread, and I was going to try to increase the lead so he could win...I wasn't starting in the second half so I was walking over to the other side of the field...but then I had to get back to the game, and I threw a touchdown pass even though all the men in front of me were taller.
MR. B. (*associations*): I am putting myself on the winning team...not the biggest but the best man...I'm about average height...even though I am bigger than my father now, of course I wasn't as a boy...used to be self-conscious about being short as a kid...in fact, I still have difficulty seeing myself as big...inferiority complex, keeps me thinking small.

ANALYST: I wonder if your dream doesn't help us understand your conflict over accepting height, prowess, success.

MR. B.: And I can perform for others too...going to make Ed a winner...you may have met him, he runs the gas station around the corner...in reality, for him I don't need to be successful or a winner...just a hell of a nice guy...trying to repay a friendship.

ANALYST: Am I involved with this move toward success and friendship?

MR. B.: You do care about my growth.

Although there are other sections of the dream that relate to working through a variety of conflicts, what is crucial for a review of analysis at the 40th birthday is Mr. B.'s assumption of manly prerogative now that he is at "halftime" and his move toward a more loving image of adult males, that is, the owner of the gas station as the analyst/father through displacement. In the last session of this first week following his birthday, Mr. B. reported a dream of oedipal success.

MR. B. (dream): At work with the partners, around a table at the cafeteria...discussing applications for new men...I was advocating certain people...but the senior partner had only trivial bullshit cut downs and then I walked off for lunch with his wife.

MR. B. (associations): Actually, it has occurred to me recently that I'll be senior partner when he retires in 3 or 4 years...it is the part of me that is still sorting out manhood...it doesn't come from my father's wife...although in the dream I'm confident enough to have her...(later in the session)...I don't think I am looking to replace my wife anymore...I used to be...I enjoy life more with her.

Second Week after the Birthday

In the first session, Mr. B. mentioned for the first time that he was now handling the family finances (his wife always had before), and he reported a dream.

MR. B. (dream): I was trying to comfort this old woman...I was hugging her, and she was crying on my shoulder...I wasn't sure why.

MR. B. (associations): The closer I get to my wife, the happier she is, but the more she cries...we have gone through a lot...and I guess she really is still mourning over her parents' death...I can't change someone else's sorrow...but I love my family and home is fun again.

In the second session, Mr. B. mentioned for the first time that he was building an addition on his house.

MR. B.: As a family room...it's about time...why didn't I do it 5 years ago?

Comments on the Birthday Clinical Data

In this material, concerns over age, stage of life, loss, and growth were everywhere. The patient accepted his 40 years with anguish and ambivalence—"Forty candles are too many." Although the new pool, the joys as husband and father, and a successful profession were some compensation for aging, his mood was more one of acceptance and resignation than joy. Jacques (1965) reports on a man in analysis for 7 years who gradually at 36 developed an awareness of the finality of time (along the way to resolution and termination 18 months later) that "introduced a new quality of earthly resignation."

Assignations, not resignations, are what we much prefer to hope for. Mr. B. was overtly gleeful earlier in the analysis while expressing counterphobic grandiosity or passive-aggressive acting out of derivative childhood and adolescent wishes. Childhood wishes, no matter how disguised or distorted, still carried the hope of great pleasure—fusing with mother and her eternal nourishment, becoming father and enjoying his omnipotence, and so forth.

Objective adult pleasures pale next to childhood wishes in much the same way that earthly joys pale next to anticipated heavenly delights, which include, of course, the promise of immortality. Nevertheless, with the help of analysis, Mr. B. decided that he might as well enjoy "the nice group of people" that were with him at 40. On balance, the adult condition was more pleasurable than his childhood fantasies and illusionary adult reenactments. References to the aging process largely disappeared over the 8 months of further analysis prior to termination. He focused instead on his pride of family, success in career, and how he could do more for those around him than was done for him. While serving many functions, his adaptive narcissism and altruistic inclinations also served to deny his ultimate death and irrelevance.

THEORETICAL COMMENTS ON BIRTHDAYS

If birthdays hurt so much, why do we celebrate them? Why celebrate aging? Why acknowledge death? Some past cultures and present subcultures have no birthday traditions. Among possible conjectures, this may relate to the relative absence of accurate calendars, a lack of relevance in human life as only the god-king has importance or from a total belief in immortality or reincarnation. The American Witness Christian sects do not acknowledge birthdays or death partly for these latter reasons.

For Western culture, where all human life is defined as precious and the hereafter is culturally doubted, birthdays may paradoxically mark success. Woody Allen is reputed to have said that to live forever is the only immortality he is interested in. We celebrate longevity perhaps because we are still alive. Although birthday celebrations also evoke reflections on aging and death, these are usually by-products and fleeting if adaptive (defensive) processes are functional. Less consciously, birthdays help focus the developmental challenge of aging (Colarusso & Nemiroff, 1981).

Mr. B.'s midlife analysis and birthday reflections also prompt a broader look at developmental theory. Erikson, in his eight stages of development, takes a positive view of aging. With considerable psychological effort, we develop the resources for intimacy, generativity, and wisdom. Yet, every expansion of psychological resource is also a posture for undervaluing or justifying the inevitable demise. We learn to give successfully so that some part of ourselves might survive, through the germ plasm, through the culture. Yet, all around us is biological and archaeological evidence that nothing survives forever.

IMPLICATIONS FOR TECHNIQUE

Review of the course of the general analysis as well as of the month around Mr. B.'s 40th birthday highlights a number of clinical issues pertinent to the understanding of adult development and the facilitation of progressive adaptation to aging.

The Patient

It seems clear, at least in the case of Mr. B., that although his struggle with time and aging helped facilitate a shift in the transference that most likely would have taken place in any event, the conflict of aging *per se* is not "in" the transference. Age in the adult frame of reference as a "race against time" is not an awareness in childhood or in early adolescence and so is not directly experienced in the transference relationship with the analyst. The unconscious is timeless, and so is the relevant part of the child's world. Colarusso (1979) has reviewed and helped formulate the nature and development of time sense for children.

Children have never seen anyone grow up. Parents are peers. *Older* has a limited frame of reference. Analyzing the transference (childhood emotional experiences) in the adult patient's extraanalytic world or examining the persistence in the patient's adult world of childhood conflict derivatives is not on a time axis for the same reason.

Time movement is an adult addendum, an addition, like the secondary elaboration of a dream in the recalling. In fact, because much significant transference material emerges from the first two decades of life, this nontime material may be used as resistance to the awareness of the ongoing adult aging process. Certainly, for much of the analysis, Mr. B. chose to have sex with his girlfriend "as a kid" and attacked his wife, partner, and analyst as if they were parent surrogates. His wishes and symptoms were more related to his nontime child/unconscious world than to adult-time realities. The gradual resolution of the transference neurosis seemed to be accompanied by, and may have been partly responsible for, the patient's increased awareness of time and aging. Only as the transference neurosis moved toward resolution did Mr. B. feel that time had flow and aging had impact.

When aging is faced, and partly acknowledged, a broader psychological reworking of the adult self and world begins. As Mr. B. moved toward the resolution of the transference neurosis, the here-and-now flow of time and the quest for ongoing real pleasure and pride took a central place in the material. He began to look for meaning in the present rather than in the past.

An attuned therapist who assumes that, along with other conflicts, his or her patients are conflicted over aging will seek the meaning for the patient of his references to time and age as exploratory therapy evolves and follows the material where it leads. A more adaptive series of consolidations and compromises that acknowledge life as having meaning then emerges.

Aging for the Therapist

If we take as a general proposition that human beings deny the aging process and that full awareness of the finiteness of life is not maintained for very long, the therapist must deal with a powerful source of therapeutic blindness that could lead to the underanalysis of the conflict of aging in almost all patients. Certainly, it is difficult to face in others what we face in ourselves only with great pain. This blindness is very much like that commonly involving patient oedipal material when the therapist dreads his own awareness (Grunberger, 1980).

In fact, the case material with Mr. B., which was conducted before the analyst gained his present perspective, offers a very clear example of this countertransference blindness. Although there was a lot of good exploratory and interpretive work during the birthday weeks presented, beyond what was presented for present purposes, the analyst, at the time, clearly underplayed the significance of the birthday and the patient's efforts to accommodate adaptively to the realities of aging.

Although there were a number of references to aging, the analyst never wondered to himself or to the patient what age meant for Mr. B. When the patient announced that he had a birthday coming up, the analyst did not question its significance. Then, again in the first session after the birthday when Mr. B. reported his surprise birthday party, the analyst wondered what upset him about the tears of a woman at the party instead of questioning the patient about his own feelings.

But the clearest example of the denial by the analyst of the aging process was his response to the "halftime" dream. On no occasion did he wonder about the detail. Limited by his own denial, perhaps heightened by his own hoped-to-be-forgotten birthday arriving a month hence, the analyst, as noted in the clinical section, chose to respond to other aspects of the dream. Peers and senior colleagues who also heard the material around the 40th birthday at various clinical presentations also did not wonder about the significance of halftime.

Although Mr. B. adapted rather well to the realities of turning 40 and was able to move toward a successful termination in analysis, there might have been yet further gain in his perspective on the adult challenges and meaningful pleasure he faced if the analyst had wondered on any number of occasions about the significance of the aging process.

In addition to the inevitable partial denial of the aging process by the analyst, the analytic procedure itself predisposes analysts to underplay the importance of the flow of time. Analysis has a unique time frame in that the unfolding of clinical material occurs most productively in an open-ended, not time-limited, setting. Most vocational activities have deadlines. Only analysts, and a rare artist, work on open-ended time. This open endedness itself, however, may restrict our awareness of the rapid time flow for our patients and limit our focus on the conflicts attendant upon aging.

For both the middle-aged and older analyst and his or her patient, thoughts and feelings about the finiteness of time and personal death, although disguised, are rarely absent. Both partners in the analytic process deny on various levels the clinical and developmental significance of this objective time frame. This is complicated by the immersion in a transference–countertransference relationship where the nontime frame of reference of childhood often prevails as part of a technical procedure that is not defined by time parameters. Perhaps an increased understanding of adult developmental processes will provide a conceptual bridge between these different time references.

References

Camus, A. *The myth of Sisyphus.* New York: Vintage Books, Random House, 1960. (Originally published 1942.)

Colarusso, C. A. The development of time sense—from birth to object constancy. *International Journal of Psycho-Analysis,* 1979, *60,* 243–251.

Colarusso, C. A., & Nemiroff, R. A. *Adult development: A new dimension in psychodynamic theory and practice.* New York: Plenum Press, 1981.

Grunberger, B. The oedipal conflicts of the analyst. *The Psychoanalytic Quarterly,* 1980, *49,* 606–630.

Jacques, E. Death and the mid-life crisis. *International Journal of Psycho-Analysis,* 1965, *46,* 502–514.

Neugarten, B. L. Time, age and the life cycle. *American Journal of Psychiatry,* 1979, *136,* 887–894.

Schopenhauer, A. *Essays and aphorisms.* England: Penguin Books, 1970. (Originally published 1851.)

Soddy, K. *Men in middle age.* New York: Lippincott, 1967.

Discussion

ROBERT A. NEMIROFF AND CALVIN A. COLARUSSO

In early childhood *every* birthday is a momentous occasion signifying the unambivalent wish to grow, to mature, to be older. As childhood passes into adolescence, certain birthdays take on more meaning than others, but all still signify the attainment of new privilege and status. Sixteen—"and never been kissed" 18—"I'm an adult now; I can vote and go to war, ha!" and 21—"No more faked I.D. cards, I can drink, legally!" These are examples.

As the 20s—"Twenty five, God, that's a quarter of a century!"—pass into the 30s—"Thirty, I guess I can't even pretend to be a kid anymore. Is it true that you can't trust anyone over 30?" Birthdays become a source of ambivalence because they mark the passage of time that no longer signifies growth and the attainment of privilege but now demarcates aging and loss of the endless future of youth.

And then comes 40, the watershed birthday, the unequivocal indicator of middle age. "I never thought I'd be 40; now that's really old!"

By studying an individual's reaction to his or her birthday, the therapist-observer may learn much about his or her patient's intrapsychic response to the engagement and mastery of major, phase-specific developmental tasks.

A brief outline of a developmental line of time sense, originally described in Chapter 4 of *Adult Development*, may put some of these ideas into perspective. In the timelessness of the unconscious, we are convinced of our immortality. The first half of life is characterized by a tendency to deny the inevitability of death. In childhood and adolescence, the denial is bolstered by the immaturity of the psychic apparatus,

117

limited awareness and understanding of the concept of time, and the progressive physical and psychological forces that characterize early development. There is little in the anabolic thrust of the developmental process to indicate a personal end.

The experience of time begins to change in late adolescence when emotional and physical ties to parents are partially severed. A distinct sense of past (childhood), present (young adulthood), and future (middle and late adulthood) is observed (Seton, 1974). The concept of time as a limited quantity gradually emerges in young adulthood but is warded off by new beginnings in work and relationships and by the awesome experience of creating new life—and thus new quantities of time.

But in midlife, the normal adult is increasingly confronted with his or her own finiteness as he or she recognizes and accepts the signs that confront him or her from every side—physical signs of aging, the deaths of parents, the maturation of children into physiological adulthood, and the growing realization that not all of life's ambitions and goals will be realized. The race against time has truly begun.

The case report by Dr. Hassler provides a rare, in-depth account of one man's psychological and emotional response to his 40th birthday as observed through the magnifying glass of psychoanalysis. In addition to illustrating the psychic importance of the passage of time and the need to pay close attention therapeutically to temporal issues in middle-aged patients, the clinical material vividly demonstrates the resistances to doing so in *both* analyst and patient.

Mr. B.'s symptoms, particularly his depression, coincided with his daughter's pubescence. From an adult developmental viewpoint, both parent and child are in the midst of significant developmental change, not just the adolescent. And conflict and symptomatology may be precipitated in either by their individual struggle with current, phase-specific developmental tasks and by interaction with each other. Because of current and past experience, Mr. B. reacted symptomatically to his daughter's pubescence. Hassler's careful developmental history and account of the transference neurosis that emerged in the analysis clearly demonstrate how the patient's depression was precipitated by current developmental conflict and interaction with his pubescent daughter and was linked to genetic determinants from all previous developmental phases, particularly adolescence and the oedipal phase where a significant infantile neurosis was experienced. This is an example of our developmental conceptualization of transference, presented in Chapter 4, in which neurotic transference and symptomatology are understood to be the resultants of experience with the infantile neurosis during the oedipal phase, which is then elaborated and modified by conflict in each subsequent phase of development, is shaped by current developmental experience, and presented by the psychic apparatus of the present.

As the transference neurosis emerged in midphase, the interrelation between current and past developmental experience and the infantile neurosis became clearer and clearer. For example, in Mr. B.'s dream (described on page 102) in which he takes his daughter hunting, she turns into his sister, and they engage in oral sex. The patient's sexual interest in his adolescent daughter, the current precipitant for the dream, was unconsciously linked with actual sexual experience in his own adolescence with his sister and her girlfriend. Further analysis related the sexual wishes for the sister directly to the patient's mother. Thus, there was an unbroken line in the unconscious from daughter to sister to mother. The depression thus can be understood as an expression of the intrapsychic conflict over sexual wishes toward all three.

Therefore, we are suggesting that adult developmental conflict may precipitate symptom formation and add a dimension to the symptom picture that is not based on the past. However, the analysis of these factors always leads to the recovery of determinants from adolescence and childhood that remain undiminished in importance. The psychoanalytic tenet that behind every adult neurosis lies an infantile neurosis remains firmly in place.

In the section on the patient's intrapsychic response to his 40th birthday, we see him first attempt to deny it and then gradually accept its meaning and eventually effect change in significant relationships. As the birthday approached, Mr. B. mentioned that he did not want a cake. Reacting initially to his surprise birthday party with indifference, he was aware internally of mild annoyance at his age—"forty candles on a cake are too many." As the patient experienced anger at his age and mourned for his lost youth, he gradually integrated and accepted his new position in the life cycle and began to evaluate relationships in the face of this new sense of self. For example, his girlfriend's age suddenly becomes a factor—"there is quite a disparity between 26 and 40...the needs are different." He decided, "I don't want to start all over again," and broke off the lengthy affair and reinvested himself in his wife and children.

Our intent is not to suggest that turning 40 was the only factor or even the most important one that produced such change; clearly, much analytic work had been done in other areas. Rather, we hope to demonstrate the sequence of initial denial, followed by anger and sadness, and then gradual integration, leading to behavioral change. This sequence may be a common reaction to aging in midlife.

In concluding the presentation, Hassler forthrightly addresses his own conflict over aging, a struggle that interdigitated with the patient's and affected his therapeutic work, suggesting that a greater understanding of adult developmental processes while the analysis was in progress would have increased his understanding of the patient's dynamics and enhanced his technique. We feel this example plus an increased knowledge of the developmental line of time sense and awareness of the intrapsychic effects of the passage of time may do the same for other therapists.

REFERENCE

Seton, P. The psychotemporal adaptation of late adolescence. *Journal of the American Psychoanalytic Association*, 1974, 22, 795–819.

7

The Development of Intimacy at Age Fifty

ELI MILLER

IDENTIFYING INFORMATION AND CHIEF COMPLAINTS

When referred for analysis Mr. Z. was a 48-year-old, unmarried white male. Casually dressed and a touch overweight, he spoke in a slightly pressured, obsessively organized manner. I found myself responding positively to his wry sense of humor, intelligence, and tight-lipped grin. Except for a course of brief psychotherapy at a local clinic prior to the referral for analysis, he had no previous psychiatric history. In a somewhat cautious but serious manner Mr. Z. began to explain his reasons for wanting analysis.

> I've been on an emotional treadmill. I've tried to solve it for myself but never got much better over the last 20 years. My old attitude was: "If I'm not sick, I should solve my own problems; I'm a big boy." I'm getting older with aches and pains and approaching 50. My father died at 73 and I can afford therapy now. I want to cope and get on with a more pleasant life.

Several sessions later, he was able to verbalize his deeper concern more specifically.

> I've never had sex with someone I cared about, just bar girls in the service. I never told anyone before. My previous therapist didn't ask. I've had all the right opportunities [for sex]. I feel like an incomplete person, the Lone Ranger type. I feel they [women] expect sex, but I block and get afraid

of failure. The "Pee Shy" problem [his fear of urination in public places] still bothers me. You know some people have almost begged me to go to bed with them, but I feared failure. I played moralistic. If it was someone I cared for, I'd feel embarrassed.

Although Mr. Z. did not specifically say so, he also seemed troubled by his recent retirement from over 20 years of active military duty and the state of his mother's health—she was dying from a chronic illness.

DEVELOPMENTAL HISTORY

Preoedipal Years

Mr. Z. was a second son, born to 30-year-old parents. Following an uneventful, full-term pregnancy and birth, he was raised by his mother and a full-time governess. According to his mother, Mr. Z. was a healthy, happy, bottle-fed infant. Before and after Mr. Z.'s birth, his mother frequently accompanied his father on business trips, leaving her son in the care of the governess.

> I spent more time with her than I did with my mother. It was hard on me when she left when I was 6.

During the evaluation, Mr. Z. described his toilet training, which was probably carried out by both mother and governess.

> I remember a small pot and being told that I would have soap stuck up my rear as a suppository if I didn't go to the bathroom. Enemas were popular then, and the rule was for me to have a bowel movement in the morning.

Apparently, he responded to such pressure by training easily. There were no lapses of bowel or bladder control after age 3. When, as a young child (post-toilet training) he lived in Europe with his family, he was horrified to see children defecate on the street and have well-dressed women take out toilet paper and wipe them. Mr. Z. was told that he was a happy, compliant toddler who developed a large vocabulary and was even tempered. He was very attached to his mother and missed her when she went on his father's frequent business trips.

The Oedipal Phase and Latency

Mr. Z.'s loving attachment to his mother and governess continued throughout the oedipal years. He recalled with great warmth the considerable amount of time spent alone with either or both of them. By contrast, the patient remembered his fear of his father, who was very strict and was usually preoccupied with business matters or his health.

> I remember once, I must have been 5 or 6, I lit a match and put it near a thermometer to see the temperature. It shot through the top. I worried all day about what my father would say but he didn't say anything.

A strong infantile neurosis was much in evidence. Mr. Z. was very frightened of the dark and would only sleep with a nightlight. He was frightened of robbers and ghosts and needed frequent assurance.

> My earliest memory is of going to see a Walt Disney movie about the three little pigs. The wolf scared the hell out of me for a long time after...I think I was overprotected as a kid from both disease and danger.

When Mr. Z. was 6, his parents did "the unthinkable" and sent his governess away. Strong feelings of resentment remain to this day.

During latency Mr. Z. attended a private boys' school where he was a model student and was well mannered and cooperative.

> I tried hard; I worried if I didn't do well.

In addition to playing sports such as soccer and baseball, Mr. Z. developed a love for music that continued through his adult years. He had friends and was accepted by his peers but never as a leader or one of the most popular students.

Mr. Z. enjoyed adolescence. He had many friends and excelled academically. In addition to meticulously editing school publications and participating in sports, he continued a serious study of music.

> I stopped taking lessons when I realized my talent only went so far. I would have liked to be *world class* in music because it's a field where you can please yourself and others; it frustrates me when I cannot measure up to the excelling people. [There were some girlfriends but] I didn't have any sex with girls in high school because it was a highly puritanical area and sex was just not done. People didn't even talk about it.

Masturbation occurred regularly after puberty, particularly before a date to prevent arousal. Mr. Z. was troubled by the intensity of his sexual feelings and the details of sexual fantasies. These were heterosexual in nature and centered upon foreplay and intercourse. At age 14, he attributed pain in his lower abdomen and testicles to masturbation and a strong sex drive. With trepidation he approached a trusted family doctor who attributed the pain to "walking around in a wet bathing suit."

Young Adulthood (Ages 20–40)

After such an easy time academically in high school, Mr. Z. was shaken by the demands of college.

My brother flunked out, and I didn't want to follow in his footsteps.

Following a change of schools and majors, both with his father's approval, Mr. Z. completed 4 years of college and went on to graduate school. A minicrisis and significant turning point in the patient's life occurred upon completion of graduate work, when it was time to make a career choice.

My father suggested that I get a job, but I got chicken pox instead.

Soon after, Mr. Z. joined the military and remained on active duty for the next 20 years.

Concerns about sexual performance continued throughout young adulthood. He dated occasionally but avoided emotional involvement with the several women who expressed a serious interest. Intimacy was never achieved with anyone.

I didn't think I could afford to get married. I tried hard not to hurt anyone's feelings.

Actual sexual involvement, "which was never very satisfactory," was rare and confined to one-night stands and prostitutes. Afterward, he feared disease and sometimes developed pains, "probably psychosomatic," for which he sought treatment. Psychosomatic concerns were also expressed by the development of a mild cardiac neurosis that eventually disappeared on its own.

Middle Adulthood (Ages 40–Present)

As he approached 40, Mr. Z. had settled into a life-style that was centered around his career, friendships, and travel. He was keenly aware of the absence of intimacy from his life but was unable to do anything about it. Frequent visits to his parents were uncomfortable because he felt dominated and childlike in their presence.

His father's death when Mr. Z. was 43 was easily adapted to and accompanied by a conscious sense of relief. Then, as the decade progressed, the patient became more involved with his mother due to her failing health and incipient senility.

Mr. Z. experienced a significant adult trauma when he unexpectedly failed (likely due to performance anxiety) a military recertification examination and was not promoted. Soon after, he left the service and returned home to care for his increasingly incapacitated mother.

PSYCHOLOGICAL TESTING

Psychological testing performed during the evaluation revealed an obsessive-compulsive character structure and a Full-Scale IQ of 126. There was no evidence of a thought disorder or organicity. The tester felt that the most difficult technical issues would concern the modification of a rigid superego that dampened the affective expression in any significant emotional relationship.

DIAGNOSTIC FORMULATION

At the time of the evaluation, Mr. Z. was felt to be suffering from a severe obsessional neurotic character disorder. Strong anal conflict was indicated by the concerns about neatness, perfection, cleanliness, and organization. Rigid toilet training, stringent discipline, frequent maternal separations, and precocious ego development were the factors most obviously related to this preoedipal fixation.

Mr. Z.'s severe sexual inhibitions were understood to be neurotic in nature. He had clearly reached the oedipal stage, engaging oedipal themes and developing an intense infantile neurosis. However, his infantile quest for phallic ascendancy was crushed by an inability to compete with a distant, demanding father and the stultifying abandonment by the deeply loved governess. The unresolved oedipal strivings persisted throughout adolescence and adulthood; they were manifested by a continuous heterosexual interest and an inability to develop loving, sexual intimacy with an appropriate partner.

The wish for treatment was precipitated by a series of adult developmental experiences (career failure, death of his father, and illness of his mother) and a growing realization of personal time limitation. If Mr. Z. was ever to experience marriage and heterosexual intimacy, he must overcome the internal forces standing in the way of their emergence soon.

For me, as the analysis began, the central question was, Is analysis a strong enough therapeutic instrument to help this man undo a major inhibition against sexuality and heterosexual intimacy that had dominated his life for nearly 50 years?

COURSE OF THE ANALYSIS

During the early hours of analysis, Mr. Z. did his best to free associate, and he gradually began to focus on fears of heart attacks, aging, and death. Other topics were a fear of public speaking and embarrassment over what he considered to be a high-pitched voice. The first major expression of anger was directed toward "my insensitive and carefree brother." Mr. Z. resented his sibling's lack of involvement in their parents' care, but at the same time he felt guilty about his own significant financial success in managing his mother's money.

At intervals during the opening phase, Mr. Z. talked about the important women in his past. He particularly remembered T., who had died of cancer several years before. Mr. Z. expressed his sadness that she had not left him anything as a memento of the feeling that existed between them. His search for sustenance from past relationships was due in part to the void experienced in his present life. While mourning a lifestyle that had sustained him for 20 years, he had little else to do but care for his mother and her affairs. Despite a deep interest in music and the arts and a friendly approach to people, Mr. Z. was suffering from a lack of social and sexual outlets.

Mr. Z. tended to reject any references to his feelings about me, preferring to focus on himself. He reported several "transportation dreams" in which the common theme was a failure to arrive safely at a designated destination. At other times Mr. Z. described himself as similar to the main character in the movie *Where's Papa*, a man caring for his comical, vivacious, but senile mother.

During the 38th session, the patient bemoaned his lack of sexual experimentation as a teenager, feeling that he was too obedient, "too good for my own good." Two sessions later he reported the following dream:

> In San Francisco Bay was a large old-fashioned sailboat with broad decks. It was sitting in the mud, permanently, like a wreck. A work boat; it suddenly had tall masts. A lot of people start hauling up the sails. I'm not doing my share. It got under way and began moving around narrow streets. I saw a high school girlfriend, B. She looked pretty. I went to ask her out, but her schedule was very busy. I wondered whether to ask her out for lunch or dinner. I gave her a choice. Lunch would be rejection. If it was dinner, it would be more like she was interested and would stay the night. She said that the evening was fine.

Mr. Z. associated to the dream.

> I was reasonably content in high school. I felt more rejection in college. In my sophomore year, I invited B. to a dance. She got ill and couldn't come; this was a real blow to me! My friends had dates and I was without one.

I thought of the boat as representing Mr. Z. floundering in the obsessional mud, needing my help to get moving (sailing) and to get his mast (penis) up.

ANALYST: The wrecked work boat becomes impressive with the sail up.
MR. Z.: Yet stuck in mud and silt.
ANALYST: A very positive dream—you may be the boat getting out of the mud and going after the girl, who says yes!
MR. Z.: I hope!

As the analysis progressed, Mr. Z. reported various obsessive-compulsive checking rituals and extreme difficulty in letting go of feelings and possessions. He was particularly afraid to ask a woman for a date. The most significant genetic material centered on Mr. Z.'s intense emotional involvement with his governess and the extreme loss he felt when the family let her go when he was 6. When Mr. Z. had a dream in which the number 6 was prominently featured, I connected it to the loss of the governess: "Hrumph," he snorted, "It was actually between ages 5 and 6, and it's hard to think the mind would trigger *that* off!" My attempt to point out Mr. Z.'s obvious rebuff of a single woman who was friendly toward him met with a similar reaction.

Soon, his mother's illness intensified, and her decompensation appeared to unearth several hypochondriacal and childhood separation fears. Childhood phobias, particularly including fears of the dark and of being alone, reappeared. Mr. Z. was also troubled by a recurrent fantasy in which he was swimming alone in shark-infested waters. He was muted in his response to his mother's deterioration, and he cried openly when a beloved cat died.

> I loved that cat more than anything in the world.

It was interesting that the pet cemetery was located on the same road where the patient's father was buried.

Transference Themes

In hour 72, Mr. Z. reported the following transference dream:

> You got ahold of this stack of this stuff of mine. You said, "Aha! What have we here!" It was like I was hiding basic stuff; like what does this stuff mean?

In association to the dream, Mr. Z. wondered about topics that he might not be ready to bring up in the analysis. He mentioned that he was trying to be honest and associate to the best of his ability.

MR. Z.: I don't have all that much to hide; not that I'm malicious or want to hurt others or that I'm carrying great guilt!
ANALYST: Yet it is like I found you out.
MR. Z.: I guess, but I'm not quite able to find myself out. I torture myself with stuff!

In this same period, Mr. Z. also communicated that he perceived the loss of the governess as "negative for my emotional development. I resented that my parents did not realize that fact!" He described the governess as an interesting and capable woman who was later hired by a rich man with several children. He knew she had subsequently died of cancer.

Gradually, with continuous resistance, additional transference themes began to emerge. When I noted that he seemed to be avoiding eye contact with me at the beginning and end of sessions, he replied:

> I'd rather almost not have contact outside of the session or know about you. I'd rather have it on a clinical basis.

Soon after, Mr. Z. was frightened by a large frog that was in his leaking frog pond.

ANALYST: When you clean the fish pond aren't you going to have to look that big frog in the eye just like me?
MR. Z.: Oh, I'm not afraid of him! If he hops around I'll get rid of him. I don't like to kill things, so I'll chase him to the grove.

During this period of time, when Mr. Z. was increasingly preoccupied with his age and health, he began to diet and exercise. His fears of being alone in the house at night were repeatedly surfacing, and he began to notice his style of holding grudges and in general of having trouble "letting go."

As Mr. Z. approached his 49th birthday, negative transference appeared around a vacation. He mentioned that he did not like the feeling of being forced or obligated to come to analysis. He began to express concerns about how I felt about him and wished that I would say that he was an "OK guy."

> I really want to change! Where there's a will there's a way.

Concern about his appearance and baldness followed.

MR. Z.: People wouldn't say "you're a fat slob; take off 100 pounds," or "You are wrinkled." A woman said to Don Rickles: "Don, why do you comb your hair up that way?" It's OK if I know the person likes me a lot. It's a problem with new relationships. I hate to force myself on people.
ANALYST: I don't really buy that!
MR. Z.: Yeah, if they come on to me I feel something is wrong with them, because they want me.
ANALYST: Groucho Marx once joked that he refused to be a member of any club that would take him.

When I pointed out that, despite what he felt were mild imperfections in his appearance, he was often approached by women whom *he* rebuffed, he replied:

> Yes, if they come on to me I feel something is wrong with them because they want me. The unobtainable is more desirable.

Mr. Z. recalled the fraternities at college; the ones that wanted him were "second best"; and therefore he refused to join any of them. The analyst was no exception.

> The way you accepted me so quickly for analysis didn't make me feel so good either. You must not have had a full case load. I would have felt better if you had put me on a waiting list.

During those first 100 hours of the analysis, as a transference neurosis was forming, Mr. Z. struggled with a growing recognition of his position in relationship to the developmental tasks of midlife.

> I feel mine is a midlife crisis but a little different. Most of the men I heard about have situations involving children and a wife. My fear is a fear of life passing me by and my becoming old and lonely. Every problem I have is associated with the feeling that I'm not of a normal range of sexuality. We could talk for 10 years, and all these other things would be just beating around the bush. I've only had sexual relationships a few times in my life, and I'm afraid to start with someone else; it's that abnormal. People lose interest after marriage, or some men give up. I feel I'm missing something vital.

His specific fears about sexual performance included concern about partial erections and premature ejaculations. Enjoyable sex might bring back the pains he experienced in his testicles as a teenager. Mr. Z. emphasized that "satisfactory sex gives one an exuberance, vitality, and a desire to get things done."

Mr. Z.'s wish for more meaningful human contact and the desire to complete his masculine identity by producing offspring became more urgent as he considered his age.

> At the core of the problem I can get along with people quite well or explain why I'm not married or dating. But I don't seek new friends; I'm not in the mainstream. I'm aloof towards other people and I have a fear of be-

ing in the house by myself. I could invite girls over if I wanted, but I can't make myself take the first step...It all gets down to sex! I don't even know if I'm sterile or not at 49 years of age.

As the positive transference grew, Mr. Z. viewed the analyst as the firm and critical but supportive and caring father figure. He was less anxious and depressed and was increasingly drawn to associations about his mother and the governess. It became clear that all women were seen as a composite of these two women—loving and involved but certain to abandon him sooner or later.

Mr. Z.'s Mother's Death

In hour 125, Mr. Z. reported with very little affect that his mother had finally died of her long illness.

Now I'm to a *turning point.* I do feel very relieved.

During the session he repeatedly strayed from the subject in an attempt to deny intense feelings about her loss. In the following hour, in response to making funeral arrangements he spoke more openly.

Mother was more of an appendage of my father. She read and cooked; she was a good wife and mother, amusing and witty.

He expressed anger about being primarily cared for by the governess. When I queried Mr. Z. as to whether he was treated more as a loved possession by his mother than someone to be interested in for himself, he replied:

This is possibly why I have trouble getting emotionally close to people. I give the impression that I'm cold and I'm not. ...I would feel guilty if I told someone this, as if it were weird, but I felt more anguish with the cat and its dying than my mother.

Mr. Z. rationalized his lack of feeling by suggesting that he had done his mourning during the long course of his mother's illness. Sympathy notes from family and friends produced momentary feelings of love and sadness that were quickly dissipated. Mr. Z. began to plan frequent vacations as another means of avoiding his feelings, his fear of staying alone, and the analysis.

In the sessions following his mother's death, Mr. Z. considered a wide range of topics. He wondered why his closest friends were two to three decades older than he. Surprisingly, he felt closer to his brother and sister-in-law and decided to invite them to dinner. Warm memories of his cherished governess flowed more easily into consciousness.

> Like she could control the world and make things pleasant. All things were good with her. It was like a sense of order; *like at one time I had it!*

At the end of August in hour 137, Mr. Z. returned from his vacation hale and hearty, well tanned, and relaxed. He sensed a positive attitude change; he was less uptight, but still very concerned with relying on himself.

Despite conscious reluctance, Mr. Z. returned to feelings about his mother through the following dream.

> I'm leaping off into space. I don't have a body. A hooded figure is walking up a ramp toward me, pulling something on a sled. I fly over them to some water. I'm a good swimmer, so it doesn't bother me. I materialize and have a body again. [Brief associations to his mother's death followed.] A woman is telling me something about not being married. It was a girl named T. from high school. She wasn't very popular, but she liked me. I was nice to her. In the dream she's explaining that I came from another existence with another relationship I'm committed to...[Mr. Z. again associated to the hospital where his mother died.]...Now I'm in a room. There's some black gauze on the floor and a body underneath. Somebody else said you can't. I thought I recognized the face on the corpse. Then somebody said the person was just pretending to be dead. I'm glad you moved here near a hospital [I had recently moved my office]. Less traffic, but it does give me negative feelings about illness and death...I once had a dream of a ruptured appendix. For a moment in the dream I felt I had the answer to the world's questions but I woke up and couldn't remember the answers.... Flying was fun. I have a friend who likes to fly. He has success and control of his life...He's now president of his own company. The dream is a bunch of nonsense!

Mr. Z.'s feelings about his mother were heightened by her death.

ANALYST: In the dream you're not married; yet you're connected to someone in another world.

MR. Z.: The girl, T., never had anything to do with me. It was just a high school crush on me.

ANALYST: Could she have been a symbol for something or someone else?

MR. Z.: No.

ANALYST: Yet dreams contain symbolism.

MR. Z.: Yes, we talked of that! In South America. An odd family; my first cousin's parents. Kids with birth defects. I don't know why. They had a couple of kids with birth defects.

ANALYST: Didn't you say in the past that the birth defects might have resulted from incest.

MR. Z.: Yea, I did. I didn't think of that.

ANALYST: I wonder what that association tells us about the dream. [Mr. Z. refused to consider the idea that the association had anything to do with the dream. Later I returned to the theme of his mother.]

ANALYST: The dream appears connected to your mother's death.

MR. Z.: You mean because of the hospital?

ANALYST: Yes, partially.

MR. Z.: (firmly) I don't dwell on it!

ANALYST: I understand, but the dream tells us that your unconscious may be working on the mourning.

MR. Z.: I'm missing the cat more at home. Animals can tell I like them. I hit it off better at times with animals than I do with people. (sadness, near tears)

ANALYST: You're sad now?

MR. Z.: I think so.

He began the following session by return to the warded off incestuous association.

MR. Z.: The incestuous connection in the dream. What does it have to do with my dream? I don't feel incest is evil. What would trigger such an oddball dream? You used the word incest as if it was an intriguing sexual experience.

ANALYST: Do you think the association may refer to your mother?

MR. Z.: I was worried you'd say that! That I have sexual feelings for my mother? In another world; obligated to someone else! I never felt that close to my mother. It's not part of my mental make up. Are you trying to say I'm obligated to a dead mother? I don't see it that way! I absolutely don't think so!! I'm actually freer since she died. It's the opposite now. I'm not obligated to her!

The Urge to Travel

As Mr. Z. began to discuss plans for additional vacations and travel, some of the dynamics behind this new interest began to emerge. Although he was phobic and frightened at home alone, particularly at night, he was very comfortable alone in public places or when on trips.

At those times Mr. Z. experienced a sense of control, largely because he did not have to deal with familiar people. He hated intrusions beyond his control. I interpreted that to mean that Mr. Z. might be feeling intruded upon by his feelings for me and my comments in the analysis.

> True! If I care I open up and I might get hurt.

He then expressed the fantasy of being a king who could command people to be there only when he wanted them. Mr. Z. was aware that he was reneging on the analytic contract, but he saw positive reasons for his behavior.

> I feel so strongly I want to do it [travel]. It would be counterproductive not to. I shouldn't deny myself at 49 years of age what I want to do! Yet, I know that I should concentrate on the analysis more.

I understood the analytic work to this point in the following manner: Mr. Z. felt that as a young child he had been trapped in relationships that had hurt him and left him vulnerable to the wishes of others. He feared a repetition of this pattern in other significant relationships. This conflict was being recreated in the transference as he felt emotionally involved with the analyst and began to react against these feelings. He appeared to be attempting to master his feelings of being "left" by his mother and governess by continually leaving the analyst. Outside of the analysis, he was able to titrate emotional involvements by avoiding women his own age and by spending most of his time with friends in their 70s and 80s. Because Mr. Z. saw these elderly friends as asexual, he was more comfortable with them, a common bias that strengthened the defense.

In hour 155, Mr. Z. spoke of recent contact with a woman he had known many years ago. This woman, P., aged 47, was in the process of obtaining a separation and possible divorce from her wealthy husband. Mr. Z. was attracted to her and enjoyed her company. Like him, she had been in treatment and accepted his analytic effort. He mentioned casually that she had had an unsuccessful pregnancy at age 44. Soon after, Mr. Z. was invited by P. to spend Christmas with her. To his surprise, he wanted to accept the invitation.

> Before you ask, I'll tell you, there's been no sex! I wonder if sex with P. would have helped. I think she is as screwed up as I am in terms of rela-

tionships. A relationship with her would be a disaster! She's *so* into her problems; she couldn't possibly understand my problems!

He began to ruminate about being 50 and wondered if any woman would be suitable for him.

After the December holiday break with P., Mr. Z. returned with increased self-esteem and an open desire to date. As he began to consider an active sex life, he decided to have a sperm count done.

> Before it was beyond my realm of reality to do something like that. Even making the appointment would have been hard to do!

The normal result from the sperm count greatly increased his feelings of potency and masculinity. Mr. Z. lamented his 30 adult years of sexual inhibition. "What a terrible waste," he said.

Mr. Z. soon spoke of another woman, G., a divorcée he had known for many years

> I've seen her off and on over the years. I held off or backed off with the sex.... This year I called her at New Year's. She knows my voice immediately. She cares. I told her to come down.... This time, if she wants sex, she'll get it!! Maybe the sperm count helped! I'm less inhibited.... She could be my surrogate.... The fact I can say this, that is considerable progress!!

He gave many examples of incidents in which he had backed off from sexual relationships. In hour 175, he again reported concern about being late to analysis, disliking his sense of obligation. He associated to his father's punctuality and the pressure his father put on the family members to adhere to *his* time schedule.

Significant Life Changes

Mr. Z. began to change his life. He planned to move out of his parents' home into one of his own. Over the years he had collected piles of records and knickknacks. They had to go! A friend had suggested a blind date with a lawyer. Would she find him unattractive, too heavy? When Mr. Z. actually began to clean out the clothes from his parents home in anticipation of a move, he found himself unable to give away a number of his father's old hats. He initiated a ritual burning of them instead.

Throwing them out would be like putting pieces of father in the garbage. It's like a tattered flag. . .how hard it is to get rid of things!"

Shortly thereafter, he bought a home of his own. As Mr. Z. began to take more interest in his real estate purchase and dating activity, he experienced an upsurge in hypochondriacal concerns and increased negative transference. These continued to center on money, time away from the analysis, and missed analytic visits. Mr. Z. made a plea to cut the analysis to 2 days a week.

I dislike being preoccupied with the analytic appointments. This thing permeates my whole day. It's becoming my whole life. In some ways it's ruining my life.

Mr. Z. was very angry about the "possibility" of having to pay for sessions that were missed beyond what the original contract stated. He said that, even though he was not planning to take off nearly as much time in the near future, he hoped to vacation with the feeling that I wished him a good time.

After expressing a willingness to be flexible, I interpreted the following:

ANALYST: You're using frequent vacations to avoid experiencing and analyzing powerful feelings—some of them are sexual, some are about your mother's death, and others are about me.
MR. Z.: A person has to be weak to stay in analysis for a long time. I want to graduate from here, like I did from college. I think travel does me good. I feel stronger then. I tie up a lot of loose ends before I go, and I seem to have additional energy during the trip.

Despite our work, Mr. Z. went off on another vacation. Upon returning, he reported being thrown into a semidating situation with a middle-aged German woman. He was dismayed with the interaction, describing her as a "single, dumpy, cheapskate." She reminded him of his great aunts in their late 60s. Following associations to his father's "standards" and lectures on meeting one's obligations, I interpreted (again) Mr. Z.'s belief that his father—and I—would strongly disapprove of his having an active, satisfying sexual life. He responded:

MR. Z.: It's true. You know, I yearn for the old days. When we lived in the country when I was a kid, life was simpler. You could leave your keys in the ignition without fear of burglary.

ANALYST: And you didn't have to worry about a sex life when you were a kid.

Mr. Z. reported a "key breakthrough" in hour 215. After a comfortable evening with another old girlfriend, he had finally taken the initiative, with some help from alcohol, and slept with her, although they did not actually have intercourse. The girlfriend, B., was described as a personable, uninhibited, divorced, 44-year-old career woman who had known the patient since he was 10 years old. For years he had thought of her as a sister.

MR. Z.: I feel a lot better about the analysis. I never would have had this positive situation with B. without the experience of psychoanalysis. I would have done the same old pattern and just gone back to my own bed!
ANALYST: What got you off the diving board [into bed and sex]!"
MR. Z.: Too much to drink! (*laugh*) I can't remember. All of a sudden it was the right thing to do! I know she likes me.

Mr. Z. started the next session as follows:

> If I get the sexual hang-up out of the way, what's next on the agenda? It has to end sometime; possibly I'll come two times per week. I *am* making some progress.

The possibility of an ongoing sexual relationship brought back fears of performance anxiety and sexual inadequacy. Mr. Z. was pleased that B. was not "uptight about sex," because this made the sexual relationship easier for him. But he became notably more anxious as the sexual relationship progressed. In hour 218, he had a preoccupation with his pulse and various pains. I helped Mr. Z. see that his sexual experience in addition to producing much pleasure was causing him concerns about his health and a sense of guilt expressed through a fear of impending doom. He acknowledged this, but he felt positive that this girlfriend, who was very attracted to him, liked him "as I am."

In hour 222, some sadomasochistic fantasies were introduced, including a memory of spanking games during childhood. Mr. Z. wondered if there was some sort of sexual thrill associated with spankings from parents. He mentioned reading a recent article on sadomasochistic behavior and how it was becoming much more acceptable. He read of a woman who supplied sadomasochistic sexual gratification to men of the upper class.

It's bizarre! It wouldn't appeal to me, although some people do like to be spanked!

Mr. Z. continued to get more involved with his new girlfriend. He wanted to take time off from the analysis to spend a long weekend with her:

> Having to keep the schedule makes it difficult. I want *no* schedule with anybody! I want to do exactly as I want to do.

Despite continuing (though lessened) hypochondriacal concerns and feelings of guilt, Mr. Z. was exhilarated by his new relationship.

A New Chapter at Middle Age

> I want her to know I care for her; that it's not just therapy for me. It's a new lease on life. At 50, sex is routine to a lot of people, or they don't do it anymore. A new lease on life at 50! A new chapter at middle age! Not routine, that's good.

Mr. Z. continued to view B. as nearly the ideal woman, and at this point he told her that he loved her.

> Two years ago I couldn't imagine talking to anyone about erections or what went on with a woman overnight. Never in my wildest imagination!

In hour 230, Mr. Z. began making comparisons between his old girl-friend, P., who was very rejecting, with his new, very accepting girl-friend, B.; he compared his warm German governess of childhood with his less demonstrative mother. As the relationship with B. deepened, Mr. Z. reported the following dream:

> The Japanese royal family comes out. (The real empress is dowdy.) I'm wandering around sight-seeing. The empress is in a geisha outfit and is very attractive. I was talking like I knew her. The emperor was not around.

MR. Z.: I was examining a silk-screen print from B. just before I went to sleep.
ANALYST: Didn't you recently give B. a Japanese gown before her trip to the Orient!
MR. Z.: (*with surprise*) Er…yes, I did! I'd forgotten that. The Japanese give gifts, mementos.

ANALYST: Did you feel the gift would be kind of sexy?
MR. Z.: Oh, yeah! An above-the-knees gown.

As his relationship with B. deepened, Mr. Z. reported that he was now looking forward to his upcoming 50th birthday.

> I was fortunate I found B., she's uninhibited. I'm more inhibited in the way I act...it's not just a short passing thing with her...I feel fortunate. I had never looked forward to being 50 before. It's nice to have something fresh and new at 50. I'm still searching; yet now I'm a little bit more optimistic.

Mr. Z. became more responsive to B. and others as well. He was more open, warm, physical, and communicative with friends and family. For the first time in his life, Mr. Z. kissed relatives and female friends on the cheeks. He began to entertain more often and expressed a desire to have a closer, "regular" group of friends.

He spoke of his relationship with his brother.

MR. Z.: Maybe I'm too hard on him?
ANALYST: He appears to like you.
MR. Z.: I know he does. It's not that I don't care. I feel guilty, like they have better feelings for me than I do for them, like with my parents!

Now that he felt fairly secure about his relationship with B., Mr. Z. began to explore his traveling and past gravitation toward elderly people as a means of isolating himself from women his age. He also began to communicate with a male friend about sexuality.

> I told him B. was uninhibited, and it was good for me. I can talk to another man about sex without being embarrassed. It opens new dimensions for me. You know, I had it in my head that women were more prim and proper than they are!...When I first told B. I loved her it seemed to bother her. Now she said: "I do love you!"

Each step forward seemed to be accompanied by new anxiety and more productive analytic work. In hour 238, Mr. Z. spoke of his episodes of testicular pain during adolescence. The anxiety erupted in the following dream.

> I'm in a clinic to have these spots taken off. Mrs. G. is there as a receptionist. I'm undressed except for my terry cloth shorts. A lot of people are in the room, and she said it was a "pants-off room" and pulled mine off.

I didn't like that. And then she was trying to give me a rectal with her finger. It was hurting, and I said I'd just had that done. I said that I didn't need that and that it was embarrassing. Other people were around.

Mr. Z. associated to a recent experience in which he had the thought that his girlfriend's vagina was too tight to penetrate. Later, he again brought up his fears of performance during intercourse. After further associations were forthcoming, I told Mr. Z. that one of the main themes in the dream was his fear of being damaged by sex. He began associating to his testicular pains during adolescence and said:

It was the root cause of all my fears about health.

He recalled experiencing the testicular pains when he was 14 years old, subsequent to finding out about a friend whose mother had died of cancer. Mr. Z. emphasized that "the root cause is that I feared something was wrong with my testicles. Sometimes they hurt all day long. It was a terrible trauma."

As his associations continued, the patient wondered if the testicular pain had anything to do with masturbation. One of his key fears as a teenager was developing cancer of the testicles.

ANALYST: You did masturbate.
MR. Z.: Yes. I never admitted I did. The kids said it was not supposed to hurt you. But the pain was from *something*; so I thought it was my just desserts for doing what I'm not supposed to!

Mr. Z. initiated another vacation and did not return to the analysis. He called, saying he had married B., was happy and "free," and had gotten what he wanted from treatment. He wished to stop without any further exploration of his actions or feelings. Mr. Z. seemed to fear further analysis would ruin his dream come true. There had been signs during the previous several months, particularly in regard to the travel issue, that Mr. Z. might bolt from the analysis. He had expressed the magical fear that analyzing his new relationship would cause him to lose it. He feared engulfment by the analyst-mother and, unconsciously, by the girlfriend-mother. Yet, on the positive side, he had loosened his obsessional stance and was expressing feelings and opening himself to friends, both old and new. The fear of aging, the loss of his mother, a responsive new woman, and the analysis appeared to combine to allow a partial developmental reworking of oedipal and preoedipal fixations and a subsequent freeing of developmental progression. Mr. Z. had now moved past a lifelong fixation toward partial oedipal success and more gratifying intimate relationships.

Discussion

ROBERT A. NEMIROFF AND CALVIN A. COLARUSSO

Can dynamic psychotherapy or psychoanalysis help an individual approaching age 50 to achieve an active sexual life and heterosexual intimacy for the first time? That was the question Dr. Miller had to consider as he listened to his prospective patient, a 48-year-old seemingly confirmed bachelor, express his complaints. Freud's pessimistic comments about the effectiveness of analysis after 40 must have echoed in his ears as he listened.

A study of Miller's careful developmental history of the life cycle, which includes the adult as well as child developmental phases, reveals that Mr. Z. was raised in an intact family and received adequate early care, albeit not without complications. There is evidence of considerable oedipal involvement, a strong infantile neurosis, and positive development along several developmental lines, despite a major arrest in sexual development in both childhood and adulthood.

As Jellifee (1925) noted over 50 years ago, chronological, psychological, and physiological age are not equivalent. The adult developmental approach to diagnosis suggests that an assessment of psychopathology should be based primarily on dynamic and developmental considerations rather than on chronological age. Using such a conceptual approach, Miller determined that his patient was essentially neurotic and was suffering from a severe obsessional character disorder. He was well motivated for analysis and was driven by a strong desire to achieve mastery of the adult developmental tasks of sexuality, intimacy, and marriage before time ran out. His uniquely individual "race against time" was also

143

stimulated by the poignant death of his father and the impending demise of his beloved mother.

Early in the analysis, it became increasingly clear that Mr. Z. had been sustained during his adult years by his deep attachments to his mother and his military career. Although he did not say so, the desire for treatment was probably related to the loss of both these supports as much as the desire for sex and intimacy. Mr. Z. was at a critical juncture in midlife; he was desperately in need of a new occupation to provide purpose and direction and new object relationships to provide love and warmth.

But before such a transition could occur, the patient had to deal with his emotional response, or lack thereof, to his mother's death. His inability to mourn was striking; the therapist had to confront the patient repeatedly with the denial of such feelings. Through the transference, Mr. Z.'s ambivalent attitude toward his mother and his deep-seated fear of, and hostility toward, women gradually became accessible. Only then (still with difficulty) was he able to grieve. The dynamics in this case are a striking example of George Pollock's ideas on the centrality of the mourning-liberation process and the need for the therapist to be alert to the relationship between incomplete grief work and neurotic inhibition and symptomatology.

It is interesting to note that chronological age was also no barrier to the emergence in the transference of aspects of the infantile neurosis. As his sexual interests and attachments to his dying mother became conscious, Mr. Z. developed fears of the dark and being alone—symptoms that were prominent during childhood. These fears were also related to other aspects of the positive oedipal conflict as was evidenced by a growing transference fear of the analyst, who was initially portrayed as a menacing frog and later as a dangerous paternal predator. Gradually, the paternal transference focused on wishes for love and support and fears of disapproval and castration. In time, Mr. Z. became proficient in the use of dreams, another dimension of the analytic work undiminished by age. A vivid example is the Japanese royal family dream in which the love for the oedipal mother and wish to exclude the oedipal father are clearly portrayed.

An interesting comparison might be made between Mr. Z. and Dr. Hassler's patient (Chapter 6). Whereas the 40-year-old Mr. B. successfully denied and avoided the intrapsychic implications of turning 40, the same defenses could not be used as effectively by the 50-year-old Mr.

Z. His engagement of the midlife developmental tasks of time limitation and personal death was too powerful to be denied, and it became a potent force influencing his efforts at change and integration in the face of profound loss. In *Adult Development* (Colarusso & Nemiroff, 1981), we suggested that such awareness could be a stimulus to forward development.

> Confronting this quintessential adult-human experience can lead to ego functioning and integration of the highest order and produce the profoundest awareness of what it means to be human. (p. 77)

How does this stimulus work?

> Gradually the adult personality, stimulated by the awareness of time limitation and personal death, may reorganize along a positive line. For example: (1) Increased awareness of physical retrogression can lead to a redefinition of body image and act as a stimulus to developing new physical and nonphysical means of gratification appropriate to a realistic level of physical competence. (2) The sense of time limitation can be perceived as a stimulus to redefine goals and channel existing energy and resources into *obtainable* objectives that gratify the self and loved ones. (3) The conscience may be affected by the deaths of parents (Steinschein, 1973) and by increased demands for gratification of impulses that were held in check when time was thought to be plentiful. (p. 78)

Despite Miller's efforts, Mr. Z. left analysis precipitously but not before achieving *his* major goal: a sustaining, intimate heterosexual relationship. Should the therapist be as satisfied as the patient and restrain his therapeutic zeal in the face of such obvious change? We think not; older patients can analyze as thoroughly and completely as younger ones. Unless this is recognized, the older patient's wish to terminate prematurely may provoke a countertransference response in the therapist. In an attempt to ward off awareness of the patient's—and his own—fear of death, the analyst may avoid completeness and thoroughness as a defense against his own race against time.

REFERENCES

Colarusso, C. A., & Nemiroff, R. A. *Adult development: A new dimension in psychodynamic theory and practice.* New York: Plenum Press, 1981.

Jellifee, S. E. The old age factor in psycho-analytic theory. *Medical Journal Records*, 1925, *121*, 7–12.

Steinschein, I. (Reporter). The experience of separation-individuation...through the course of life: Maturity, senescence, and sociological implications (Panel report). *Journal of the American Psychoanalytic Association*, 1973, *21*, 633–645.

8

Short-Term Psychodynamic Psychotherapy with a Sixty-Two-Year-Old Man

Jill E. Crusey

Historically, the mental health profession has shown minimal interest in therapy with older adults. Such treatment has been regarded by many mental health practitioners as a drain on the already strained fiscal and psychological resources of the profession. Too often, these professionals suggested that this age group was depressing and difficult to work with, incapable of improvement or growth, and therefore unlikely to yield satisfaction for the therapist.

However, careful studies of older patients have shown that the same wide range of disorders is found among young patients too. These studies also demonstrated that, as in earlier stages of growth, the process of aging is accompanied by its own unique developmental and psychological issues. One interesting observation that emerged from these studies was the large number of older men and women who had functioned well throughout youth and middle adulthood but developed psychological difficulties in later life. This phenomenon will be illustrated through the case history of an older man who, at 62, experienced acute psychological distress for the first time and undertook short-term psychodynamic psychotherapy with a 31-year-old female therapist.

INTRODUCTION

Mr. D. suffered a myocardial infarction at the age of 62. After surgery, he remained in the hospital for several weeks for rehabilitation. A social worker assigned to the rehabilitation unit visited Mr. D. and learned of several stressful life circumstances that she considered detrimental to his recovery. His doctor and social worker suggested that if he returned to those conditions, a relapse was probable. Psychotherapy was offered to him as a way of understanding the reasons for his prior strenuous pace and consequent psychological distress.

The most recent stressful circumstance occurred 2 years prior to Mr. D.'s myocardial infarction. At that time, his wife of 38 years suffered a stroke that left her partially paralyzed and incapable of caring for herself. With some assistance from a home health care agency, Mr. D. assumed responsibility for his wife's care. Between the demands of his job as an administrator of a large firm and the nursing responsibilities his wife required, Mr. D. had two full-time occupations. These pressures contributed to his own physical decline. Before Mr. D. returned home from the hospital, his doctor instructed him to place his wife in a convalescent center.

DEVELOPMENTAL HISTORY

Infancy

At the insistence of his doctor, Mr. D. made an appointment for a psychological evaluation shortly after his discharge from the hospital. When we met for our first session, Mr. D. hesitatingly shared some information about his current health problems and those of his wife. Within the first 15 minutes, he acknowledged that the myocardial infarction jolted him into recognizing that he had a "limited time left to live."

> I never believed this would happen to me. I've always thought of myself as a healthy person. I guess I've never seriously considered my own death. Somehow, I always thought my clean living and farm-boy background would keep me alive forever. I can't believe I've done this to myself.

In the course of our sessions following the initial evaluation, a detailed developmental history was presented. Mr. D. was the first of three children born to a midwestern couple in their 20s who farmed many acres of grain and had livestock. Mr. D. recalled that his mother wanted to have a large family but seemed prone to first-trimester miscarriages. Although Mr. D. was carried to full term, his mother experienced several miscarriages before and after his birth.

With the assistance of a midwife, Mr. D. was delivered at home without complications. His normal birth was greeted with much relief and excitement. Mr. D.'s mother was extremely protective of her newborn son and was reluctant to accept assistance offered by several sisters and cousins. Her choice to breast-feed her son prevented her from fulfilling her responsibilities on the farm. Consequently, the father took over the additional chores which left him little time for his new child.

As Mrs. D. was settling into the routine of child care, her own mother suddenly moved in with them. Her husband, after 27 years of marriage, had abruptly abandoned the family and moved to Australia with a younger woman. Mrs. D.'s mother refused to discuss the situation with anyone and insisted on staying with her oldest daughter. Mrs. D., angry and bitter, made only infrequent comments about her father's hasty departure. So little was said about it during Mr. D.'s upbringing that only during his 20s did he learn the whereabouts of his mother's father.

Mrs. D.'s mother quickly adapted herself to household and farm duties, a situation that allowed her daughter to spend more time with her growing son. According to Mr. D., his early childhood was average. He recalled that his mother regarded his sleep patterns, weaning, sitting, walking, and interaction with others as normal and on time. However, Mr. D. apparently demonstrated early signs of his ability to accept responsibilities. He "mastered" toilet training within a week and language and motor development occurred 4 to 5 months earlier than usual.

Mr. D.'s first memory was of himself at approximately three years of age. He was entrusted with the responsibility of gathering eggs and feeding some of the small farm animals.

> I guess I was a responsible person even then. About that time, my father purchased more land. Consequently, there were more things to do, and everyone had to chip in. Even my father's father, who lived down the road, helped with the chores. That's the way things were done in those days.

It was no surprise to learn that Mr. D. was involved in farm tasks as a preschooler. His mother regarded her son as a quiet, even-tempered, friendly child. He was not particularly aggressive but was rather obedient. "You just did what you were told to do. You never asked questions. That just wasn't done." Mr. D. felt that his parents' attitudes toward discipline were reflective of the era in which he grew up.

> My mother and father didn't have to ride hard on me. I regretted the few times I stepped out of line. At those times, my father seemed like an awesome man.

There were few opportunities for Mr. D. to get into trouble. The distances between neighbors and to the nearest town were considerable. The little contact the family had with others took place at weekend church meetings.

> It was drummed into me that family was the most important thing. We did everything together. When I was growing up, separate vacations or social lives were never considered.

By the time Mr. D. was ready to attend school, his mother had assumed an even greater protective posture.

> I couldn't step outside the front gate without mother checking my work and appearance. I couldn't wait to get to school just to get away. That was the only time I had to play with friends.

Outside of school, Mr. D.'s time was consumed by farm chores and family duties. "I wished I could spend more time with the kids from school, but I knew I had to do my share of the chores. What good would complaining have done?"

Sexual Interests

Mr. D.'s earliest memory involving sexual overtones related to the birthing process of the family's cows.

> I was quickly indoctrinated into the world of sex. When you live on a farm, you can't ignore all the copulation and conception that goes on. Somehow, I never thought much about it in relationship to human beings. My family was rather prudish about sexual matters. I can't remember mother or grandmother any way except fully clothed. Sexual matters weren't discussed among family members.

An exception was a conversation Mr. D. had as a 6-year-old with his grandfather. This was a conversation Mr. D. felt had a dramatic impact on his sexual life. His grandfather began to explain the "birds and bees" to his grandson who interrupted him to let him know he already knew all that. However, Mr. D. told his grandfather that he was curious about the night and morning erections he experienced and the pleasure he felt exploring his genitals. His grandfather assured him he would not have to worry about erections and masturbation once he grew up and found the right woman to marry. "Unfortunately, I took my grandfather literally and stopped masturbating when I married my wife."

These earliest memories prompted Mr. D. to elaborate on his parents' overprotective attitude toward sexual issues.

> My parents never said much about sex, and I didn't ask many questions. The few times I approached my mother with questions, she told me I was too young to understand. I took her word for it as she was the one in charge.

Mr. D.'s father, however, impressed upon him that girls and sex did not belong in his son's life until he finished high school. The senior Mr. D. was a religious man who believed that sex happened between two married adults in the privacy of their bedroom. Except for holding hands on the way to church, Mr. D. could not recall his parents ever displaying affection in front of the family.

At the age of 7, when Mr. D. was enjoying newly found abilities to read and draw, he rushed excitedly into the bathroom to show one of his creations to his father. He halted abruptly at the sight of his father standing in front of the mirror naked and larger than life.

> I was frightened by my father's physical stature, particularly the size of his penis. I remember I ran off as fast as I could. My father didn't have a chance to scold me for barging in.

As he described this incident, Mr. D. admitted he felt uncomfortable. When questioned further about his feelings, he acknowledged his lifelong fear of his father.

> My dad was a highly respected man in the community. When he wasn't working the farm, he was busy with church and civic activities. I assumed it was my responsibility to take care of things at home when he was ab-

sent. Although I didn't enjoy being stuck with chores day in and day out, I couldn't see any alternative. My mother would remind me that, when Dad was away, I was her little man. I would enjoy that position when my efforts were rewarded with an apple pie. Other times it would drive me crazy because I didn't want to be Mom's little man.

This "little man" role prevented Mr. D. from participating in opportunities generally available to young boys. While his peers were enjoying hobbies and games, Mr. D. was occupied with family responsibilities. When he was 8, these responsibilities increased after his mother gave birth to his brother. His mixed feelings of excitement over a new playmate and resentment over increased duties resulting from the new arrival remained unresolved. To Mr. D., it appeared as if his mother invested herself in her new son and excluded him.

I can't remember when my mother spent time alone with me after my brother's birth. From that point on, I became the built-in baby-sitter as well as the "little man." I felt my brother would be more of a nuisance than a possible companion.

During this period in his life, Mr. D. became committed to his schoolwork and appeared to enjoy the rewards of good grades. In retrospect, he felt his appetite for learning was motivated by a desire to leave the farm. Good grades and hard work on the farm seemed to be the only way to get closer to his father who seemed proud of his son's scholarly accomplishments. Because of his father's obligations, Mr. D. could not spend as much time with him as he would have liked. However, he thoroughly enjoyed weekend church-related activities that brought his father and him together for recreational reasons.

Adolescence

Preadolescent years are recognized as a time for mischief; they are a period of testing the limits of authority and building a sense of conscience. For Mr. D., participation in any pranks was unthinkable. Defiance of parental authority was equated with severe punishment. Although Mr. D. had not experienced much parental wrath, he felt no desire to precipitate it. On a few occasions, he witnessed his father lose his temper at the dinner table. The intensity of the rage coupled with his father's strength and size frightened the entire family. Although Mr.

D. was tired of chores, schoolwork, and his brother, his fear of his father's anger deterred any complaints.

A year after his brother's birth, his sister Lydia was born. She quickly became the pride and joy of the family. His mother took extreme care with her, treating her as if she were a fragile doll. Mr. D. felt removed from his sister's earlier years due to his mother's protective, possessive attitude. By the time Lydia was old enough to become involved with other family members, Mr. D. was preparing for high school. He never felt resentment or responsibility for the care of his little sister because his mother or grandmother assumed greater responsibility for Lydia's development. The older he grew, however, the more fortunate he felt to have a sister. Nonetheless, this feeling did not deter him from describing the D. children's split in age as dividing the family into two.

Mr. D.'s adolescence was not fraught with the turbulence traditionally ascribed to those years. Disagreements with parents or authorities continued to go unexpressed. It was at this developmental transition that Mr. D. became acutely aware of the opposite sex. Mr. D. reluctantly described several occasions when his mother noticed him having spontaneous erections regardless of what he was doing around the house.

> I felt so embarrassed when she came into my room where I was doing schoolwork and noticed my excitement. I couldn't help it. It just happened. Sometimes she would ignore it, and other times she would scold me. Once she accused me of dirty thoughts, which, unfortunately, I wasn't thinking. She reminded me that involvement with girls would come soon enough. Mother believed that any girls who wanted to "play around" weren't nice. I was convinced that if I followed my inclinations and disregarded my religious background and rather strict parents, I'd be labeled an eternal sinner.

Although a few classmates teased him about his school accomplishments, Mr. D. felt accepted and enjoyed good relationships with boys his age. Most of them lived closer to the school and the town where social activities took place. Consequently, Mr. D. dated less than his friends because of the distance he had to travel between home and social functions. With financial resources limited to an allowance given by his father, Mr. D. concentrated on sports activities.

As a lanky adolescent who felt more graceful, coordinated, and confident by his 2nd year in high school, Mr. D. did well in track and swimming events. Although he was quite strong, he was not muscular in stature. This was, he felt, a disadvantage that undermined his attempts to attract girls. Once again, he invested himself in schoolwork, hoping to earn a scholarship to a university as well as the attention of girls interested in socializing with the brightest boy in class.

Mr. D. could not recall when he began sexual explorations with his infrequent dates. The only sexual contact he would allow himself was kissing and a little fondling. If he tried to do more, he was stopped by a feeling of impending doom. Usually, an image of his mother scolding him came into focus. This image was compounded by his Episcopalian religious training that forbade sexual activity until marriage.

Without conscious acknowledgment, Mr. D. organized his energies toward leaving the farm. His proclivity for mathematics and higher levels of abstract design conceptualization were rewarded by a local engineering firm that sponsored outstanding male high school students through college. Mr. D. felt very fortunate to be able to leave his small town environment for a new life at a large midwestern university. After the limited existence of farm life, Mr. D. felt like the country cousin heading off to life in the big city.

After several months away, his high hopes for a different kind of life were overshadowed by feelings of loneliness and anxiety.

> I wasn't prepared for the demands of school. I was so shy that making friends became a burden instead of a pleasure. I suppose that's one reason why I married so soon.

Young Adulthood

After 2 years at university, Mr. D. married and moved to the west coast where his wife's family lived. Because of his in-laws' contacts, he was offered a job with an engineering firm. Despite his preference to settle in the Midwest closer to his family, he was persuaded to accept the position because his wife wanted to live closer to her family.

Initially, Mr. D.'s marriage was emotionally and sexually gratifying. Prior to this relationship, Mr. D. had never experienced a liaison of any length or intensity. After 2 years of marriage, however, Mr. D. recognized that his wife seemed more preoccupied with herself and less interested in their relationship. Her demands for more material goods, clothes, possessions, vacations, and his attention increased considerably.

Mr. D. felt that his wife's demands conflicted with his wishes to explore professional and personal goals outside of the marriage. At this particular juncture, Mr. D. was establishing himself as an industrious and creative employee and making friendships with colleagues. Although he argued with his wife about her possessiveness, he gradually gave in to her endless demands to avoid further confrontation. His hobbies, extracurricular professional activities, and friendships diminished in proportion to his wife's demands. Sexual intercourse diminished also. The issue of children was repeatedly avoided because Mrs. D. insisted that a home and a substantial nest-egg were prerequisites for starting a family.

Mr. D.'s contact with his own family in the Midwest became less frequent. Because his wife did not enjoy the family reunions, he rarely visited home. Mr. D., therefore, saw little of his brother and sister who had both married in their early 20s and started families several years later. At this point, when Mr. and Mrs. D. were in their early 30s, owned a home, and had some savings, Mr. D. tried to reopen the issue of children. Mrs. D. was adamant. She wanted to enjoy the fruits of their efforts and felt that children would saddle them with problems and responsibilities. "I guess I just went along with her notion that children would disrupt our lives. We didn't want children just to have someone to take care of us in our old age." Sensing that his marriage was stalemated, Mr. D. immersed himself in his job as he had done as a young boy in school.

Although Mr. D. recognized his envy of his siblings' growing families, he felt helpless to change his life circumstances.

> I know mores have changed, but when I was growing up divorce was unheard of. If there were problems, you just made the best of things. I suppose my family background and religion contributed to my hesitation about leaving.

Middle Adulthood

According to Mr. D., his wife experienced a difficult "change of life." In response, her sexual appetite decreased from seldom to never. She became more domineering, controlling, and jealous. The amount of attention Mr. D. devoted to her was never enough. She constantly accused him of neglect and infidelity. In an attempt to give his wife less ammunition, Mr. D. relinquished all outside activities such as his monthly golf game and card playing. However, the accusations persisted and then increased following Mrs. D.'s stroke. With much resignation, Mr. D.

relayed this information and asked, "What can you do with a sick woman anyway?"

Mr. D. may not have been the decision maker at home, but at work his problem-solving skills and diplomacy were rewarded with merit increases and promotions. As supervisor of 50 employees, his position provided status and satisfaction. At this stage in his career, he was reaping benefits from the company's stock share-holding plan and began making financial arrangements for his eventual retirement.

As Mr. D. concluded our evaluative period with some general information about his current symptoms, he casually mentioned his father's death 3 years prior to Mrs. D.'s stroke. He discussed the loss of his father with little emotion. His major focus and concern, however, appeared to be his mother's welfare. At his father's funeral, his mother subtly reminded him of his position as the eldest in the family. He understood her overtures to mean that he was still the responsible (i.e., loved) son.

TREATMENT COURSE

Mr. D. agreed to participate in weekly intensive psychodynamic psychotherapy sessions for at least 5 months. He expressed interest in wanting to decide, during this time, whether or not to place his wife in a nursing home.

Within a relatively short period of time, the first of several transference postures became apparent. When asked how he felt about seeing a young, female therapist, Mr. D.'s readiness to please was evident in the reply:

> That's no problem. I like women. I guess I never thought a doctor could be so young and attractive. I'm not worried. In fact, I kind of like it.

For the fourth session, Mr. D. arrived tastefully dressed. He opened the session with new information about his feelings toward younger women. He spoke of his sudden involvement with a young, divorced nurse whom he met during his rehabilitation at the hospital. Eventually, they expressed their mutual attraction. As the session continued, Mr. D. made several obscure references to his desires and fears regarding sexual contact with the nurse.

At this point, I suggested that he might have similar sexual feelings toward me. Mr. D. became very quiet and embarrassed.

> Well, I didn't think it was right to say anything about such feelings for you. I'm not here for that kind of thing. You're here to help me with my problems. If I talk about those kinds of things, you'll think I'm a dirty old man, and then you won't help me. I respect you, and I know that you wouldn't want me to say those kinds of things.

I responded to Mr. D.'s candidness by assuring him that such feelings are often an expected aspect of therapy in general. I suggested to him that examination of these feelings might help us to understand him and the sexual issues involved in his other relationships. This clarification seemed to reassure him for he surprised himself by continuing his candid discussion about his sexual feelings. For the first time, he elaborated on the sexual deprivation in his long-term marriage and his fears regarding performance with someone new. He felt that, in the past, guilt had prevented him from seeking sexual gratification outside of his marriage.

I felt it was of paramount importance to Mr. D's therapy that his sexual attraction and possible oedipal feelings toward his therapist be addressed within the context of therapy. His sudden involvement with the young, divorced nurse suggested that these feelings were being enacted outside of the transference relationship.

In the next session, Mr. D. apprehensively described a dream.

> I was on the back porch with my mother who was shampooing my hair. She promised to give me some strawberries if I didn't fuss too much while she washed my hair. We had just finished when my father walked in and started yelling at my mother for giving me the last of the strawberries. She was supposed to save them.

Mr. D. was visibly perplexed and upset by the dream. I asked why he felt so much discomfort. He immediately described his fear of incurring his father's wrath. His position as the oldest child carried with it the responsibility of being a good model. If he was disrespectful, his punishment was used as an example for the others.

The Timeless Unconscious

The dream and Mr. D.'s fears concerning his father dramatically reminded me of the fixed, neurotic quality of his conflicts. I was listening to a man close to my grandfather's age who held a responsible, authoritative position in a major firm and was discussing difficulties of an infantile nature. How timelessly intact the unconscious had remained! As a newcomer to the treatment of older patients, this timelessness of the unconscious was an important concept for me to keep in mind. With this concept, I was able to appreciate and work with Mr. D.'s sexual feelings without his being as frightened by them. His previously described dream suggested that he recognized some resemblance between his mother's image and that of his therapist. If I had shown discomfort with his earlier sexual remarks, the dream might not have surfaced in treatment.

The oedipal dream appeared to open the door to repressed material that provided some genetic understanding of Mr. D.'s issues.

> My mother's father, after 27 years of marriage to my grandmother, ran off with a younger woman. You know, I haven't thought about that in 50 years. No one in the family ever discussed it. My mother was very upset by it. She hated her father. She felt humiliated by him. Our town was so small that everyone knew about it. Maybe that's why our family never talked about sex. Anytime a reference was made to someone's nakedness or intercourse, it was quickly dismissed.

During the 2nd month of treatment, Mr. D. pondered his grandfather's infidelity with a younger woman. He questioned how his grandfather could run off with a younger woman when his grandmother was a beautiful and loving lady. He also described his own mother as a very "handsome" woman. "Kind of like you," he added. At this moment, observing my wedding ring, Mr. D. mentioned my marital status for the first time. "I can't ever imagine your husband's leaving you."

When asked if he had any particular feelings about my marital status, he replied, "Yes. I'm disappointed, but if you weren't married, I would have wondered why. Maybe it interferes with my fantasies, but don't worry, they're just fantasies." I suggested that just as my husband interfered in our therapeutic relationship, vis-à-vis my marriage, then perhaps his father interfered with some fantasies he enjoyed about his mother, vis-à-vis the dream.

Mr. D. responded to this suggestion with silence. When he spoke, he rejected the idea of a sexual attraction to his mother. He felt that, although she was a nice-looking lady, that just wasn't possible. Suddenly, he began discussing his ambivalent romantic feelings toward the young nurse. He confided that she had called and asked him to lunch. He felt flattered and rejuvenated by her interest. "Oh, how nice it was to be chased."

Although I felt my previous interpretation concerning his sexual feelings toward his mother may have been a little premature, I raised the issue again in response to his enjoyment of "the chase."

"Perhaps you wish I would make some obvious gesture of attraction toward you as well; then the risk of sharing your feelings of attraction wouldn't be so difficult." Mr. D. responded by confiding that he had never made the first move in any relationship. His wife, in fact, had proposed to him. If she had not, he did not feel certain that he would have asked her. Risk, it seemed, was a frightening prospect. So frightening, perhaps, that he disowned any sexual feelings toward his mother.

Mr. D.'s previous recollections of his grandfather's infidelity provided him with the insight to understand more clearly some of his own ambivalence concerning extramarital sexual relationships. Such ambivalence had been expressed concerning the potential for an affair with the young nurse. However, he acknowledged a sense of being in limbo because of his wife's obvious sexual inabilities and the loveless state of their relationship.

> It's like being divorced but not really being divorced. My wife needs someone to feed, clothe, and care for her. There isn't even a possibility of a sexual relationship with her. She can't even talk.

A Sexual Triumph

I shared with Mr. D. the observation that one of the feelings he appeared to be concerned about was the reawakening of his sexual being. Perhaps he felt that, as a 62-year-old man, he should know how to manage these young feelings and was promoting a premature decision about whether or not to have an affair before we had a chance to explore this issue. He disagreed with the observation and suggested instead that his marriage complicated his decision.

> You just don't do such things when you're married, regardless of the circumstances. Somehow, I can't reconcile myself to having a sexual relationship outside of the marriage even when my wife's own brother has encouraged me.

Shortly after this, Mr. D. opened another session by excitedly proclaiming a sexual triumph.

> For the first time, I've made love with the nurse I've talked about. I can't believe how often she wanted to make love. It's absolutely great.

He continued to boast in an adolescent manner about his sexual victories. I suggested that although he was enjoying the emergence of a new appetite and new feelings, perhaps he was trying to show his therapist that "he could have a younger woman."

Mr. D. responded angrily to this interpretation. He questioned how I could suggest something so ridiculous. He reacted as if I'd reprimanded him for such acts and forbade him future contacts. When asked if he felt that I had scolded him like a mother or punished him like a father for his newly acquired drives, he remained silent. Eventually, he described feelings of disappointment; disappointment that it was not his therapist with whom he was sexually involved and disappointment that a man was in my life with whom he could never compete.

This disclosure prompted me to suggest that he may have experienced similar feelings as a young boy. He may have felt then that his abilities to attract his mother's attention were inadequate. Once again, a suggestion related to feelings for his mother was met with silence. Although there were several minutes left in the session, Mr. D. departed.

The following week, he apologized for his "impolite and childish" behavior. He explained in great depth the anger and hurt he felt the previous week.

> Before last week's session, I saw you smiling and laughing with a male colleague. I felt angry. I thought I wasn't interesting enough or that you wouldn't have time for me.

At this point, I felt it was important to reflect upon an earlier statement Mr. D. had made about "mother's rewards" and how his father seemed to "reap the harvest" of her gifts. Although Mr. D. was hesitant to state his feelings of envy toward his father, he introduced the emotion through his observation of my discussion with a colleague.

> I wanted to be the one you were talking and laughing with. You seemed so relaxed and sociable with your colleague. I was jealous just like I used to be because my mother made the entire apple pie for my father. I got just a small slice.

I suggested to Mr. D. that he might be concerned that I would not attend to his needs and that my time would be devoted to my colleagues or my husband.

> I feel like a child saying this, but all I really wanted was some special attention, someone to appreciate my efforts. My father seemed to get a lot of attention and appreciation. I'm sure you appreciate your husband.

This was a pivotal therapeutic juncture in Mr. D.'s treatment. At this time, depression surfaced in such a manner that we agreed an increase in sessions would be beneficial. Through the security of more frequent contact, Mr. D. felt he could examine his rage and competitive feelings for his father without rejection or retribution from me. The depression appeared to lift when he felt more confident about coping with his intense feelings. The "little boy" fears he expressed in the initial phase of treatment seemed to recede in significance.

At approximately the 4th month of treatment, Mr. D. expressed a sadness about his relationship with his father.

> The irony is that my father is gone, and I've spent all these hours telling you about my jealousies. I really wish he was still alive so I could share my accomplishments with him. For all my fears about not doing good enough, I've really done quite well.

Simultaneously, the nature of our transference relationship shifted. The degree to which Mr. D. sought my approval and permission diminished. Despite himself, he was sharing a wide range of emotions that were previously unexpressed. He spontaneously discussed his longing for attention and affection from his mother, wife, and therapist.

> When you suggested that our sessions be increased, I was frightened that you thought I was crazy. Now I feel as if you care about me and want to see my problems through to the end.

Disappointments in Women

From this point forward, the session material focused on his disappointments with the women in his life: mother, wife, girlfriend, and therapist. He felt that these women, particularly his mother and wife, imposed stringent controls on him. With these two women, he sometimes felt like less than a man.

Serendipitous to Mr. D.'s treatment was the fact that his sister became a new grandmother. He was simultaneously happy and jealous of her new role. He acknowledged his belated wishes for offspring while assuming a greater paternalistic posture toward me. Mr. D. appeared to utilize his therapy as a developmental stepping stone by changing my role from mother to lover to daughter. His concerns for me were now expressed in terms of my family, my professional goals, and my future.

As a result of Mr. D.'s newly realized confidence, treatment sessions were reduced to weekly visits. At this time, he decided that his wife required nursing care that only a convalescent center could provide. In addition, his girlfriend presented him with a no-strings-attached option of producing offspring. He felt this was absurd.

> I'm an old man. I couldn't begin to provide the physical and emotional things a child would need. In fact, I'm not even married to this woman, nor do I want to be. I know mores have changed but I still believe in the family unit.

As therapy was coming to a close, Mr. D.'s interest in my life took on a familial feeling. He asked whether I planned to have children, whether my health got top priority, and whether my husband could support a family. His questions made me feel like I was home again.

At this juncture, Mr. D. introduced the subject of terminating treatment. His major concern about leaving involved the life changes I would experience of which he would not be a part. "I know that I've missed a lot of life. I just want to know that you won't." He then requested the opportunity to contact me to see how I was doing. At this point, he also assumed an active interest in his sister's new granddaughter.

By the last month of treatment, he had immersed himself in several old friendships. The relationship with the young nurse had diminished in importance. A month after our last session, Mr. D. called. "I just called to say thanks. I've returned to work on a full-time basis for a short time. I'm going to start planning for retirement."

DISCUSSION

Mr. D. entered therapy as a result of the emergence of infantile neurotic conflicts that prevented him from entering the mainstream of adulthood. Consequently, such adult developmental tasks as intimacy, parenting, and grandparenting were not negotiated.

Why did Mr. D. live a relatively adapted life until this time and then, as an older adult, suffer psychological difficulties? Much has been written about the losses accompanying the aging process: loss of bodily vigor, loss of employment, and loss of continuous relationships. These losses have been considered by older people as well as mental health professionals to be irreversible. Prejudices about the aging process have apparently prevented professionals from examining these losses and/or occurrences as changes. Only in earlier developmental stages have losses been referred to as changes.

Mr. D. initially suffered the loss of his physical vigor as a result of the myocardial infarction. This attack on his bodily integrity also impacted on his limited, rigid sense of self. He called upon his former coping mechanisms to handle these changes without much success. Fortunately, the sensitive rehabilitation worker recognized that Mr. D. might benefit from psychodynamic therapy through which he could explore his old defenses and acquire new and more appropriate ways of coping at this stage of his development.

Initially, Mr. D. required the assistance of the physical rehabilitation program in his attempt to reconcile the impact of the myocardial infarction. After leaving the rehabilitation program, he desired emotional care and concern in response to his trauma. His infantile and adolescent oedipal conflicts resurfaced with great intensity at this time. Because he had always found it difficult to request help, he felt relief at the social worker's suggestion of psychotherapy.

Previously, Mr. D. had turned to his mother and wife for approval and attention, but his fantasies and desires were not gratified. Now, his need for approval and attention was brought to light by the concomitants of the physical and emotional aging process. As his therapist, I partially provided the attention and affection of which he had felt deprived of formerly. With those desires partially gratified, Mr. D. could express the past rivalry and conflict that he had experienced with his father and that which he was experiencing more currently within his therapy in terms of my colleagues and husband.

Throughout the course of treatment, Mr. D. accepted the limitations of his relationships as a young boy to his mother, as a husband to a paralyzed wife, and as an older male patient to a young female therapist. His ability to resolve these issues allowed him to separate from past and present idealized relationships. As he acknowledged his disappointments across the life cycle, his low self-esteem was revised.

Mr. D.'s definition of self was formerly built around control, propriety, and achievement. Most of his dependency needs were externalized.

In response to these dynamics, his limited marriage served as a means of protection. His wife, perhaps, expressed some of his oedipal rage and competitive feelings through her jealous accusations. Ironically, Mr. D.'s wife's stroke may have triggered his psychological difficulties. The emergence of developmental pressures for greater dependency appeared to have been surfacing at this time.

Psychodynamic psychotherapy assisted Mr. D.'s entry into the mainstream of adulthood. Parenting and grandparenting were no longer taboo subjects. Retirement became a goal toward which Mr. D. worked. He spoke of the time he had left to live and his desire to make it a productive, lively period. An important goal was his desire to leave something behind that reminded himself and others of his existence.

I was gratified to have been involved with Mr. D. as his therapist. His candid approach and motivation to work were a therapeutic benefit that is not often presented by younger patients. I attributed his commitment to therapy in part to the "time remaining" in his life. Younger counterparts have "the time" to procrastinate. He did not. In addition, Mr. D. never discussed the prospect of prematurely leaving therapy, a move that is so frequently made by younger patients. The patience and perseverance he demonstrated were unique attributes of the aging process.

Mr. D.'s considerable flexibility impressed me. It was almost as if he had decided to "go for broke" and take risks within the context of therapy. He expressed the notion that he had nothing to lose but everything to gain if we were successful. He reported that older colleagues and friends were very supportive of his psychotherapeutic efforts.

My surprise and admiration for Mr. D.'s approach to therapy suggested to me that I still retained some prejudices about older patients' dynamic potential. Mr. D.'s situation vividly reminded me that the psychic structures of any period preserve the primitive demands of the personality; yet Mr. D.'s demands changed in priority and intensity according to his developmental stage and age.

Transference and Countertransference

The countertransference feelings stimulated by a young female therapist working with an older male patient provided one of the most interesting aspects of this case. Early in the treatment process, Mr. D.'s sexual feelings emerged. His well-groomed appearance and adolescent-like nervousness in the first half of our sessions prompted a little discomfort on my part. My concern was how to engender respect and develop a therapeutic alliance with a patient who approached each session as a date, particularly a patient who was old enough to be my grandfather.

After my own transition period with Mr. D., which entailed obtaining a thorough developmental history and background information, I recognized that I was conceptualizing a diagnosis and treatment approach that I would use with any patient, regardless of age or sex. Once I confronted my stereotypic tendency to treat an older person by manipulating his external world, I engaged more readily in his internal world.

Many young colleagues have difficulty with the notion that oedipal issues remain unconsciously fixed. It is as if they imagine the unconscious diminishes in its intensity just as physical strength diminishes with age. I suspect that my young colleagues, despite their own life experiences and psychological training, still wish to regard their older authority figures as developmentally stable.

Apparently, it is difficult for a young colleague to imagine that he or she and a parent may have a similar infantile conflict to resolve in spite of a 30-year age difference. Somehow, I wanted Mr. D. to be all grown up, devoid of issues with which I may be grappling with also. However, Mr. D. taught me that to ignore the psychodynamics of his conflicts would be to sentence him to a premature death.

In the many transference postures of our therapeutic relationship, I was the domineering mother, the seductive lover, and the unborn daughter. Mr. D.'s age uniquely impacted on the treatment in each of these situations. As the domineering mother, I needed to juxtapose Mr. D.'s feelings about being a good little boy with his very real adult circumstances and accomplishments. Similarly, it was important that I respect the healthy sexual drives of a 62-year-old man while simultaneously understanding the adolescent oedipal impulses toward his seductive lover. Finally, the transference relationship of the unborn daughter provided Mr. D. with the opportunity to care for and mourn the loss of the opportunity for his own child while we maintained the boundaries of our therapeutic relationship.

Each of these transference situations stimulated the question, How would I feel if it were my father in treatment working through such issues? I found it illuminating to be reminded that he too may have psychological conflicts.

Mr. D.'s case demonstrates the dynamic capacity an older person may have for psychotherapeutic work on a short-term basis. Changes in his later life precipitated the opportunity to achieve a new and healthier homeostasis. I would like to think that our work together was, in fact, expedited by my youth and gender as opposed to being inhibited by these circumstances. Mr. D. dramatically confronted his realistic limitations and attempted to accept his losses, something each patient must do at any stage of development.

Discussion

ROBERT A. NEMIROFF AND CALVIN A. COLARUSSO

In her opening paragraph, Dr. Crusey comments that practitioners have often suggested that older adults are "depressing and difficult to work with, incapable of improvement or growth, and therefore unlikely to yield satisfaction for the therapist." Her case study convincingly reflects these ideas by describing the considerable intrapsychic power and drive, investment in the therapeutic process, and capacity for change in her 62-year-old patient. As a therapist, she found herself confronted by an eager patient who quickly developed a powerful erotic transference and promptly acted it out. This is certainly a challenge for anyone's therapeutic skill. Further, the age difference of 30 years between patient and therapist added a unique dimension to the transference and countertransference.

In each developmental phase, there are central developmental tasks that must be engaged. Individual experience in the present and past determine whether the encounter leads to developmental progression, regression, or fixation. In middle and late adulthood every individual must deal with time limitation and the idea of personal death. Because of excellent physical health and stable, albeit neurotic, relationships and life circumstances, Mr. D. had traversed middle age with the following conscious assumptions: "I've always thought of myself as a healthy person. I guess I've never seriously considered my own death. Somehow, I always thought my clean living and farm-boy background would keep me alive forever." This illusion was shattered in his late 50s and early 60s by his father's death (he still minimized the importance of this enormously significant event at the time of his evaluation), his wife's stroke,

167

and his own myocardial infarction at age 62. Within the first 15 minutes of the initial interview with Crusey, he revealed that the infarction jolted him into recognition that he only had "a limited time left to live."

Mr. D.'s initial response to his wife's illness and his own was pathologic; he developed symptoms and a pattern of activity that endangered his mental and physical health. However, awareness of a limited time left to live also acted as a stimulus to enter treatment, and it resulted in a dramatic, positive change in his intrapsychic and real world. For this man, the "race against time" became a stimulus to change long-standing neurotic patterns and enjoy life more fully.

In the developmental history, we learn that Mr. D. was the firstborn, especially prized because of his mother's multiple miscarriages both before and after his birth. A deep attachment and control by his mother continued until age 8 when a brother was born. His father was there throughout; he was seen by the patient as bigger than life, distant and demanding. Mr. D.'s neurotic response to his sexual wishes toward his mother and his fear of his father was to become an unusually responsible, nonrebellious boy. This pattern continued throughout childhood; indeed, throughout life. However, despite his neurotic inhibitions, he was able to achieve considerable success along many child and adult lines of development—making friends, achieving academically and in his career, and effecting a physical, and to a degree psychological, separation from his parents that was soon followed by a stable and restricting marriage.

This history demonstrates clearly how the neurotic residue from one stage effects the engagement and resolution of the developmental tasks of the next. Because of neurotic conflicts over sexuality and unresolved attachments to his parents that were experienced consciously in late adolescence as loneliness, Mr. D. rushed into a marriage (meeting his needs for attachment and sex) that prematurely short-circuited the sexual experimentation and the striving for emotional independence and individuation that are an integral part of a healthy late adolescence and young adulthood development. In the process, he exchanged one set of neurotic dependent attachments for another. Mr. D.'s choice of a wife also determined, in part, his response to other central developmental tasks of young adulthood such as career achievement, friendships, and parenthood. In each area, she stifled (with his conscious and unconscious concurrence) his adult development.

Such a developmental interpretation of Mr. D.'s history helps explain why his wife's stroke and his own subsequent myocardial infarction produced such a crisis in his life. His lifelong pattern of dependent relationships with his parents and then his wife and her family were ended abruptly. The neurotic equilibrium was shattered, producing acute distress.

When treatment began, surprisingly, the sexual transference was immediate, powerful, and promptly acted out through a sudden, completely uncharacteristic affair with a young nurse. A basic point about therapeutic work with older patients, which is evident in this case and many others in this book, is that they develop erotic transferences toward their therapists regardless of age, their own or that of the therapists, just as younger patients do. Further, such transference is based on the same genetic constructions as those in younger patients and is brought into the treatment in similar ways. For example, as soon as Crusey acknowledged the therapeutic legitimacy of discussing the patient's sexual feelings for her, he produced a patently oedipal dream about his parents and himself. As stated eloquently by Crusey, ''I was listening to a man close to my grandfather's age; he was a man who had a responsible, authoritative position in a major firm and was discussing difficulties of an infantile nature. How timelessly intact the unconscious has remained.'' The therapist who is unprepared to accept the undiminished intrapsychic sexuality of the older patient and its continued representation in the transference will be severely limited in his or her work with this age group.

Technically, as was demonstrated by Crusey, both current representations in the transference and genetic reconstructions can be used to help the older patient understand the present (the involvement with the young nurse) and the past (the patient's feelings about his parents), even when the past events occurred nearly 60 years ago.

Later in the therapy, Mr. D. established a father–daughter transference with Crusey. This tendency on the part of older patients of either sex to treat a younger therapist as their child and to work out themes and issues related to parenthood through the transference paradigm is a common phenomenon and may occur in everyone because the experience of parenthood, real or fantasized, is such a central developmental theme in adulthood. Although one may not actually have become a parent, as Mr. D. did not, *every* adult intrapsychically engages the concept of parenthood, relating it to other developmental tasks such as sexual identity (becoming a parent confirms one's sexual identity and completes one's sexuality) and time and death (one achieves a measure of immortality through one's biological offspring). Through his paternal interest in Crusey and in his sister's new grandchild, Mr. D. sublimated his wish to be a parent and mourned not having children. He also accepted his position in the life cycle and refused his girlfriend's offer to have his child. "I'm an old man. I couldn't begin to provide the physical and emotional things a child would need. In fact, I'm not even married to this woman, nor do I want to be."

In her own discussion Crusey raises an important point. Older patients have been seen traditionally as rigid, unmotivated, and incapable of significant change. The therapist could expect the treatment to be primarily focused on supportive issues and not be particularly dynamic or interesting. As all the cases in this book demonstrate, older patients may be very motivated and work diligently and with considerable flexibility. Crusey relates Mr. D.'s motivation to his feelings about time to his recognition that time was precious and in limited supply. If he were going to achieve anything meaningful in therapy, he needed to cooperate as much as he possibly could. Thus, the race against time can serve as a stimulus for therapeutic motivation and action.

Countertransference takes on a special character in working with older patients. A recurrent theme in younger therapists is expressed with clarity and apprehension by Crusey. How could she "engender respect and develop a therapeutic alliance with a patient who approached each session as a date, particularly a patient old enough to be my grandfather"? She relates her anxiety and discomfort to internal conflict over infantile sexual issues, in herself and the patient, despite the 30-year age difference separating them. Defensively, she, like many others in young adulthood and midlife, may have had a need to see those in late adulthood as mature and asexual because such an image contained the idea that one day, she, too, might be free of infantile wishes and conflict. When the therapist accepts the dynamic nature of the mind and the continuation of basic developmental themes throughout the life course, therapy with older patients becomes meaningful and exciting and provides the therapist with new understanding not only of the patient but of himself or herself as well.

9

New Beginnings at Seventy

A DECADE OF PSYCHOTHERAPY IN LATE ADULTHOOD

GARY A. LEVINSON

PRESENT ILLNESS

Mrs. A. presented for treatment at age 63 as an obese, white, twice-divorced woman. The mother of three, she lived alone, supporting herself on social security disability payments. The patient described herself as suffering from "neurotic fears" about her health; she was experiencing blurred vision, dizziness, and an unsteadiness in gait, all of which made her feel "nervous" and "in turmoil." The patient assumed these symptoms to be "neurotic" because she had been diagnosed as such at a midwestern clinic some 20 years previously. Mrs. A. also believed that her recent myocardial infarction had intensified these concerns.

The immediate reason for referral from the patient's internist, who assured me that the somatic complaints were not organic in nature, was marked obesity. He described her 220-pound weight as life threatening. The weight gain had all occurred during the patient's 50s, probably resulting from her role as caretaker of an increasingly debilitated and senile mother. Until that time, the patient was very interested in her appearance, highly valuing her slimness. At present, however, she saw her weight as of no consequence because she was "old and hopelessly ugly."

Following her mother's death 3 years prior to beginning treatment, the patient began living with a brother and his wife. He died 3 months before her own myocardial infarction (9 months before the treatment began). Mrs. A. had weathered both of those losses without serious emotional consequence, and only now, as she confronted her own mortality, did she experience recurrent feelings of depression, alienation, and

171

isolation. One of her worst fears was of becoming an invalid, confined to a wheelchair while living in a "sleazy nursing home."

Mrs. A. was also preoccupied with "guilty feelings about the past." Increasingly, she experienced recurrent, intrusive thoughts about how "I screwed up the past," especially in relation to a lack of responsibility toward her children, siblings, and parents. The patient lamented the fact that her son from her first marriage (who was at that time in his 40s) had totally rejected her after she left him with his father at the time of the divorce. She had not seen him for approximately 30 years and was crushed when he emphatically refused a rapprochement at the time of her mother's death. Even more heartbreaking were recurrent memories of two daughters from a second marriage (now in their 30s) who had been spirited off to another country by her foreign-born husband. She had last seen them when they were latency-age children. Mrs. A. feared that she was remembered by them as an alcoholic, uncaring mother who had deserted them in their time of need.

Whereas most of her life had been spent in a free-wheeling, adventuresome manner without a thought about tomorrow, she now found herself confronted by a bleak, limited future and a cruel past. Her inner pain was mirrored in the deprivation present in her current life. Until recently, she had been financially secure, provided for by trust funds from her parents. Because she had spent freely, these monies had run out. Although Mrs. A. longed to resume her life of travel and pleasure, she could not because of her financial circumstance and phyical limitations. "I'm trapped, my own worst enemy."

Whenever the patient had been confronted with limitations and restrictions in the past, she had merely left that situation, moved to another locality, and began life anew. The inability to run made Mrs. A. more aware of the importance of others. Fear of alienating her few friends prompted her to monitor actions and limit opinions. This resulted in uncharacteristic attitudes of compliance and dependence. She asked if therapy could help her feel less "blocked and nervous."

FAMILY HISTORY

The patient was the first of four children born to a stable midwestern couple. The family moved to the South when Mrs. A. was 5 and returned to the Midwest when she was 15. This move followed a severe business reversal. Of three male siblings, two became professional men, and the third was a chronic schizophrenic. The oldest brother, her favorite, had died a year before treatment began. The patient described him as a man constantly searching for his place in life but never finding it. In his later years, he abused alcohol and was prone to depression. The middle brother, her mother's favorite, raised a family and developed a successful professional practice. The patient always resented him, feeling that he was spoiled and constantly trying to embarrass her. They had little contact over the years; their last meeting was at their mother's funeral when he accused her of treating their mother poorly. The patient's youngest brother had been the least favored of the children. In his early 20s, after dropping out of college, he joined the service and become floridly psychotic. He has been hospitalized or institutionalized consistently since that time. The patient recently found him in a board-and-care home in another community and was taking steps to have him moved to a facility near her apartment when she entered therapy.

The mother was described as a hypochondriacal, domineering woman who always had the patient's best interests in mind. At best, their relationship was an ambivalent one: The patient alternated between attitudes of deep attachment and rejection. During the patient's preschool years, her mother worked in the health profession and was seen as a respectable, outgoing, capable woman. She came from a well-to-do, aristocratic family who felt she "married down" and "lived beneath herself." From the time the patient was age 8 until her midteens, her mother was hospitalized several times for hypochondriacal symptoms and depression.

The patient's father, whom she described as a "wonderful tyrant," was the principal person with whom she felt allied during her latency and preadolescent years. Although he was short tempered and difficult, he favored the patient. After the severe financial reversal when Mrs. A. was 15, he became severely depressed and was hospitalized for 2 to 3 months. Thereafter, she remembered him as prone to recurring periods of depression and alcohol abuse. When the patient was in her midthirties, her father died in a fire that he accidentally set in a drunken state with a lit cigarette.

DEVELOPMENTAL HISTORY

Mrs. A. remembers being told that she was a planned and wanted child. Her mother's pregnancy and delivery were described as uneventful. She was breast-fed and reportedly accomplished her developmental milestones of crawling, walking, and talking within the usual expected framework. She does not know when she was weaned or toilet trained but believes it was done in a "strict fashion," which was her mother's style.

Throughout the patient's preschool years, her mother was an active, outgoing socialite who spent little time at home; she entrusted the patient's care to a series of maids. Mrs. A. fondly remembered her adored maids, who easily carried out the mother's directives. One of the patient's earliest memories is from approximately age 4, when she was taken home by one of the maids; there the maid's father sexually molested her. It was unclear exactly what he did other than fondle her genitals. She was never able to tell her parents about this episode but remembered feeling embarrassed and "dirty."

The patient did not recall nightmares or other symptoms of an infantile neurosis. She did describe a very close relationship with her father that began "before I started school" and intensified especially after her mother began a series of psychiatric hospitalizations when Mrs. A. was age 8. Her teasing, bantering antics with her father were both exciting and pleasant until he would "get to be too much." Teasing would turn into needling, "Can't you do it better than that?" Then she would feel criticized and angry. At age 8, during her mother's recurrent hospitalizations, the patient found herself in constant conflict with the nuns at the parochial boarding school where she had been sent. These battles led to transfers to other parochial schools, some that were far away from home. Mrs. A. was an excellent student who was outgoing and popular. Many of her friends were boys. Her relationships with girls and, later, women were always fraught with conflict, because she felt that they might be jealous, turn on her, and be untrustworthy. Menarche was a difficult time. There was no one to turn to because her mother was weak and unreliable, and the nuns were cruel and overly moralistic. Mrs. A. remembers herself as quite irritable and withdrawn prior to the onset of her menses at age 14. Afterward she began to date and was more outgoing and comfortable. After her father's financial reverses and hospitalization, the patient returned home. The conflicts intensified until, at age 17, she impulsively ran away with a boyfriend.

ADULT DEVELOPMENTAL HISTORY

The patient's first husband, whom she married soon after leaving home, was an itinerant musician who traveled the country during the big band era. The patient enjoyed accompanying him, spending days and nights in different places, seeing and doing "different things." Soon, she was episodically drinking to excess. When her parents began having serious marital problems, Mrs. A. invited her mother to travel with her, her husband, and infant son, a pattern that continued for almost 7 years.

By the time the patient was in her late 20s, the excitement had gone out of the marriage. Mrs. A. still wanted to live her adventuresome life, but without the constant nagging and constraints of her mother and husband. She therefore divorced her husband, who took custody of their son, initially in conjunction with the patient's mother. This produced a major rift between mother and daughter, after which Mrs. A. impulsively left and went to a foreign country.

A new era began in the patient's life as she traveled back and forth between continents. She felt free, unrestricted by family or responsibility, able to be carefree and to give "free rein" to her feelings. At that time, Mrs. A. described herself as attractive and outgoing, a woman who easily made friends and attracted interesting men. She was slim, well-built, and the center of attention.

At age 33 she married her second husband, a foreign businessman. After several years and two children, she began to experience him as overbearing and dominating. Further, the patient was torn between her husband and children and her mother who by that time was having recurrent periods of depression and asked the patient to come home and take care of her. Mrs. A. began to make frequent trips to her mother's side. On one such occasion, after a stay of 3 months without her daughters, her husband initiated divorce proceedings. A long legal battle resulted in a divorce and paternal custody of the children. Mrs. A.'s first serious bout of depression, during which she took an overdose of pills, followed.

When the patient was in her early 40s, she first developed hypochondriacal symptoms of dizziness, nausea, and unsteady gait. Menopause occurred at age 46. Her mother insisted that she go to a midwestern clinic where she herself had been treated on numerous occasions. There Mrs. A. saw a psychiatrist who told her that she suffered from a neurosis for which psychotherapy was indicated. After refusing his advice, Mrs. A. returned to the maternal home, dismissed her symptoms as unimportant, and began to work for the first time as a salesperson in a local women's clothing store. This was interspersed with occasional trips out of the country to escape feeling cornered and being dominated by her mother, whose health gradually deteriorated to the point of dementia, requiring placement in a nursing home.

Through the remaining years until her mother died when the patient was 58, Mrs. A. continued to use alcohol and occasionally barbiturates. Her involvement with men, which had been one of recurrent "flings," became less frequent. With advancing age and rapid weight gain, the patient no longer saw herself as an attractive, seductive woman, and she increasingly denied the significance of this change. She found herself "not caring" about her appearance because "it didn't matter anymore." Her body was now experienced as "a convenience that had lost its usefulness."

Mrs. A. reacted to her mother's death with considerable sadness and social withdrawal. These feelings were heightened by the accusatory attitude of her middle brother who berated her for "taking advantage of mother and using up all her money." After settling her mother's affairs, Mrs. A. moved closer to her oldest brother. After his death, she traveled for the last time to another continent and had what she described as "my final fling." It was at that point that she had her myocardial infarction.

MENTAL STATUS EXAMINATION

Mrs. A. presented as a tall, obese woman who dressed neatly in out-of-style floral print dresses and walked with effort. Her face, when not hidden by sunglasses, was that of a younger woman, perhaps in her early 50s. She had an attractive vitality about her despite her weight. As Mrs. A. settled with difficulty into the low, overstuffed chair, she spoke clearly and lucidly. A mildly depressed affective state was evident behind the pleasant exterior. Associations were always intact, with no evidence of a thinking disorder. The patient acknowledged suicidal ideation in the past but none in the present. She was oriented as to time, person, and place, and she had an intact memory for both recent and past events. Her judgment was good, and her intelligence appeared to be in the superior range.

DIAGNOSTIC FORMULATIONS

My initial evaluation of the patient indicated that she was suffering from a neurotic depression with hypochondriacal features and alcoholism, which was now in remission. (She had stopped drinking approximately 2 years prior to starting therapy.) In addition, there was considerable evidence of arrest along those young adult developmental lines related to intimacy, marriage, and parenthood. When the patient entered midlife, she reacted symptomatically to the aging process in herself and to her mother's death, becoming hypochondriacal and later obese.

I believed that Mrs. A. had not come to grips with issues from multiple levels of development, particularly those from the preoedipal, oedipal, and young adult phases. However, I was intrigued by her keen intellect and curiosity. She was a woman who suddenly recognized that her itinerant life-style had caused her to "race through life" without experiencing many of its most significant pleasures—particularly a lasting (and sustaining) relationship with children and grandchildren. How could that have happened she asked. Was it too late to do anything about it? Here was an introspective bud that might blossom in a conducive therapeutic setting. Could it happen in one so old? I decided to try.

THE THERAPY

For the first 3 years of treatment, Mrs. A. was seen once or twice per week. Thereafter, treatment continued every other week (except for occasional weekly visits when periods of crisis arose) to the present. Because the patient had no financial resources of her own, the treatment was paid for by Medicare and Medi-Cal.

Opening Phase

The initial psychotherapy sessions were dominated by the patient's hypochondriacal concerns about her dizziness, blurred vision, weakness, and anxiety. This soon led to consideration of the major change that had occurred with her life following the myocardial infarction. Never having experienced any physical limitations, Mrs. A. now tired easily and found herself occasionally short of breath. She lamented:

> I haven't adapted to old age...old age is ugly...I'm on my way down and out; this is just an anticlimax to an interesting life, and there is nothing left for me anymore.

She did not believe that there was any way that she could adapt to these new limitations, and she felt at the end of her "lifeline." Besides her failing health, the patient was confronted with a bleak financial picture. She had always had what appeared to be an endless supply of money from her parents; but as her mother's illness lingered, these resources were used up, leaving the patient feeling abandoned and nearly destitute.

A number of sessions during the first 6 months of therapy revolved around her initial lack of reaction to the myocardial infarction and subsequent recognition of its staggering impact. She would say, "I'm a different person now; I'm so vulnerable and helpless." Mrs. A. was especially bothered by the sense that her condition was permanent. Increasingly, she felt that she had lived her life and had no future.

Gradually, we reconstructed the experience during the myocardial infarction. Mrs. A. described the crushing pain that took her breath away as a very frightening experience—this was in sharp contrast to her response at the time of the infarction. Then she ignored the pain, believing it to be due to indigestion. In the hospital she was "the ideal patient" (according to her cardiologist), who never complained and went along with all procedures and recommendations. I interpreted to the patient that her current hypochondriacal symptoms were in part a defense against the terror, panic, and loss she sustained at the time of the infarction. Subsequently, as the hypochondriacal symptoms subsided, Mrs. A. was better able to accept the limitations imposed by the heart condition.

As she came to see herself as someone who had, indeed, had a myocardial infarction, the patient began to work on her sense of "getting old." She began to read extensively about psychotherapy, psychiatry, and psychoanalysis. During this second half of her first year of therapy her introspective curiosity grew by leaps and bounds. "I've always wanted to find out more about myself, but I was afraid that no one would ever be able to figure me out. I never could before this." As the transference developed, Mrs. A. expressed fear that I would tire of her and get rid of her like the other men in the recent and distant past.

By this time the patient was thoroughly enjoying the therapy sessions and began reporting dreams and memories about her past relationships with parents, siblings, and husbands. She became fascinated with the idea that there were "hidden meanings" that had motivated her over the years. As she spoke of her pattern of "being on the move," I pointed out that her wandering appeared to be precipitated in part by "strong emotions" from the past. When I suggested that we might be able to understand this more clearly, she responded with a flood of associations about her autocratic father who dominated every action and thought, and many memories of the strict, at times vindictive, nuns at the boarding

schools. I was eventually able to interpret that one of the "strong emotions" that motivated her frequent moves was repressed anger toward
her father (and others, like the nuns) that was stimulated in situations
(marriages) in which she felt dominated. Mrs. A. responded with further memories of rebelliousness but then focused, mournfully, on how
shocked she was by the realization that this option was no longer open
to her. She realized she had never taken time to reflect on her impulsive behavior, let alone control it for any length of time, until she was
forced to do so by the myocardial infarction.

Middle Phase

Slowly, she began to idealize me as a caring, stable, knowledgeable
father who could be trusted with her innermost thoughts. In addition,
I became a father-protector. Mrs. A. would bring me medical questions
about her physical status that had been "inadequately explained" by
other physicians. For instance, whenever the internist would advise her
to stop smoking or go on a specific type of diet, she would immediately
come to me and try to find out "the real truth" about why this might
or might not be indicated. She began bringing me baked goods in various shapes and forms, especially at holidays or other times when she
was feeling particularly close to me. The transference was one of me as
the all-knowing, good father who could protect her and, at times, dominate her. Initially, I felt surprised that this older woman would see me
in a paternal role because I was 30 years her junior; feeding me was
much more what I expected. I had to be continually aware of my own
countertransference wishes to be taken care of by a mother or grandmother. This, of course, was also an expression of the patient's unfulfilled needs to mother and be mothered.

At the beginning of the second year of treatment, however, I was
perplexed by her frequent self-berating and self-critical comments. Only
after a period of time did I realize that she was expecting me to be much
like her critical, dominating, father who would punish her for her rebellious and free-wheeling attitudes and behavior. When I did not respond
like him, she unrelentingly attacked herself until her harsh superego had
been assuaged. After I interpreted her expectation that I would attack
her much as her father had done, especially during her teen years, she
felt both surprised and relieved; she was grateful that this masochistic
pattern of behavior could be understood.

Gradually, the patient became more outgoing, slept better, and began to lose weight. At this point in the therapy, she began the quest to have her institutionalized youngest brother moved from his board-and-care facility in another city to San Diego so that she could visit him regularly and deal with the injustices that she imagined were being inflicted upon him. When Mrs. A. ran into the resistance of the board-and-care operator, who did not want him transferred, she enlisted my aid to learn more about patients on conservatorship and their rights as well as the treatment facilities that might be available for her brother in San Diego. Over a period of 6 months, the patient's attentions and activity were mobilized and directed toward the goal of having her brother transferred. I wrote a letter to the conservator indicating that Mrs. A. was competent and interested in her brother's welfare and could serve as a suitable conservator.

After the bureaucratic haggling was finished, her brother was transferred, and I saw him in consultation for my patient to help her understand how to best meet his needs. He had a chronic organic brain syndrome, which was apparently secondary to repeated insulin shock treatments with prolonged coma. Filtering through the organicity were paranoid ideation on a fixed, grandiose delusional system. In general, he had the appearance of a back-ward state hospital patient. I educated Mrs. A. on the proper care and treatment of someone with a chronic organic brain syndrome (the need for structure, predictability and clarity of information, etc.) and maintained him on the psychoactive medications that had been started some years ago.

As the years passed, his condition deteriorated progressively to the point that he could no longer be managed in an open board-and-care home. I therefore facilitated his transfer to a longer term, locked facility. In 1981 he died.

During 1975 and 1976, when her brother was the center of Mrs. A.'s attention, an ample opportunity was available for the reworking of similar feelings toward her mother and next-younger brother with whom she had similar relationships—albeit with more intact people. The ambivalence experienced toward her brother caused much distress; Mrs. A. feared that her anger would have a devastating effect. This led to a discussion of similar wishes toward her mother whom she both loved and wished dead, particularly during the long final illness. This burden of unresolved guilt and grief for her mother and brothers was repeatedly worked through in therapy, resulting in Mrs. A.'s feeling less conflicted about her own aggressive, hostile impulses toward those she loved and outlived. She was thereafter more able to tolerate her ambivalence and accept her longevity. The connection between ambivalent feelings toward loved ones and its effects on attitudes about personal longevity played a central role in this therapy and may be of similar importance in the treatment of all elderly persons.

Thus, a major therapeutic focus, as Mrs. A. watched her brother's downhill course, was a continuing adaptation to, acceptance of, and working through feelings about growing old. Through his death, she confronted her own advancing age and mortality. For example, several years earlier, when Mrs. A. had thought of bringing her brother to San Diego, she felt "strong and secure, the big sister." Now, she had "shot [her] wad" and felt incapable of confronting the entrenched bureaucracy surrounding his transfer. Becoming "too angry" might precipitate another heart attack and death. I helped the patient see that, whereas previously she had enjoyed strong feelings, she now saw them as dangerous and life threatening. Again, her life had been dramatically changed by this sense of fragile emotional equilibrium, due to her cardiac condition and advancing age.

Another layer of the overdetermined nature of her fear of strong emotion, especially anger, was related to her living longer than her next-younger brother who died at age 60. The patient experienced survivor guilt; he had died from his infarction and she had not. "Fate must have missed me. I should have died. I lived such a bad life," she said. Thus, not only aggression and hostility might lead to another heart attack; she might be punished for allowing her emotions such free rein throughout her adult life.

At about that time, as Mrs. A. was grappling with the authorities about her brother, she related a dream in which she went to see him. As her brother was in a dental chair getting dentures, the patient realized it was someone else. A nurse in a white uniform threatened to give her brother electroshock unless she, his sister, left him alone. The patient lunged at the nurse and began to choke her. Abruptly she awoke. She associated to hating women; they had always put so many obstacles in her way, limiting access to money, time, and love. Mrs. A. felt that women had often choked her to death and wanted to bite back, especially her mother. But now, turned white with age, she was weak and toothless like her brother. Enraged by her impotence, she wished to attack the woman in white who represented her aged self.

When her brother was moved to San Diego, the patient was surprised by his debilitated state. "He's old. So am I. We're both ugly. It's all finished." We explored the equation she had made between youthful beauty and expensive clothes on one hand and strength and power on the other, particularly the power to attract men. Now, overweight and poorly dressed, she felt powerless and hopeless. This led to further associations about being old and weak and having to depend on others, such as myself. Mrs. A.'s dependence on me became a major aspect of the transference. When I went away on vacation that year, she developed symptoms of staggering and lightheadedness. We began to explore her feelings that I was now the major source of power in her life; through an alliance with me she could borrow my strength and protect her brother and herself from life's insults and the ravages of old age.

In a dream, later in the 2nd year of therapy, I was represented as the hated middle brother, a successful professional, who had decided to try a new fountain-of-youth drug on the senile brother. In her associations, the patient described her own fears of dying. In her youth she had tempted death by living a wild, adventuresome life. Now in old age, death had the upper hand. Perhaps, like her brother in the dream, I had a magic potion to restore youth. Although the patient wished me to have such power so she could survive, she hated me for possessing it.

Our intense work began to produce adaptive changes. Toward the end of the second year of treatment, Mrs. A. decided to take a genealogy course. As she discovered unknown ancestors, in a sense gaining thereby new objects and conquering time and death, her attitude toward her known relatives softened. In Eriksonian terms, Mrs. A. was coming to terms with the relationship between her own life cycle and those who had preceded her. Later, after taking all the genealogy courses that were offered at the various adult schools, the patient returned to an earlier interest, painting. This activity had powerful transferential implications because Mrs. A. knew that my wife was an artist. In an attempt to gain my love and approval, she began to bring her paintings to our sessions, acting in some ways like a 5-year-old trying to seduce her father.

As time passed, Mrs. A. became increasingly aware of another complication of aging, arthritis of the hands, knees, and hip joints, described by an internist as degenerative. She feared that she would become crippled and bedridden, then placed in a nursing home like her mother. As a result of our earlier work, she was able to understand this fear as a partial identification with her mother. In addition, she berated herself for being less active but soon saw this as a defense against accepting the reality of another limitation that had come with age.

At the beginning of the 3rd year of treatment, the patient related an upsetting dream in which she was busy packing for "a final trip" to visit her mother whom she knew was dead. She awoke in an anxious state with a sense of loss and finality. How could she go on any trip, feeling the way she did. If only she could travel again, as she did so easily for most of her life, she would go out of the country and find her abandoned children. Like the mother in the dream, they too were "dead," lost to her. The wish to seek out her children began to increase in urgency. In another dream, Mrs. A. went to a doctor's office and was told that she would have to scream before she could see her children. Later, at another session, she wondered what price she would have to pay for a reunion. Was she being deprived of this possibility as punishment for abandoning them?

On Turning Age Sixty-Five

During the 3rd year of therapy Mrs. A. turned 65. Now she was "officially designated as old," a "certified old lady." Reaching this milestone heightened her feelings of insignificance and inadequacy because her "grand plan for life" had not produced any money, friends, or substantial material possessions. At times the patient felt angry and cheated, discontent and unhappy with her lot in life. There was no one but me to turn to for support and solace. In part, her complaint was a transferential wish for greater attention from me. She had become friends with an older woman who was unfamiliar with the complexities of American life, and their friendship continues to the present.

My efforts in psychotherapy were directed toward helping Mrs. A. recognize the magical thinking surrounding turning 65. She realized that it was quite unreasonable to believe that "the bottom would fall out" just because she had a birthday, but she had always believed that people aged 65 were "finished." As we focused on her capabilities, Mrs. A. became more accepting of her status. After all, now that she had been "declared old," she was entitled to certain rights and privileges. In addition to being freed from the obligation to work because 65 was the official retirement age, Mrs. A. noted that she "knew a thing or two about life" and could advise the young and foolish (as she now saw her youth) about the pitfalls ahead. Being younger, I, too, could benefit from her wisdom, particularly about life in foreign countries. Within the transference, I became her lost child, young, naive, and inexperienced, learning about the world from a wise, loving mother/grandmother. At those times, as I listened attentively, in the countertransference I felt protected and mothered.

During the 4th year of treatment, Mrs. A. continued to be concerned about her aging, as was manifested by her tiring more easily and a new concern—"I'm getting forgetful," particularly about names and dates. As the patient's 66th birthday approached, time was "speeding by" and her age was "hard to believe."

Soon after her birthday, Mrs. A. related a dream in which I was talking with her brother. In the dream, Mrs. A. resented my firm statement that I did not have to explain to her what was going on; her brother would do so. Associations were to being disappointed and angry with me for not giving her useful answers to questions about her brother and herself. She wanted to be "cradled" and taken care of like him. She was not getting enough from me. I interpreted this transference dream as containing a wish to be taken care of in the present, like her brother, and at the same time to be a child, young again, "cradled" in a loving, protecting, parent's arms. She tearfully nodded in agreement, but then stated with resolve, "but it can't be so; I'll do the best I can with what I have." Not much later, her brother deteriorated to the point that I placed him in a long-term, closed geriatric center. Mrs. A. mourned her brother's progressive deterioration and deeply missed the opportunity to take him out of the hospital on weekends.

Becoming a Mother and Grandmother

Later, in the 4th year of treatment, Mrs. A. received a letter from an old friend in a foreign country. Its arrival further stimulated her curiosity and concern about her children, who were still there. She was quite reluctant to find out more about her daughters and eventually, after much procrastination, did write a letter to this friend, asking about them. This occurred after we had focused extensively on the overdetermined nature of her reluctance to "open up the old wounds." It was my belief that on one level she again feared punishment for sexual and aggressive impulses expressed through "flings with men" and the eventual abandonment of her children. Such retribution might take the form of another heart attack or a stroke. Further, she feared that her daughters would reject her overture with abuse and ridicule. Another layer of this reluctance was exposed when the patient associated to the ambivalent relationship she had with her own mother. "What if I turn out to be as terrible a mother as she was?" As Mrs. A. worked through her fears of motherhood via identification with her own mother, she felt comfortable enough to write again to her friend to ask about her daughters.

This working-through process took about a year. In the 5th year of treatment Mrs. A. summoned her courage and wrote to her children. To her amazement, she received an immediate reply; they wanted to meet her! Within 2 weeks both daughters came to San Diego for an anxiety-filled but joyous reunion. Because I saw growth along the adult developmental lines of parenthood and grandparenthood as essential to the patient's mental health, I accepted her invitation to meet the family. Her older daughter, age 32, a bright, interesting woman, was very supportive of her mother. Unfortunately, the 30-year-old younger daughter suffered from chronic paranoid schizophrenia. Again, I took the role of advisor and resource person, reviewing the daughter's care over the past 10 years during which she had been recurrently hospitalized and treated with various medications. I gave Mrs. A. and her daughter a list of board-certified psychiatrists in her country, one of whom eventually saw the daughter.

Mrs. A.'s life was now significantly changed. Overnight she became a mother with one successful child and another with major problems. Contact between mother and daughters was continuous—the children called frequently and visited four to five times a year. When the grandchildren came to see her, Mrs. A. again proudly brought them to meet me. They were active, inquisitive children who enjoyed being pampered. The patient's newly found happiness was marred by the death of her brother in February 1981. Mrs. A. mourned his death but felt that he had died for her in 1978 when his dementia had become so severe that meaningful communication ceased. "I found my daughters again just in time. Now that my brother is gone I'd be completely alone if it weren't for them."

Turning Age Seventy

Mrs. A. approached her 70th birthday with a considerably more positive attitude than she did on her 65th. Although feeling "old and on my last lap," she energetically engaged her daughters and grandchildren on their frequent visits. Her role as mother and grandmother—"I feel needed again. I have a purpose in life"—was clearly energizing and tended to put psychosomatic preoccupations into a more manageable perspective.

DISCUSSION OF THE CLINICAL PRESENTATION

Mrs. A. sought treatment at age 62 for the relief of psychosomatic symptoms (and obesity) that developed after a myocardial infarction. The symptoms were similar to ones the patient had experienced approximately 20 years earlier that were related then to failure to master a number of midlife developmental tasks. Then Mrs. A. had responded to two failed marriages, the abandonment of her children, and a dawning awareness of the limitations incumbent in the aging process by a regressive return to mother. In a sense, the developmental process up to that time had been dominated and skewed by unresolved, intensely ambivalent infantile feelings toward her mother that blocked adult separation and individuation. By her 40s, the patient was obviously suffering from a severe adult developmental arrest. The infantile surrender to her mother was initially punctuated and modulated by the well-established patterns of frequent travel, involvements with men, and excessive use of alcohol. Thus, for several years, the patient's conflicted feelings about dependence versus independence were managed through alternating periods of caring for her mother (and through an unconscious reversal, herself) and abandoning her.

The adaptation worked until time and reality finally caught up with the patient in her early 60s. Then the myocardial infarction, obesity (another expression of the wish to be nurtured), death of mother, and limited financial resources blocked the previously utilized means of obtaining gratification. A depression with somatic ruminations followed. The presenting symptoms were thus understood to be the culmination of a lifetime of pathologic development and a response to the difficult developmental tasks of late adulthood.

The psychotherapeutic strategies that I employed in the treatment of Mrs. A. emphasized the developmental crisis of old age. Because so much of the therapeutic work revolved around real and imagined concerns about physical well-being, I worked in close collaboration with the other physicians involved in Mrs. A.'s care. There were sound therapeutic reasons why such activity was required in this case—as in most psychotherapeutic efforts with older patients. First, I needed to have a detailed understanding of the reality of her physical problems (and that reality was constantly changing) in order to help the patient understand and accept the limitations involved. It was also necessary to differentiate for the patient and myself the organic aspects of her condition from those that were primarily psychogenically determined. Further, like all older patients, Mrs. A. had to integrate a rapidly changing body image with powerful feelings from the past about physical appearance and well-being; in this patient, her physical beauty and slimness had been corner-stones of her self-esteem for most of her life. As the treatment progressed, another aspect of my therapeutic role in relationship to Mrs. A.'s physical care evolved. It was extremely important that I serve as an ally and translator, bridging the gap between the recommendations of the medical/surgical specialists and her understanding and acceptance of their treament. In the absence of our relationship, it is highly unlikely that the patient would have been able to participate meaningfully in her own care.

Such therapeutic flexibility and activity was also focused on another developmental task that is central to the aging process—the maintenance of family ties. As Mrs. A. entered old age, she sought to reestablish, through her chronically disabled brother, ties to the family of childhood. Because I understood the importance of this developmental process, I facilitated the transfer of her brother to this community and took on an educational and caretaking role for both. Mrs. A.'s reinvolvement with her long-lost brother produced feelings of wholeness and well-being and a sense of longitudinal connection with her "roots." The relationship with her brother stimulated the patient to analyze conflicts about being a mother and led eventually to greater acceptance of that adult role. The resumption of a meaningful relationship with her children and grand-children was seen as a resolution of a major developmental task of late adulthood.

At the inception of psychotherapy, I was Mrs. A.'s sole support: friend and family rolled into one. Gradually, her brother was brought into this matrix; then her daughters and grandchildren. My facilitating role in the resolution of Mrs. A.'s identity as a sister, mother, and grand-mother required significant flexibility, according to the needs and con-flicts that she was dealing with at the time. For instance, on occasion I was the knowledgeable, authoritative parent who could educate her about her brother or ill daughter, whereas at other times I was the ad-vocate, battling the bureaucracy to effect her brother's transfer.

A very poignant experience for the patient and me occurred when I saw her and her daughters and grandchildren as a group. Here I was functioning in the mode of a family therapist helping the members deal with the crisis of reestablishing multigenerational bonds. Sessions with the patient and her healthy daughter have continued intermittently to the present as they evolve and deepen the bond between them.

A chronological consideration of the treatment process will clarify some of the transference and late adult developmental issues. As therapy began, Mrs. A. transferred her quest for a strong, loving parent to me. As the transference evolved, I became the powerful preoedipal mother and the "wonderful tyrant," the father of the oedipal phase and adolescence. As we analyzed these themes, it became clear that the harsh, archaic aspects of the powerful mother and tyrannical father were internalized in the superego. This became very evident as the patient repeatedly saw me as hostile and berating, or tried to provoke me to attack. Much subsequent effort reworked the issues revolving around her strong ambivalence toward her mother. Mrs. A. began to see herself as capable and worthwhile; she began to lose weight and cooperate more easily with her physicians. The next step in the caring process involved "mothering" her brother and herself. Later, she actually became a functioning mother and grandmother.

Much work was done on the issues of aging. As Mrs. A. mourned the loss of her youthful beauty, physical endurance, and past life-style, she came to understand the neurotic components of her fear of mortality, particularly the idea that she would become "too emotional" and cause her own death. As she turned age 65 and then 70, we explored the magical connections between birthdays and death. As feelings about aging became less conflicted, they were sublimated into interests in genealogy and painting. Not surprisingly, the developmental task of accepting aging was deeply connected with other themes. For instance, the pastoral scenes that Mrs. A. chose to paint were of the countryside around her mother's childhood home.

SUMMARY

This case illustrates the interaction of the normative crises of aging with earlier developmental psychopathology and demonstrates how psychoanalytically oriented psychotherapy, even once weekly, can be effectively used to treat both. The clinical material further demonstrates the capacity of an elderly patient to utilize dreams, free association, and transference to effect significant emotional and behavioral change. Working with such patients requires an understanding of the developmental processes of late adulthood and a therapeutic flexibility that encompasses the patient's physical condition, real life relationships, and intrapsychic world.

Discussion

ROBERT A. NEMIROFF AND CALVIN A. COLARUSSO

After giving his diagnostic formulations, Dr.Levinson says of his patient, ''I was intrigued by her keen intellect and curiosity. She was a woman who suddenly recognized that her itinerant life-style had caused her to 'race through life' without experiencing many of its significant pleasures—particularly a lasting (and sustaining) relationship with children and grandchildren. How could that have happened? she asked. Was it too late to do anything about it? Here was an introspective bud that might blossom in a conducive setting. Could it happen in one so old? I decided to try.''

Many therapists would share Levinson's initial skepticism, assuming that the ''introspective bud,'' if it was observed at all, would not flower, and despite their best therapeutic efforts would be dull and boring, consisting mainly of support techniques and chemotherapy.

But as Dr. Levinson goes on to demonstrate, despite her years, Mrs. A. was quite capable of producing a brilliant flower from that therapeutic bud. By the end of the first year of treatment ''her introspective curiosity grew by leaps and bounds,'' and she participated actively in the dynamic work, sometimes leading the effort rather than following.

We do not believe that Mrs. A.'s introspective capacity is either unusual or rare for a patient in late adulthood. Similar capacities are demonstrated to varying degrees by Crusey's 62-year-old man (Chapter 8) and Cohen's 80-year-old woman (Chapter 10) as well as the patients of Hildebrand (Chapter 11), Notman (Chapter 12), and Kahana (Chapter 14). We hope that this wealth of clinical material suggests that therapists should routinely include in the diagnostic evaluation of older patients an assessment of introspective capacity and therapeutic approaches, just as they would with younger patients.

189

This case material also illustrates another dimension of diagnostic work with elderly patients: The presence of organic disease (the myocardial infarction and chronic obesity) does not rule out and may actually precipitate psychosomatic and/or neurotic symptomatology. A thorough diagnostic study, which includes close cooperation with the patient's primary physician(s), will assist the therapist in demonstrating and understanding the complexity of etiological factors, organic and psychological, from childhood and adulthood.

Levinson tells us that Mrs. A. had considerable guilt about the past. Older patients tend to focus on the past because of (1) diminished capacity for involvement in the present and future due to the loss of objects through death or distance, personal illness, and so forth, and (2) the need for a life review, the evaluation of the past in the face of advancing age and the prospect of death. Either can lead to a sterile, unproductive focus that does not facilitate change. But not all preoccupation with the past is unrewarding. We shall see that Cohen's patient (Chapter 10) began her treatment in this manner but quickly shifted to greater preoccupation with the present and future. Perhaps because she had more to feel guilty about, Levinson's patient continued to consider the past for a longer period of time with a dramatic and surprising result: She reestablished contact with her children after nearly 30 years of estrangement. These cases seem to suggest that in the opening phase of treatment with older patients, the therapist should allow the patient to use the past (and the life review) as they wish until it is clear whether such an interest serves therapeutic progression or resistance. No singular approach to the past should be expected in older patients in general or in the course of therapy with a single individual.

Just as in younger individuals, sudden interference with one or more lines of development may precipitate regression and/or symptom formation. Within a relatively short period of time Mrs. A. had to cope with a myocardial infarction, the death of her mother, and the loss of financial security.

Several therapeutic techniques should be considered by the therapist when confronted by such circumstances.

1. Efforts should be made to address directly those obvious factors impeding ongoing development. For example, Levinson focused on the recovery and maintenance of good physical health, encouraged Mrs. A. to establish new and strengthen old object ties following her mother's death, and discussed money management and new means of financial support.

2. Particular attention should be paid to those developmental interferences that undermine basic character patterns. For instance, Mrs. A. particularly valued her motility, which was now diminished by physical illness and financial limitations. The symptoms that arose in her 60s were in part necessitated by her inability to use the long-standing character defense of running from painful situations. Because the patient could no longer use travel to avoid or reach out to loved ones, Levinson demonstrated admirable therapeutic acumen by helping the patient bring her children and grandchildren to her.

3. Many times an impending crisis can be anticipated and approached prophylactically. As Mrs. A.'s brother gradually decompensated, Levinson addressed her avoidance of him, facilitated an active involvement in his care, and then helped her mourn his passing. Because she was involved in his life in a loving way in his last years, the patient felt less guilty when he did die and tolerated the loss without significant regression.

The family history is usually thought of as referring to the family of childhood. In *Adult Development*, we spoke of the need to pay close attention to the course of adult experience with the family of childhood as well. Because of her unresolved infantile conflicts, particularly those revolving around separation themes, Mrs. A. remained extremely involved with the family of childhood, particularly her mother, throughout midlife. These problems clearly had their origin in childhood and youth. They also, however, had an adult course that compromised ongoing development, particularly the young adult tasks of the achievement of intimacy and parenthood, because Mrs. A. eventually left both her husband and children, returning to her mother. We are suggesting the therapeutic need to *explore and connect* the infantile and the adult experience, leading to resolution of past conflict from all stages of development, and to promote healthy involvement with parents and siblings who may still be alive.

As in Crusey's (Chapter 8) and Cohen's (Chapter 10) cases, Mrs. A. developed complex transference attitudes toward Levinson, demonstrating again reversed or multigenerational transference. The therapist who works with older patients is the recipient of powerful transference feelings from all stages of the life cycle. This fascinating experience is a therapeutic challenge requiring a developmental understanding of transference and considerable empathy and therapeutic flexibility.

For example, Levinson states, ''The transference was one of me as the all-knowing, good father who could protect her and, at times, dominate her." This is clearly a variation of a fairly typical father transference. But as therapy progressed, the transference picture changed. "Within the transference, I became her lost child, young, naive, and inexperienced, learning about the world from a wise, loving mother/grandmother." Here Mrs. A. was transferring feelings from her adult past about her experiences as a mother. Son or daughter transference appears to be a common experience in the treatment of older patients. In our opinion, it is neither a variation of, nor a replacement for, traditional versions of transference emanating from childhood; it is, rather, a manifestation of transference unique unto itself, emanating from experience in living during the second half of life.

Levinson speaks of his countertransference wishes to be mothered. "At these times, as I listened attentively, in my countertransference I felt taken care of, protected, and mothered." We understand such feelings to be a common and expectable response to reversed or multigenerational transference that requires the same kind of self-analysis as any other form of countertransference. Positive or negative, traditional of reversed, erotic or maternal, as with younger patients, transference and countertransference remain the cornerstones of the dynamic treatment of the elderly.

Mrs. A. also provides us with another powerful reaction to a birthday. When she turned 65, she saw herself as "officially designated as old," a "certified old lady." Observance of this milestone stimulated additional life review and facilitated the mourning process for unrealized goals and wishes. However, the patient responded to this marking of chronological time very concretely, as though the passage of time magically dictates life's events and attitudes. Time is experienced as a pursuer, a depriver, as tyrannical. Mrs. A. keenly felt that she was losing the race against time. But, as the subsequent pages of the case history demonstrate, she had many rewarding, even new, experiences ahead of her.

Such despairing attitudes toward time may be shared by an older therapist because he or she, too, is becoming increasingly aware of a personal race against time. Ongoing self-analysis is necessary to minimize the tendency to deny the passage of time or identify with unrealistically morose attitudes in the patient.

Shifting roles in the course of his work with this patient in the absence of other family members, Levinson not only helped his patient arrive at a decision about what to do with her dying brother, but he also arranged for his placement in a geriatric center, again demonstrating the need for great involvement and therapeutic flexibility in treating the elderly, as Cohen will be seen to have done with his 80-year-old patient in Chapter 10.

But the greatest example of therapeutic flexibility and ingenuity was Dr. Levinson's involvement in the patient's reestablishing a real relationship with her daughters and grandchildren after 30 years. The concepts of adult developmental lines and adult developmental arrest (Chapter 3, pp. 49–54) helped Levinson understand the nature and importance of Mrs. A.'s feelings about motherhood and grandmotherhood. After helping her analyze the deeply conflicted feelings about her own mother of childhood, which contributed to her leaving her own children and precipitated the adult developmental arrest, he raised the possibility that a rapprochement might still be possible. His conceptualization of motherhood as a critical function in all phases of adulthood and his respect for the ongoing nature of the developmental process led to a natural consideration of its resumption despite the passage of three decades. Once the family was reconstituted, the new therapeutic task became the facilitation of its evolution and integration.

10

Psychotherapy with an Eighty-Year-Old Patient

GENE D. COHEN

Psychodynamic aspects of treatment for older adults have long been misunderstood or underappreciated. Such has been the situation with the elderly in general and those of advanced age in particular. Part of the explanation for this repeating scenario is simple. Psychiatric experience and psychotherapeutic approaches with older patients have been sparse. Moreover, case reports in the literature have been too few, and comments about such efforts have sometimes been contradictory. Consider, for example, the divergent impressions of Sigmund Freud and Karl Abraham. In 1905 Freud indicated that,

> The age of patients has this much importance in determining their fitness for psycho-analytic treatment, that, on the one hand, near or above the age of fifty the elasticity of the mental processes, on which the treatment depends, is as a rule lacking—old people are no longer educable—and, on the other hand, the mass of material to be dealt with would prolong the duration of the treatment indefinitely. (p. 264)

Approximately 15 years later, in a classic paper entitled "Applicability of Psycho-Analytic Treatment to Patients at an Advanced Age," Abraham (1979) wrote:

> In my psycho-analytic practice I have treated a number of chronic neuroses in persons of over forty and even fifty years of age. At first it was only after some hesitation that I undertook cases of this kind. But I was more than once urged to make the attempt by patients themselves who had been treated unsuccessfully elsewhere. And I was, moreover, confident that if I could not cure the patients, I could at least give them a deeper and better understanding of

their trouble than a physician untrained in psychoanalysis could. To my surprise a considerable number of them reacted very favorably to the treatment.
I might add that I found some of those cures as among my most successful
results. (p. 313)

Freud's comments on the educability of older people and the elasticity of their mental processes around age 50 are ironical; this is especially
true because he wrote this when he was nearing his own 50th birthday
during a productive and creative phase of his life and work in which he
seemed most educable and elastic. There is further irony in that Freud's
view of the greatest masterpiece of all time was a work done by a play-
wright in his 8th decade. Sophocles was 71 when he wrote *Oedipus Rex,*
the drama that was likely perceived by Freud as a brilliant literary vali-
dation of his concept of the oedipus complex in his then-developing and
pioneering psychoanalytic theory. Perhaps too, the mass of material that
Freud was concerned would prolong treatment was the same body of
knowledge and perspective that permitted the aged Sophocles to achieve
his great masterpiece, his great insights (Cohen, 1981).

Confusion about the capacity for change and the significance of time
in later life have played a part in clouding views about the applicability
of psychotherapy for the elderly. Curiously, paradox surrounds both
these areas and is captured by Somerset Maugham:

When I was young, I was amazed at Plutarch's statement that the elder Cato
began at the age of eighty to learn Greek. I am amazed no longer. Old age
is ready to undertake tasks that youth shirked because they would take too
long. (Comfort, 1977, p. 83)

The matter of time, or time left, is intriguing, because, by age 65, one
is a survivor with an average life expectancy moving toward 20 years—
ample time for both life and treatment. Moreover, averages do not speak
to the individual, and the number of individuals reaching age 100 continues to grow.

Although there are conceptual questions about goals, process, and
techniques in psychotherapy with elderly patients, there are also less
spoken concerns about how interesting and challenging such work
would be. And all these issues emerge yet larger when the focus shifts
to the "organic" older patient. In the following case example, some
aspects of work with "functional" psychiatric problems as well as "organic" mental disorders in later life will be looked at in the same subject.

CASE STUDY

Mrs. C., an 80-year old childless widow, living alone in an apartment, came to the outpatient clinic (in which both internal medicine and psychiatric services were provided) with complaints of both depression and anxiety. She described feelings of despair, discouragement, and uneasiness; her appetite was diminished; difficulty falling asleep and early morning awakening were reported. There were nightmares characterized by an ominous feeling or by scenes in which she was being chased by a frightening man. She looked somewhat despondent and agitated and displayed perspiration on her forehead and hands. No delusions or hallucinations were described. Stream of thought was appropriate. Affect was consistent with content of thought. There was no mental status evidence of an organic mental disorder. Otherwise, her appearance was of a physically attractive and well-dressed elderly woman. Her most immediate concerns were about the recent death of a close male friend and how she would adjust now that she would be so much more alone. No previous treatment with a mental health professional was described; this was her first psychiatric visit. Nonetheless, she described periods of despondency dating back to adolescence. Except for mild hypertension, controlled by diet and the use of diuretics, her medical history was otherwise unremarkable. She had no surviving siblings, and the only relatives with whom she had contact were two nieces and two nephews, all of whom lived out of state. She had one close friend in her apartment building and several others elsewhere in town.

Mrs. C. was the youngest of three sisters, and she grew up in a rural southern town. Her mother was a housewife to whom Mrs. C. was close, but the mother died of tuberculosis when the patient was 15. Mrs. C.'s father worked as a clerk at a small factory and was described as being periodically moody and extremely critical of her. She had always been physically striking, even as a young girl, but her father never complimented her on her beauty; at the same time, he conveyed distrust of her dating behavior. Mrs. C. was skillful at practically everything she did and was particularly talented in skating, winning various awards. She described both disappointment and resentment at her father's taking little interest in this endeavor or in others in which she demonstrated excellence.

When the patient was 15, both her mother and a sister died of tuberculosis. The patient recalled first becoming depressed at this time, and she subsequently became symptomatic herself: Largely through the support and encouragement of a young doctor at the sanatorium where the patient stayed, she kept her will to live.

A couple of years later, Mrs. C.'s older sister married and left home. Shortly thereafter the patient and a friend, not being able to find satisfactory work in their home town, moved to a northern city where the friend's cousin had landed a good job. The three made plans to share an apartment. That summer she traveled with her friend across the country, eventually arriving in California where she had a romance with a man several years older. Her girlfriend returned to the East, whereas the patient took a job as a hostess in a restaurant, rented a small apartment, and soon discovered she was competing with Mary Pickford for the beau; Mary Pickford won. The patient felt mildly despondent for a while, but shortly thereafter she met another man, a vaudeville performer who was 12 years her senior. They married. It was never basically a romantic relationship, but the patient felt secure and enjoyed the traveling they did as her husband performed around the country. Around that time her father died.

Mrs. C.'s marriage gradually became less gratifying and was not helped by the fact that she and her husband were unable to have children. During subsequent periods of attraction to other men she felt anxious and moody and would suffer disturbing dreams. Eventually, Mrs. C. and her husband moved to the Baltimore–Washington area, and she began work as the assistant manager of a small clothing store for women. She continued this work for 30 years and was regarded an exemplary worker. Her husband died when she was 60, and her remaining sister died shortly thereafter. The patient moved to an apartment when she was 65. Around that time she was losing interest in her job and was struggling with sporadic bouts of feeling sad and lonely. She then decided to do something totally different. Drawing upon her outstanding skills as a driver, which were developed when she and her husband traveled a great deal, she decided to become a chauffeur for elderly rich ladies. She took to this job with the same diligence and dedication that she applied to all her endeavors. Out of her concern to assure the protection of these rich ladies, Mrs. C. secretly carried a pistol. She was extremely well liked and appreciated by these women, but after several died and she herself got older, Mrs. C. decided to retire.

Mrs. C. was in her early 70s when she began dating a man in his mid-80s. He was very generous, and the patient began to live in a better style than she ever had. One day her dear friend fell, broke his hip, developed a severe infection, and died. He had planned to revise his will to her benefit, but he had not done so. In addition to her loss of this most important relationship, the patient, now 80 years old, was suddenly thrust into a situation where, without her friend's financial support or will, she would suffer an immediate decline in her standard of living as well. She became depressed, agitated, and quite disturbed by her troubled sleep and nightmares. At that point, she thought of seeing a psychiatrist and came to see me.

Mrs. C. responded quickly through emotional catharsis and the sense of support she felt in the therapeutic alliance; her pessimism and malaise both diminished. Her appetite improved; her sleep became less broken; and nightmares waned in frequency and intensity. Early discussions dwelled on disappointments across the decades, but by the end of the first month talk about positive life events had become common. It was about that time, too, that Mrs. C. announced she was having an easier time with personal resources. She had polished an old talent for card playing and had joined the Later Life Ladies Poker Club; she often came away a winner.

In looking back over their lives with older patients, issues about the pros and cons of life review techniques come up. Butler (1963) described the life review approach as a therapeutic use of reminiscing to resolve, reorganize, and reintegrate what is troubling or preoccupying the patient. It is an effort to facilitate the capacity of older people to reconcile, or come to better terms with, the meaning of their lives. Others, however, emphasize that questions of when and for whom to use this technique must be raised because some older people will look at past life experiences not as they have been, but as they might have been and in the process experience guilt and a profound sense of loss. Weinberg (1976) addressed this point when he wrote about adding insight to injury. Still, Grotjahn (1955) has pointed out that resistance against unpleasant insight is frequently lessened in old age as the demands of reality, which in younger people are considered narcissistic threats, finally become acceptable.

During the first few months of therapy Mrs. C. would frequently say something to the effect that I was like a son to her. As therapy progressed, the transference changed. She started to talk more about her relationships with men and took noticeably more care in her appearance around me. In one of our sessions she brought in a framed 9- by 12-inch photograph of her in her 20s that was designed to stand on a table. I was sitting behind a desk, and she beside the desk on that occasion. While talking about the photograph, she placed it on the desk in such a manner that it partially blocked my view of her. It seemed that she was trying to get me to see her physically as a younger woman. The next session led to her looking back at the men she was attracted to during her marriage, recalling again the anxiety, moodiness, and bad dreams she suffered around that time. An association followed where she wondered in retrospect if the distrustful feelings with which her father had hurt her in adolescence had come back to haunt her when she fantasized about affairs during the time in which she was married. She then asked me what I thought of a married woman having thoughts about other men; I thought to myself that the transference had again changed and that she was attempting to place me into a paternal role.

Berezin (1972) reminds us that transference by definition is unreal, unconscious, and not time related. In this sense, it is also consistent with the concept of timelessness. In treatment, transference reactions do not follow chronological calendar considerations. This is not to say that the age of the patient or the age of the therapist has no dynamic impact on transference or countertransference phenomena. The point is that age may or may not make a difference. The therapist may be seen by the older patient as a grandson or granddaughter, son or daughter, sibling, or parent. Such a range is certainly reflected in the case of Mrs. C. Similarly, the therapist may find himself or herself relating to the older person as one would to an elder; at other times he or she will relate as to one in his or her own cohort group; and on yet different occasions the therapist may act in a parental mode. Sometimes the therapist will act in all three ways with the same patient.

After several months in therapy, the patient's apartment was robbed; her most valued personal possessions were stolen. This resulted in a particularly untimely setback for her. Mrs. C. had been in the process of renewing her driver's license, and because of her age had to retake the driver's test, including the written part. Passing the driver's test was particularly important to her self-esteem. The robbery caused Mrs. C. to become depressed and anxious, and suddenly she found it difficult to remember the answers to several of the questions on the practice driver's test. She also reported that, for the first time, she was losing at the poker table. This clinical picture was noteworthy in illustrating the way that problems with memory and concentration in the elderly are commonly symptoms of depression as opposed to dementia. Gradually Mrs. C.

came to terms with the theft and losses, and her recent-onset symptoms subsided. She resumed winning at poker and easily passed her driver's test, getting 100% on the written part.

After approximately a year and a half had gone by, Mrs. C. came in smiling and with an expression not unlike that of the cat who had caught the canary. She eventually divulged she had a new boyfriend, giggling that she had "done it again." "Done what?" I asked. "Gotten involved with another older man," she said. Her new boyfriend was 97! She suggested, too, with mixed humor and insight, that perhaps this was her way of still trying to deal with the problems she had with her father.

Therapy continued for another 6 months. Mrs. C.'s relationship with her new friend was going well, she was feeling much better; and she thought that perhaps it was no longer necessary to see the psychiatrist. After exploring her feelings about stopping psychotherapy, I agreed, and with mutual satisfaction we said goodbye.

In reviewing what had transpired during the course of my work with Mrs. C., I felt that there had been several dimensions to the therapeutic process. The psychotherapy began with crisis intervention marked by a release of intense emotions of mixed grief and rage. She had suffered the loss of a man close to her, but at the same time she had been severely let down by that man, (e.g., not having been taken care of in his will, which was symbolically reminiscent of the way her father did not take care of her emotionally). Had Mrs. C. not responded so soon and so significantly to psychotherapy alone, the additional use of antidepressant medication would have been considered because, when indicated, this type of medication can be a useful adjunct. As the transference progressed, I was eventually put in the role of her father where it appeared that some corrective emotional experience transpired. Also going on in this phase of the psychotherapy and related to the transference dynamics was a process of reconciliation with past disappointments on Mrs. C.'s part. My major concern at termination of therapy was how Mrs. C. would respond if her latest relationship was disrupted or came to an end.

I felt my efforts with Mrs. C. illustrated a number of other aspects of psychotherapy with the elderly. Certainly, the capacity for growth in dealing with emotional conflict knows no end point in the life cycle. Moreover, light was shed on the course of illness with aging. In this regard, the concept of exacerbation and remission of illness, especially with the elderly, seems less well appreciated with psychiatric than with medical disorders. When someone with diabetes or congestive heart failure has a flare-up, family and physician expect that a remission is likely to follow with proper treatment. An aggravation of a psychiatric disturbance, however, is more likely to be met by others with greater impatience and disappointment or a sense of futility. Such reactions can be magnified when the patient is an older person. But the fact remains, as in the case of Mrs. C., that mental disorders do remit and do so throughout the life cycle; old age is no exception. Working with Mrs. C. also illustrated the unique opportunity the therapist has in psychotherapy with the elderly to look back with the patient at the course of early life conflicts and problems across the life cycle and to examine in one person the interplay of development and disorder over a period of decades. It is as if we have a chance for a 60-, 70-, or 80-year follow-up of disease in an individual. By looking at an illness over that period of time—in this case, depression—we might gain a better understanding of that illness that could be applied in treating patients with the same disorder in other age groups. The opportunity to gain new perspectives on the human condition is also a possibility in working with those who have a long perspective on human experience.

Three years later I received most distressing news. Mrs. C. had suffered a major stroke, leaving her severely demented—with cognitive impairment similar to that of an advanced stage of Alzheimer's disease. I went to see her in the nursing home. When I arrived I was stunned with what I witnessed. Rather than the strikingly appealing person she had always been, it seemed she was the ward pest or pain. Her intellectual dysfunction, agitation, and high level of disability had made her quite difficult to manage. I was also struck by the matter-of-factness with which the staff passed by her with minimal visual contact—this was in such contrast to the attention she had commanded throughout her life.

I realized at that point the double tragedy experienced by Mrs. C. in relation to her history, her identity. Mrs. C. had not only lost touch with her personal history, but she had also lost her ability to convey her own history to others. In this regard, we all have a compound history, a two-faceted history—a history of ourselves as we know it and a history of ourselves as others know it. Not to be known by others, to be in effect without a history by being unable to convey one's past, puts a person at a severe disadvantage in eliciting the understanding and empathy of others; a competitive edge has been lost. Here, the therapist can be enormously helpful in conveying the individual's personal and dynamic history, his or her clinical biography. I then attempted to restore some of this competitive edge, this most interesting human phenomenon—Mrs. C.'s history, her biography. Scrapbooks, photos, news clippings, and other personal items of memorabilia were gathered in the process of trying to portray a sense of the patient's past to the staff dynamically. The impact was pronounced. When I returned the next week, there was considerably more verbal and non-verbal engagement between the staff and Mrs. C. And, as more time passed, it became apparent that in addition to the staff's feeling more in touch with the patient because of their knowledge of her personal history, fragments of disjointed thoughts she would express were somewhat better understood due to the enlarged frame of reference in which they were heard.

The problem of imparting Mrs. C.'s history was a much more complicated idea than what has been described. This was because of the dual problem of there being more than one shift of personnel during the course of each day and substantial staff turnover (particularly nursing assistants at nursing homes) during the course of the year. How, then, can one practically convey the patient's history in the dynamic manner described for each shift and for ongoing new staff? Certainly, it is difficult to achieve this effect with a typical chart history; the length involved might preclude many from reading it. It was felt then that one could take advantage of the new technology of audio- and videocassettes and record the history on one or the other of these media. For some institutions there would be the resources to develop a program of audiovisual histories. In other settings, the costs might be prohibitive, but audiocassette histories could still be feasible. Staff at all shifts might be much more likely to obtain these histories due to ease of access—listening to or watching a cassette presentation as opposed to pondering over a chart. Family members could also assume an important role here and probably derive much satisfaction by contributing to the information and presentation on the cassettes. Especially if a given family member is a good storyteller, they should be involved in giving the patient's biography. The experience could be rewarding all the way around. And, in this case example, it might be appreciated that in patients with severe dementia the role of biography can be as important as that of biology in the overall approach to treatment.

The elderly as a whole present mental health practitioners with a wide range of problems and therapeutic considerations (Cohen, 1982). In the case of Mrs. C., we see the potential clinical diversity that sometimes can occur with a single older person.

REFERENCES

Abraham, K. Applicability of psycho-analytic treatment to patients at an advanced age. In H.C. Abraham (Eds.), *Selected papers on psychoanalysis.* New York: Bruner/Mazel, 1979.

Berezin, M.A. Psychodynamic considerations of aging and the aged: An overview. *American Journal of Psychiatry,* 1972, *128,* 1483–1491.

Butler, R.N. The life review: An interpretation of reminiscence in the aged. *Psychiatry,* 1963, *26,* 65–76.

Cohen, G.D. Perspectives on psychotherapy with the elderly. *American Journal of Psychiatry,* 1981, *138,* 347–350.

Cohen, G.D. The older person, the older patient, and the mental health system. *Hospital and Community Psychiatry,* 1982, *33,* 101–104.

Comfort, A. *A good age.* London: Mitchell Beazley, 1977.

Freud, S. On psychotherapy. In J. Strachey (Ed. and trans.), *Standard edition 7:257.* London: Hogarth Press, 1905.

Grotjahn, M. Analytic psychotherapy with the elderly. I: The sociological background of aging in America. *Psychoanalytic Review,* 1955, *42,* 419–427.

Weinberg, A. On adding insight to injury. *Gerontologist,* 1976, *16,* 4–10.

Discussion

ROBERT A. NEMIROFF AND CALVIN A. COLARUSSO

Dr. Cohen tells of an 80-year-old childless widow who sought psychiatric treatment for the first time because of the death of a close friend and increased concerns about loneliness. We suggest that this was as appropriate a time in life for an initial psychiatric contact as any other because the need grew out of feelings generated by a major developmental theme of late adulthood and led to the onset of symptoms, primarily anxiety and depression.

This patient had a lifelong capacity to react to life's traumas and losses and to create new circumstances and opportunities for growth. For example, when she was 60, both her husband and sister died within a short interval. After a period of adjustment, propelled by her loneliness, Mrs. C. decided "to do something totally different" and started her own business. The capacity for resourcefulness and adaptation to loss and change is an important diagnostic indicator in the elderly because it suggests that older patients, even at age 80, will bring the same adaptability to the therapeutic arena that they display in life.

Cohen comments on the controversy in the literature about the therapeutic use of the life review in elderly patients. In this case, Mrs. C. began the treatment with "discussions dwelling on disappointments across the decades," but within a month she was enthusiastically focusing on the present and new means of adaptation. Technically, Cohen's work again suggests that the therapist should neither initiate nor stifle an initial preoccupation with the past because in a relatively healthy patient such a life review may be short lived, self-limiting, and quickly replaced by an adaptive focus on the present. Understood in this way, the life review may become a stimulus to further therapeutic work without becoming either a major resistance or the primary vehicle for therapeutic change.

As in each of the other four cases presented in this section, Mrs. C. quickly developed a transference relationship with the therapist. In addition, as Cohen clearly demonstrates, he was seen successively as a son, lover, and father. Thus, the concept of multigenerational transference is again demonstrated.

As the erotic transference developed, Mrs. C. brought a picture of herself as a young woman to the sessions. By so doing, she attempted to attract the therapist to what she was, rather than to what she had become. This poignant vignette also illustrates that the need to mourn for the lost body of youth, described by us in relationship to midlife development in Chapter 5 of *Adult Development*, continues into late adulthood as well.

The therapist who is working with older patients for the first time may initially be surprised and shocked by such sexual interests and active expressions in one so old. But such transference manifestations, which are seen in every patient described in this book, are an expression of the human condition, regardless of age, and if accepted by the therapist, they quickly became integral parts of the treatment process and vehicles for change.

The clinical material illustrates that signs of memory loss are not necessarily the result of impending or actual dementia; dynamic conflict and situational stress can also result in memory impairment that may respond to therapeutic intervention and stress reduction.

Propelled by her therapeutic improvement and an undeniable need for significant object ties, Mrs. C. became "involved with another older man," who was 97. Having thus reestablished a meaningful heterosexual tie and feeling energetic and optimistic, she suggested termination. Mrs. C.'s criteria for termination were the same as those expressed by "younger" patients, that is, removal of symptoms and a resumption of gratifying relationships. We would add that, again like younger patients, she was able to leave the therapist and resume an active independent life. In contrast to Levinson's patient (Chapter 9), who continued in treatment for 10 years, Mrs. C. was able to terminate after a relatively brief period of time. The five cases in this section illustrate a wide range of termination experience in older patients, again requiring the therapist to react to each individual patient with flexibility and openmindedness.

One of the most innovative therapeutic techniques utilized by Cohen was to act as historian and advocate for the patient after she suffered a major stroke and was unable to communicate with her caretakers. Through his efforts, Mrs. C. became a person in the eyes of the hospital staff, resulting in a significant improvement in clinical management. In describing this innovative technique, Cohen suggests that patient biographies be presented through scrapbooks, photos, news clippings, and memorabilia. These can be organized and recorded on audio- and videotape, thus becoming available to all caretakers.

Above all, this chapter illustrates what a sensitive and skillful therapist who is not bound by stereotypes about the elderly can do to reduce incapacitating psychiatric symptoms and enhance the later years of his or her patient.

III

Critical Clinical Issues
in the Treatment of
Older Patients

Oh for one hour of youthful joy!
  Give back my twentieth spring!
I'd rather laugh, a bright-haired boy,
  Than reign, a gray-beard king.

Off with the spoils of wrinkled age!
  Away with Learning's crown!
Tear out life's Wisdom-written page,
  And dash its trophies down!

One moment let my life-blood stream
  From boyhood's fount of flame!
Give me one giddy, reeling dream
  Of life all love and fame!

My listening angel heard the prayer,
  And, calmly smiling, said,
"If I but touch thy silvered hair,
  Thy hasty wish hath sped.

"But is there nothing in thy track
  To bid thee fondly stay,
While the swift seasons hurry back
  To find the wished-for day?"

"Ah, truest soul of womankind!
  Without thee what were life?
One bliss I cannot leave behind:
  I'll take—my—precious—wife!"

The angel took a sapphire pen
    And wrote in rainbow dew,
The man would be a boy again,
    And be a husband, too!

"And is there nothing yet unsaid,
    Before the change appears?
Remember, all their gifts have fled
    With those dissolving years."

"Why, yes"; for memory would recall
    My fond paternal joys;
"I could not bear to leave them all—
    I'll take—my—girl—and—boys."

The smiling angel dropped his pen,—
    "Why, this will never do;
The man would be a boy again,
    And be a father, too!"

And so I laughed,—my laughter woke
    The household with its noise,—
And wrote my dream, when morning broke,
    To please the gray-haired boys.

Oliver Wendell Holmes (1809–1894), *The Old Man Dreams*

11

Object Loss and Development in the Second Half of Life

H. P. HILDEBRAND

Erik Erikson (1981) defines the eighth stage of his epigenetic cycle as integrity versus despair:

If, at the end, the life cycle turns back on its own beginnings, so that the very old become again like children, the question is whether the return is to a child-likeness seasoned with wisdom or (and when) to a finite childishness. The old may become (and want to become) too old too fast, or remain too young too long. Here, only some sense of *integrity* can bind things together; and by integrity we do not mean only an occasional outstanding quality of personal character but, above all, a simple proclivity for understanding, or "hearing" those who understand, the integrative ways of human life. It is a comrade-ship with the ordering ways of distant times and different pursuits, as expressed in their simple product and sayings. For an individual life is the coincidence of but one life cycle with but one segment of history; and all human integrity stands or falls with the one style of integrity of which one partakes. There is an integrating aspect, as there can be a boringly repetitive one, in the ritualistic tendency of the old to reminisce about what events and what persons made up the decisive trends of their lives. But there emerges also a different, a timeless love for those few others who have become the main counterplayers in life's most significant contexts.

And so, all qualities of the past assume new and distinguishing values which we may well study in their own right and not just in their antecedents, be they healthy or pathogenic. For to be relatively freer of neurotic anxiety does not mean to be absolved from existential dread; the most acute understanding of infantile guilt does not go away with the human evil which each life experiences in its own way; and the best defined psychosocial identity does not preempt one's existential identity. In sum, a better functioning ego does not explain away the mystery of the aware "I."

For all these, and more, reasons, the dominant antithesis comes to be now *integrity* versus *despair*—the despair of the knowledge that a limited life is coming to a conclusion; and also the (often quite petty) *disgust* over feeling finished, passed by, and increasingly helpless. The strength arising from these antitheses, however, is *wisdom*, a kind of "detached concern with life itself, in the face of death itself," as expressed both in the sayings of the ages and in those simplest experiences which convey the probability of an ultimate meaning.

The antipathy to wisdom is *disdain*, again a natural and necessary reaction to the lifelong experience of prevailing pettiness and the deadly repetitiveness of human depravity and deceit. Disdain (as rejectivity and exclusivity before) is altogether denied only at the danger of indirect destructiveness, including self-disdain. But wisdom can well contain disdain as a refusal to be fooled in regard to man's antithetical nature.

Oh yes, what is the ritualization built into the styles of old age? I think it is *philosophical:* In maintaining some integrity in the disintegration of body and mind, it can also advocate durable hope in wisdom. The corresponding ritualistic danger, however (do I need to spell it out?), is *dogmatism*, which, where linked with undue power, can become coercive orthodoxy.

Finally, we have suggested a procreative drive as a further psychosexual stage in adulthood. For (presenile) old age, I can only suggest a *generalization of sensual modes* which can foster an enriched bodily and mental overall experience even as part functions weaken and overall vitality diminishes. (pp. 45–47, italics in original)

I was gratified when I read this passage recently because I had long wished for Erikson to expand on his later epigenic life stages, which had always seemed to me to be very schematic. By chance, they coincided with my coming across a letter written by the psychoanalyst Martin Grotjahn (1982) in the *Lancet* in which he says,

For many years I had great expectations of old age. In my fantasies, I would be wise, perhaps somewhat detached from the worries of this world, beyond desire and temptation, without frustration, and therefore without anger. Finally, I would be without guilt, without obligations and duties—just alive. That would be true freedom; freedom from inner drive and outer threat. I thought that as an old man I would finally be what I was supposed to be: I, myself, and free.

Grotjahn then recounts suffering a serious heart attack at the age of 75 and its effect upon him.

But now I feel old. I do not work anymore, nor do I walk. Strangely enough I do not mind. Suddenly, 50 years of work is enough. I no longer worry about my patients, nor feel guilty because I do not understand them sufficiently or know how to help them. I feel free of the guilt that accompanies our work, the feeling of never being as good as our work demands us to be. Let others worry now! I have finished with work and worry.

I sit in the sun watching the falling leaves slowly sail across the water of the swimming pool. I think, I dream, I draw, I sit. I feel free from worry, almost free of this world of reality. I still love in a quiet way and I feel loved by my family and friends. This southern California "winter" is more beautiful than I have ever seen it before. How could I have known that I would be happy just sitting here, reading a little, and enjoying life in a quiet and modest way; or that to walk across the street to the corner of the park would satisfy me more than the long walks I took a year ago when I used to find that four hours were not enough?

I have time now. I do not know how much time is left for me to live, but I am in no hurry. I am in no hurry to get anywhere, not even to the end of time. That can wait, and when it comes I will try to accept it, although I have no illusions; it will not be easy. Right now I live in the moment and I want to sit here a little while longer, quietly. I used to think that old age was an achievement in itself. I now know better: to get sick and to live on, that is an achievement. (p. 441)

In thinking about these beautiful statements, what puzzled me was how to help my own patients achieve a state such as Grotjahn described. For some years now, I have conducted a workshop for patients in the second half of life at the Tavistock Clinic, gradually extending the age range of patients seen from the early 50s to the late 70s. In my private practice, too, I see elderly patients for psychoanalysis and psychotherapy and now feel that my colleagues and I have begun to have some understanding of the psychotherapeutic problems involved in aging.

The goals described by Erikson and Grotjahn were entirely sympathetic and appropriate to me. But, as always, in trying to work in this field I felt that, although it was easy to state goals, it was never going to be easy to achieve them. Nevertheless, I was trying to do what I could, and it seems worthwhile to share some of my experience.

I would like first to describe two patients who illustrate the difficulties in achieving the state of "wisdom" we are discussing.

Then I'll discuss another group, who are perhaps more numerous than one would expect, in whom despair has the upper hand over wisdom and to whom the analyst or psychotherapist has little to offer.

Let me first speak of a man now aged 70. I will call him William. I am his third psychoanalyst. Twenty-five years ago he went to a colleague of mine, Dr. X., now dead, complaining of anxiety and phobias. On Dr. X.'s death, he was interviewed by another colleague, who wrote of him:

His symptoms are a general sense of anxiety and insecurity manifested in fantasies about disasters happening to him and to people or animals who feel close to himself or to property such as his house. He constantly is plagued with the idea that illness, accidents, and disasters are likely to happen. It seems that outside this narcissistic world he, in fact, has little feeling for people and therefore can deal quite cooly and calmly with emotional problems in others. He feels himself to be very withdrawn from life, relating only to his wife and to his work. The only relief from his anxiety occurs when he gets back to his flat in the evening and starts drinking a fair amount of whisky. He has to use Nembutal to sleep, taking Drinamyl in the mornings and Nembutal at night. He really cannot bear change.

William had a very traumatic childhood. His mother seems to have been a very selfish and unmotherly person who doted upon his homosexual older brother. His only close tie was to his nurse who was with the family until she died. The nurse was overprotective and constantly preoccupied with the idea that her charge would develop illness. He was unhappy away from her at boarding school and lived in dread that she would one day be dismissed. When William was 13 or 14, his parents separated. He felt guilty that he did not choose to stay with his father but was terrified to tell his mother that he did not want to stay with her. Guilt toward his father for having abandoned him seems to have been strong, as was the narcissistic loss at not having had a father to identify with and idealize. He saw his father as being progressively destroyed by his very powerful mother.

After a very fearful and timid childhood, from the age of 15 onward, William lived rather wildly until the age of 40, marrying four times. His present marriage, which has lasted now for 20 years, has been stable, but before that he was very riotous with women. He felt guilty still about the ways in which he treated women and let them down.

We made good contact looking at this relationship with his father, particularly the aspect of being abandoned and the lack of a secure father with whom to identify. William found a point of view that he had not explored in his previous therapy. He was close to tears once or twice, and there was obviously a lot of sadness in him, although it would be difficult to say that this represented a chronic underlying depressive state.

Analysis had been for William a part of his life support system, something that he needed to keep going. But, in recent months, various major events occurred to make the prospect of his own death much more of a reality. First, he had two severe attacks of renal pain, leading eventually to an emergency operation for kidney stones. He also had to have two operations for hernia. Surviving those well, he regained his health. However, various friends died during this period, and he had to cope with many feelings about his own and his wife's possible deaths.

The episode that I wish to report concerns his wife's sudden illness. She had surgery for a recurrent ovarian cyst, and he became very worried. A glamorous woman friend offered to stay in their flat, and, although he had been impotent with his wife for at least 4 years, he almost immediately began an affair with the friend. William felt no guilt toward his wife and regretted that he could not go on with this relationship because of various external factors. We had long known that his compulsive sexuality during his earlier years was a way of defending against the fear of abandonment—a falling into nothingness or falling apart as Winnicott (1973) has defined it. For him, continual sexual pursuit and conquest of young attractive women, at whatever cost, were ways of keeping this fear at bay.

There was little interest in children—sexuality had little to do with pleasure but more with safety. Although William could work with and recognize all of these themes and could integrate them into his life, what he could not bear was his depression when his wife's recovery was slower than expected. Although she was plainly aware of his infidelity, her only overt response was to withdraw and refuse to look after him. He struggled against ennui, against despair, against sadness. He could not face the realization that he had entered his eighth decade, with all that implied. Although busily engaged at his office, where his work was still enormously successful, he was terrified of retirement or redundancy. A beautiful country house, stuffed with antiques, brought no pleasure because the thought of living there for more than a few days at a time horrified him. When his wife became depressed and sadness became a problem for him, he said to me, "I must get away—I'll take the Concorde to New York for a few days." I interpreted that I had become in the transference the mouthpiece of his sad, neglected, and abandoned younger self; I had become the voice of feelings that he had to defend against by a lifetime of denial—a denial in which desertion, the primal scene, and death all became identified as threats to his safety and were defended against by compulsive sexuality and by a whole series of deals. He knew very well intellectually what I was saying but could not integrate it. His response was to burst into tears and complain that I did not like him.

I, thus, became the father who deserted him and forced him to face the terrors of abandonment, sexuality, and death on his own. I pointed out that he felt his accusations were driving me away, so that I became even more invested with the lost feeling part of himself, which had to be projected so as to have it survive. Contemplation of death and feeling could not be allowed to come together; he would be overwhelmed by intolerable despair. I understand that I may have to wait, perhaps for years, before he will be able to contemplate what is before him. He cannot feel hope or trust me to help him with this lack in himself.

I will contrast this patient with another 55-year-old man, whom I shall call Dr. Socrates. An authority in his own field, he sought help for an inexplicable phobia of opening letters. Never having suffered any form of psychiatric illness before, he was bewildered by this increasingly severe fear, particularly of official-looking letters. Because his affairs were gradually getting into a bad state, he assumed, although without real justification, that he would be arrested and fined heavily by the Internal Revenue Service.

Dr. Socrates came originally from Greece, the only son of a ship's captain and a cultivated society woman. His mother had not wanted to spend much time on him; therefore his childhood was spent with many relatives in the various islands of the archipelago. When his mother subsequently had a daughter who died in early childhood, Socrates was made to feel responsible. Although one might have expected him to be schizoid and withdrawn, he had enjoyed his childhood, having related well to some of his foster parents, particularly an old couple who had spoken to him in the local dialect and encouraged his altogether striking intelligence. One of his earliest memories, from about age 6, concerned an arrangement to meet his mother at a cafe. He got there on time, only to see her ride by in the family car with a female cousin and go off on a jaunt without him.

His parents emigrated to England before World War II, and he pursued a distinguished career in medicine. Like his namesake, he had married a shrew, a brilliant classical scholar with a Greek background who created for him a life that eventually became hell. His Xanthippe was determined to fail in whatever she did, at the same time continually carping and destroying what he achieved. At the time I knew him, their children had grown up and left home, and Dr. Socrates lived a dog's life, shopping, cooking, cleaning, and looking after Xanthippe, who was almost maniacal in the violence and fury of her attacks on him. She would not allow him a desk or a study in their large family home; therefore he wrote learned papers and even books in his head and dictated them in final draft to his secretary.

As we worked together, it became clear that the precipitating incident for his unusual symptom was the death of Xanthippe's mother some 12 years before. When Socrates and his wife had been on a trip abroad with their children, the old lady had stayed in their house. An alcoholic, she'd fallen asleep while smoking a cigarette and died in the subsequent fire, which also badly damaged their house. Xanthippe blamed Socrates for her mother's death and relentlessly punished him—without retaliation or even protest on his part. It turned out that the letters represented his fear that he would be invited abroad again, with the consequence that there would be another death. It took some time before he could begin to see that the death in question would be his wife's.

After some months, he had a healing dream in which he vividly experienced an expression of redness. We gradually understood this to be a preverbal representation of intense feelings, particularly of rage toward his wife and mother. In the transference, I was positively identified as a (returned) father who helped him work through feelings by giving him a language through which to express them. I identified the way in which his (pathological) altruism worked and showed him the secret destructive rage that lay beneath all that he so carefully did for his wife and to a lesser extent for others. Gradually, he was able to become far more overtly aggressive with Xanthippe, to take appropriate steps when she attacked him physically, and to arrange for medical help when she threatened suicide or appeared to be on the verge of a psychotic breakdown. As one might expect, his symptom disappeared.

One of the most striking qualities that Socrates displayed was preeminence as a teacher. He had an extraordinary capacity to develop the skills of his students—often at the expense of his own ideas. I found him a joy to work with, not merely because of his intelligence and culture, but because I, too, found myself able to analyze in an extremely satisfying way. He had the capacity to enable me to draw on unsuspected imaginative and creative aspects of myself that caused me to think of new ideas and deeply satisfying interpretations. Dr. Socrates was operating a profound split in which he assumed all the badness in intimate situations, while projecting the creative parts of himself into others.

As we worked on this notion, his life changed even further. Until this time he'd never slept more than 3 to 4 hours a night, waking to listen to the World Service of the BBC at 4:00 A.M. Now he began to sleep through the night, assert himself, drink less, and gradually lose the quite marked depressive features that he had never acknowledged to anyone before. Most rewarding was an altered view of his own work. Dr. Socrates had regarded himself as a burnt-out volcano, with no more ideas to offer. But suddenly he began to write papers that offered new and quite revolutionary perspectives on his field, thus moving into a creative period in his later life that was deeply satisfying. Although the patient felt that he could never leave Xanthippe and might, therefore, miss a really loving and sensual relationship with a woman, life did once again have meaning. Proud of his achievements, his own man, Dr. Socrates began to enjoy its gratifications—namely, fame, travel, and grandchildren. In Erikson's sense, he moved toward wisdom and personal integrity.

The notion that helped me to understand some of the problems of these two men was suggested by Clifford Scott (1982) when I wrote to him about a patient whom we both knew. He suggested that certain crucial experiences represent symbolically primal—or if you wish, primary—scenes. They are birth, sexual intercourse, and the death of oneself or one's spouse. Each of these experiences are nodal points in life, symbolically significant experiences of tremendous importance. If they cannot be faced, thought about, and worked through, then much displacement takes place, and various defensive operations prevent people from enjoying the latter part of their lives. In later life, one function of the life review is reflection on these matters. The analyst has to be prepared to accompany the patient through this review, accepting and reflecting the various roles that he or she may need to carry in the transference.

This explains the apparent contradiction concerning transference in dynamic therapy with older patients. On the one hand, as Berezin (1972) has suggested, we need to be prepared to embody both early and adult figures in the patient's life in order to revalue and rework the past in the conventional way. On the other hand, much more than with younger patients, we have to become the embodiment of the ideal child or children whom the patient needs as the guarantors of his or her immortality and thus of the future. In the two cases I have cited, William cannot yet face his or his wife's death and remains locked into his depressive system, whereas Socrates is able to do so and recognize his own achievements. For both of these men, facing anxiety about their own death and that of their spouse is crucial to their capacity to live creatively and well as they age.

LOSS OF AN ADULT CHILD

Sadly, there is another group of older patients with whom one cannot achieve this sort of transference resolution because fate has stepped in and dealt the patient a blow from which it seems almost impossible to recover. I refer to patients who have had the misfortune to lose an adult child through accident or illness.

Mr. Woodentop

My attention was drawn to this group of people, who, insofar as I am aware, have not been reported in the literature, when I accepted for treatment a 46-year-old policeman whom I have described briefly elsewhere (Hildebrand, 1982) as "Mr. Woodentop". (*Woodentop* is a slang word for a policeman.) Complaining of depression, stress, and psychosomatic symptoms, he had lost his oldest son, James, in a motorcycle accident.

The patient described himself as having been brought up in Scotland during the 1930s in a rather impoverished family, although his father later succeeded well. He has an older sister who spent some years in a hospital with tuberculosis. It was plain that he saw himself as having had a rather deprived childhood in a lower-middle-class family with all the restrictions that involved. Mr. Woodentop found a way out by joining the R.A.F. when he was 18. Then he became a policeman because he enjoyed the street work and what he calls "the involvement and excitement on some occasions and the patience required on others."

He married young because his wife was pregnant. The relationship was almost immediately unhappy, but the couple continued to live under the same roof to the present time with their youngest child despite the absence of social and sexual intercourse. According to the patient, this situation had been going on for so long that he really does not seem to notice it. He has no interests or activities at home, apart from repairs and things of that nature, and now his social life was entirely outside the home in the physical activities that he most enjoyed.

The consultation centered around the traumatic effect of the death of his son some 3 years before in the motorcycle accident. This son, very much the apple of his eye, was brought up to be as good a cyclist as his father who, as a police motorcyclist, was extremely good. Just before the boy's death, Mr. Woodentop had seen that he was repairing his bike himself, and he had had the money to allow him to suggest to his son that he buy the part required. He had not, however, given his son the money, and a few days later the homemade repair had gone wrong and led to the boy's death. The patient went to the hospital after the boy's accident (this was on a weekend, and he was in the country sailing with some friends and not at home with his wife) and stayed with his son until he died, blaming himself for his demise. Later in the same year, he was called again to the same hospital by another policeman in the middle of the night because his second son had an accident in his car and went headfirst through the window after which he looked like "raw meat." These two episodes and the loss of a girlfriend seemed to the patient to be the causes for the acute panics of which he was complaining. These were related to dreams in which he was either flying through the sky or else unable to communicate.

The third loss has been of V., a girlfriend in her mid-20s. She was "a marvelous girl, a keen motor racing cyclist herself, with blonde hair and a powerful bike, who looked great in leathers." When V. eventually betrayed Woodentop for a younger man, he became enraged, threatening her and her new boyfriend with physical violence.

The patient presented himself as a very sensitive, understanding, and thoughtful man who was working in a job far below his real capacities. He seemed to be in touch with his feelings and able to explain to the interviewer that he was actually suffering from a midlife crisis related to guilt and unhappiness over the death of his son.

When I presented the history and a videotape of an interview with Mr. Woodentop at a diagnostic conference, a consensus emerged. Woodentop seemed to be a man who had managed to cope with the lack of genuine relationships in his life through the exercise of a well-functioning manic defense, taking the form of philobatic behavior in various important areas. He had come for help with a midlife crisis in which the identification with both his son who had died and his girlfriend who had obviously taken the place of his son had been disrupted by their respective deaths and desertion. His panic feelings and depression seemed to be the result of an intense conflict between aggression toward those lost objects and the wish to preserve them. Having spent so much of his life expressing himself in physical activities, he might not have the appropriate verbal capacities to express these conflicts in a therapy situation.

Evidence of true resolution of Mr. Woodentop's problems would be indicated by the following changes:

1. Working through his grief and guilt concerning the death of his son
2. Coming to terms with his actual chronological age and the abandonment of compulsive sexual and athletic activities
3. Maintaining a stable and satisfying sexual life rather than one in which he used women primarily as receptacles
4. Developing the capacity to behave with compassion and love toward those close to him
5. Accepting the more passive and loving side of his nature rather

than the maniacally determined aggressive impulses that seemed
to predominate at the moment

6. Accepting support from others rather than continually relying on
   himself and his exploits for solace

Specific midlife factors were prominent. Woodentop was aging. He
had reached a point where retirement from the police force was a consideration. Further, three of his children had left home and only a 16-
year-old daughter remained. Life had brought him to the point where
he was no longer the father of a young family and was therefore free,
if he wished, to leave his unrewarding marriage. Instead of being able
to identify with a much loved son and live and work out his own disappointments through that son's achievements, he had lost him. He
seemed faced with the choice of either mourning what was lost in many
different ways and finding a new beginning or else restructuring his
character around depression, anger, and emptiness and taking an increasingly paranoid view of the world.

The conference felt that therapy should be directed toward the ventilation of grief and guilt related to the son's death because if he were
enabled to do this he would be much freer to deal with the other problems outlined before. This was felt to be the appropriate focus for a brief
intervention that would promote the emergence of more developmentally appropriate coping mechanisms.

The Therapy

Mr. Woodentop began with a contract for 15 sessions with the focus as suggested above. The first few sessions were devoted to working through the very strong intellectual defenses that were sharpened
by the patient's skills as a police interviewer. He found my method of
work difficult to tolerate, particularly the absence of direct questions or
suggestions as to how he should behave. He gradually revealed himself,
however, as a man who reacted to frustration with an enormous amount
of physical violence, which could find sublimation in his work as a
policeman but which colored all other relationships.

Although I was able to help him get somewhat closer to his grief,
it quickly became clear that he felt it would be girlish to allow himself
to cry in front of me and that he had to keep up the facade of manly
strength at all costs. If we did begin to talk about his feelings, Mr. Woodentop would think himself into the actions that he took when landing

an airplane and used this as a control mechanism so as not to release his emotions.

This fear of loss of control included angry feelings as well. The patient saw his aggression and strength as extremely dangerous to those around him. He told me various stories of assaults on others and destructive acts such as breaking down doors or smashing telephones in half. The transference situation was not an easy one because he treated me as a superior officer and a rigid and unyielding father and was surprised to find that I could be human and tolerant. He felt that this was all wrong because, in my place, he would not behave in such a way. The treatment revolved around this theme of authority and control and the implied threat from him that if I said or did something that he found unacceptable he would assault me. I was more than somewhat apprehensive at times.

Some progress had been made when the 15 sessions terminated, and I subsequently left for a trip. On my return, I found that the patient had been in touch with the clinic asking for an early appointment. It became clear that he had suffered an acute depressive reaction and blind panic attacks during my absence and that the police medical officer was at his wits end to know what to do about him. The same was true for his general practitioner, who was obviously terrified of him: "I would like him under St. Thomas' Hospital with the ECT machine fully charged. I would certainly not like to cross this man; he is physically strong and could well kill someone in a rage." I felt therefore an obligation to take Woodentop back into treatment, and I offered him a further contract for another 30 sessions. At the same time, I wrote to the police suggesting that he go back on light duties. The patient was placed in charge of the communications room at a large police station near his home, where he was extremely successful and recognized as one of the pillars of the organization.

After that time, the work focused more on his midlife problem, which had to do with giving up omnipotent control over those around him and accepting the passive, giving, and generous aspects of his own nature. This placed him in some confusion: On the one hand, he felt the need to control everything and everybody; on the other, he never felt able to trust another person. Before Christmas, he brought me as a joke a cartoon of Father Christmas sitting on a chimney pot with his trousers down. This, of course, exemplified his attitude toward those to whom he gave with such generosity.

In the next year, things moved quite quickly, and the patient became much softer and gentler in his relationships with those around him. He was able to talk more about his wife, who up to that point had been a completely anonymous figure. Woodentop began to plan to divorce her (she was actually capable of living independently of him) as well as apply for retirement from the police force on medical grounds at full pension. He also planned to undertake a course of study in the area that interested him most—marine engineering.

Things seemed to be moving toward a moment when I could begin to work through the termination of the treatment when just before Whitsun he telephoned in great distress, asking to see me. I, of course, agreed to see him, and he told me that the surviving son had what seemed to be a schizophrenic episode while decorating a friend's cottage in North Wales. Woodentop immediately dashed there, fearful that the boy had committed suicide. He found, however, that he had merely wandered off and had been found by the local police and taken to a mental hospital. Fearful of his being hospitalized under an order and thereby stigmatized for life, the father persuaded the doctor to discharge the boy and brought him home. The boy, whom I shall call Stewart, felt that the machines were destroying the world and that we should all go back to nature. After he started smashing his parents' house and garden, wrenching mirrors off cars in the neighborhood, and leaving a trail of damage through the village, he was arrested and sent to a prison hospital for observation. During this time, Woodentop manically repaired all the damage that had been caused but then had to face the recognition there was little if anything he could do in the present situation. This, of course, brought us right back to the present problem of his unresolved grief over his oldest son's death and his inability to do anything about that as well. He began to use the therapy quite constructively, and, in a sense, we were able to rework the original trauma.

Over the next year, things went from bad to worse; Stewart continued ill, smashing up his parents' home so that his father had to call in his own colleagues and charge him. He spent 3 months in prison on remand and then was sent to the local mental hospital for treatment. He seemed to have stabilized on Modecate, and I felt that things had at long last begun to settle down. But last autumn, while I was away on a lecture tour in another country, Stewart, too, was killed—by a railway train after he had broken out of the hospital where he was living. On my return, Woodentop, who had not been in touch with the clinic, came into my office and said, "Stewart's dead." He then told me of the death and burial, his agony and fury with the authorities, but all in a completely unemotional way. I did all I could to help him express his grief and pain, his guilt and rage, but he still could not allow himself to show his tears in front of me. The most effective intervention I made, having seen the extraordinarily good film called *Ordinary People*, which was about a family's reaction to the death of an adolescent son, was to bring it to his attention and suggest he go and see it. He did, accompanied by his current girlfriend who was a nice and caring person. She had the kindness and humanity to hold him all night while he wept for his lost sons after seeing the film. Although he could tell me of this experience and be grateful to me for helping him acknowledge it, he could never let go enough to experience the same sadness and despair with me.

During the past year, he was tested even further because his wife, about whom he feels responsible and guilty, became seriously ill with renal failure and eventually needed a kidney transplant. The police medical service wished to retire him on medical grounds, but after discussing the matter with my patient, I wrote asking them to keep him on light duties in order to give him financial and organizational support, which they generously did. After his wife recovered, Woodentop agreed to be retired on health grounds from the force. His plan was to sell the house and split the money, setting his wife up with her half, and using his half to build a boat and sail it to the Mediterranean where he would lead a philobatic life, never staying on one place long enough to become really involved. I think that, given his despair, his continual attempt to prove that he is stronger than fate and the terrible blows that life has dealt him, like Tennyson's Ulysses he will,

> Push off, and sitting well in order smite
> The sounding furrows; for my purpose holds
> To sail beyond the sunset, and the baths
> Of all the western stars, until I die.
> It may be that the gulfs will wash us down...

I think it entirely possible that I will hear one day that he has drowned.

Helga

Mr. Woodentop is not alone in this situation. At the Tavistock, I have seen six people who have suffered in the same way. Helga, a 55-year-old well-organized social worker was another of them. She came to the clinic referred by a relative shortly after the suicide of her only son of 21. He had been assessed by us a year earlier, was considered unsuitable for outpatient psychotherapy, and was referred for inpatient treatment. A student, he had "blown his mind with LSD." When Helga was seen by one of our consultants she told him that her depression and despair were irremediable, declaring that she wished to commit suicide and would do so once her son's affairs were cleared up. He told her that we could not stop her, but that I, as the person most senior and most interested in the problems of later life, would like to work with her.

Helga was born in Eastern Europe of a wealthy family. After both parents were killed by the Nazis, she spent her adolescence bravely fighting for the Resistance. After the war, she came to England and married a man much older than herself. He had died 18 months earlier. Helga had made a good career in the social services and was an acknowledged expert on battered children. Her life had been bound up with her very intelligent only son, who carried her hopes for a brilliant career. With his death, she felt there was little or nothing left to live for. I could see that to help Helga, she and I would have to confront some fairly appalling experiences if we were to get behind her main defenses and face the depression. We worked together for about 6 months, at times at quite a deep level. I always made sure that attention was available and that the consultant who had seen her originally was on call during my absences. I was away over Christmas, so that he had been seeing her. When I returned from holiday, I learned that she had killed herself, having wound up her son's affairs. She left a note for the coroner, absolving the consultant and me of any blame. We had tried, she said, but she had not wished to continue to live.

It was clear that her son had represented her immortality and that with his death she felt that she had nothing left to live for. I certainly could not offer her hope or any material change in her appalling circumstances. All I could do was try and share her life review and work with her on trying to reconstruct her defenses. I was prepared to go through the horrors with her if she wished. I had no option but to accept her final choice, and perhaps do her the small service of containing my anger at her destruction of the creative aspects of me and her retaliation for the way life had treated her.

There is one more person to report, who was not a member of my sample. Sigmund Freud lost his beloved daughter Sophie in the epidemic of Spanish influenza at the end of the World War I.

Telling Ferenczi of the bad news, he added: "As for us? My wife is quite over-whelmed. I think: *La séance continue*. But it was a little much for one week." Writing a little later to Eitington, who as usual had been as helpful as possi-ble, he described his reaction: "I do not know what more there is to say. It is such a paralyzing event, which can stir no afterthoughts when one is not a believer and so is spared all the conflicts that go with that. Blunt necessity, mute submission." (Jones, 1957, p. 19)

Jones adds,

In the same month something happened that had a profound effect on Freud's spirits for the rest of his life. His grandchild, Heinerle [Heinz Rudolf], Sophie's second child, had been spending several months in Vienna with his Aunt Mathilde. Freud was extremely fond of the boy, whom he called the most in-telligent child he had ever encountered. He had had his tonsils removed about the time of Freud's first operation on his mouth, and when the two patients first met after their experiences he asked his grandfather with great interest: "I can already eat crusts. Can you too?" Unfortunately the child was very delicate, "a bag of skin and bones," having contracted tuberculosis in the country in the previous year. He died of miliary tuberculosis, aged four and a half, on June 19th. It was the only occasion in his life when Freud was known to shed tears. He told me afterwards that this loss had affected him in a different way from any of the others he had suffered. They had brought about sheer pain, but this one had killed something in him for good. The loss must have struck something peculiarly deep in his heart, possibly reaching even so far back as the little Julius of his childhood. A couple of years later he told Marie Bonaparte that he had never been able to get fond of anyone since that misfortune, merely retaining his old attachments; he had found the blow quite unbearable, much more so than his own cancer. In the following month he wrote saying he was suffering from the first depression in his life, and there is little doubt that this may be ascribed to that loss, coming so soon as it did after the first intimations of his own lethal affliction. Three years later, on consoling with Binswanger whose eldest son had died, he said that Heinerle had stood to him for all children and grandchildren. Since his death *he had not been able to enjoy life* [italics added]; he added: "It is the secret of my indifference—people call it courage—towards the danger to my own life." (pp. 91–92)

SUMMARY

I have tried to describe some patients whose problems and their elu-cidation in the transference have led me toward a better understanding of the developmental psychology of the last years of life. I have found useful the notion that the primal scene is not merely a sexual fantasy of parental intercourse but rather that the notion may be expanded to ac-count for the problems that many people have in facing the idea of their own death or the death of a spouse. The anger, pain, and incredulity that have to be worked through, together with the narcissistic injury involved, face the individual with as much of a problem as the notion of a parental intercourse that excludes him or her. It may well be that, just as the acceptance of a sexual relationship that excludes the child and diminishes his or her grandiose view of himself or herself may release creativity and foster independent thinking, so acceptance of death, of the reality of one's own end and of extinction, may curtail the ordinary omnipotence of thought from which we all suffer and promote what Erikson has called integrity at the expense of despair.

Older people are remarkably easy to work with in the analytic situation, but my experience does suggest a caveat as far as the special group who have lost children are concerned. As I see it, these people have suffered a narcissistic wound that can never be healed. Instead of being able to hand on the best parts of themselves to their descendants, they have to accept a real caesura, a break in the chain that in psychological terms is generally irreparable. Although the therapist can be parent, love object, or child in the transference, there seems to be no way in which we can help the patient restore and repair the lost object of his or her projections and idealizations when the child actually dies. Even for those whose children go mad, there is still the hope that they will regain their sanity. But where there is no hope, we have to accept that all that might have been potentially there can no longer be. It seems to me that these people, because they can no longer hope to immortalize themselves, throw into relief the problems that face the rest of us—the reality of our own deaths. Through the existence of our own children and grandchildren who will be the receptacles for the immortal parts of ourselves, a sort of psychological gene plasm, we hope to live forever!

REFERENCES

Berezin, M. Psychodynamic considerations of aging and the aged: An overview. *American Journal of Psychiatry*, 1972, *128*, 33–41.

Erikson, E. H. Elements of a psychoanalytic theory of psychosocial development. In S. I. Greenspan & G. Pollock (Eds.), *The course of life (Vol. I): Infancy and early childhood*. Washington, D.C.: U.S. Department of Health and Human Services, 1981.

Grotjahn, M. The day I became old: The story of a physician. *Lancet*, February 20, 1982, pp. 441–442.

Jones, E. *Sigmund Freud—Life and work (Vol. III). The last phase 1919–1939*. London: Hogarth, 1957.

Scott, W. C. M. Personal communication, 1982.

Winnicott, D. W. *Playing and Reality*. London: Hogarth, 1973.

12

When a Husband Dies

MALKAH T. NOTMAN

Mrs. G., a 65-year-old woman, was referred by a colleague who is also a friend of her family. Her husband, a well-known lawyer who was active in community affairs, had been diagnosed as having a malignancy. It was not clear what his course would be, and although he seemed to be in remission, their daughter had turned to friends to look for some potential help for her mother.

Mrs. G. presented as a trim, conservatively dressed woman with a relaxed, open manner. She had never had any experience with psychotherapy, nor had she had any recognized emotional problems. Her husband was known to have little respect for psychiatry in general and would not have felt he could support her psychotherapy under any circumstances other than those of his life-threatening illness; there was a tacit agreement between them that they did not discuss this.

He was 69, 4 years her senior, and they had been married 43 years earlier. All during her husband's successful career, Mrs. G. had been seen as an adaptable woman who was willing to move around with him, attend activities with him, and join him as he moved up the professional ladder. It was clear that she was perceived as somebody who was rather dependent and whose life was organized around her husband's choices. Her daughter felt that Mrs. G. would need some preparation for her husband's death and the period afterward. His death seemed fairly remote at the time of referral because he was relatively well, but Mrs. G. spoke freely and openly about the issues.

We began treatment with the goal of becoming acquainted and agreed to meet on a monthly basis for the time being. Although he had formally retired, Mr. G. was still very active professionally and often traveled for consultations; thus, the timing of our sessions was influenced by their plans.

Mrs. G. began by telling me about her family. She was the middle of three children and had been brought up in the suburbs of a large eastern city. At that time the area was predominantly gentile, and her parents wanted a more Jewish environment for the family; so they moved closer to the city. Her sister, who was 6 years older, had always been a bright and accomplished woman; she was married to a successful physician and lived nearby. This sister was clearly very important in Mrs. G.'s life. She had "opinions about everything," and Mrs. G. turned to her often for advice. She compared herself with her sister and felt herself to be much less ambitious and less concerned with the overt signs of success and achievement, which seemed important both to her sister and to her own husband. Her brother was an architect who lived at some distance, and their relationship was not very close.

As a child, Mrs. G. had been shy, somewhat retiring, and felt "dumb." She spent the first year of school in a large public school where she was neither very successful academically nor aggressive enough to belong to the prominent social group; she felt extremely lonely. Later she transferred to another, much smaller school where she thought the other children were not as bright as they had been in the earlier school; by contrast, she felt more competent there. She became much happier and more self-assured. She remembered vividly the growing realization that she was not "dumb" after all, but she remained essentially noncompetitive, although she was a good and well-behaved student.

After high school, Mrs. G. went to a prestigious women's college. There she did well, formed her first close friends, and began to date. She had been "going with" somebody who seemed very lively and interesting and had a sense of humor, but for some reason she did not feel ready to marry him, and when he pressed her for a decision, she broke off the relationship. She met her husband some time later. She remembers his warmth, his obviously promising future, and his overall appeal for her. Her family liked him immediately, and she herself felt they went well together. They married and to all intents and purposes had a very happy marriage. She looked back on her marriage many times during therapy and only gradually changed her view of it. At first she said that they were doing very well at the present time but that during the years when he was greatly ambitious, although she never let on, she had not been as happy. Later, she spoke of the good years when the family was young and when she felt they were closer than in later years. Later still, she developed a more positive retrospective view of the later years.

After marrying, Mrs. G. worked briefly, but she stopped working after her children were born. She did do volunteer work in a number of organizations and valued that immensely. However, she could not sustain a relationship with any organization because of her husband's frequent trips and his expectation that she would accompany him.

They had two children, one son and a daughter who was born 4 years later. The daughter had felt both that she was not as attractive as her sibling and that she was unsuccessful in gaining her father's attention as compared to her brother. She was resentful and rebellious, and only after many years and some psychotherapy felt comfortable with herself and her life. She was the person who persuaded her mother to seek help.

Mrs. G. described her life as being centered around the children and their school and community activities when they were young. They lived in a large house in an attractive neighborhood close to her sister (where she herself had spent her childhood). In actuality, she had not liked it much and was relieved when they were able to move to another suburb and a more modest house, which incidentally, was farther from her sister's. Her father had died a few years before that move. For several years her mother lived with the G.'s. Mrs. G.'s mother was very fond of Mr. G., and she regarded him as "the generous person" in the family because of his agreeing to have his mother-in-law live with him. However, he was not home much, and therefore did not have to deal with her on a daily basis.

Mrs. G.'s relationship with her mother had been fairly harmonious. She said with some surprise that they really had very few of the tensions that existed between her and her own daughter during the daughter's adolescence, or between other mothers and daughters, including those between her own sister and mother. She had also been very fond of her father and felt close to him, although he worked hard as a tailor and, as she looked back at those years, she thought he had not been very available to her.

DESCRIPTION OF THE THERAPEUTIC PROCESS

We met monthly for about 1½ years. The first sessions were spent describing the outlines of the family's life, her personal history, and filling in the details of the family's current concerns. I listened with the intent to make her feel comfortable and diminish the strangeness of the situation. When I said something that she could not fit into her understanding of things, she would say to me, "I'm not hearing you" or "That doesn't quite fit for me," making it clear that she felt reluctant to accept what I was saying, not just that she did not understand it.

In the initial session, Mrs. G. talked in some detail about her husband's illness. At first, the malignancy was thought to be confined to its primary site but later some extension was discovered. He had been treated with chemotherapy and radiation and seemed to be in remission, but at the time of the initial consultation, she had felt "low" and her mind jumped to "the worst."

She was still reluctant to think about getting some help for herself, but a good friend whose husband was also a prominent lawyer with some of the same bias against psychotherapy that Mr. G. had supported her decision. So it turned out that the patient had support from her daughter, her son, her friend, and, unexpectedly, her husband. He spoke realistically to her about his prognosis, and she realized that, although he was currently in a remission, it was unclear what path the illness would take. His denial was also probably obvious because he clung to his round of busy commitments, public appearances, and extended plans.

Mrs. G. recalled the onset of his symptoms. They had been visiting one of their children, and her husband had been scheduled to make a public appearance in another state. He had what he thought was the flu and seemed to be recovering but was not getting well as fast as he should have been. She was startled when he canceled the talk because she knew how important "those things" were for him. They returned home; he was carefully examined, and it was then that the diagnosis was made. She described his treatment in some detail and his reactions each time he had radiation or chemotherapy. It was very unlike him to express disappointment or discouragement. During all that time, she was the good wife, fulfilling a nursing, caring, and supportive role.

She talked about his past life and their relationship in some detail. He was a kind person but had really paid very little attention to the minutia of their daily life. In the first session, she hinted at the problems there had been in the marriage; for example, those deriving from her husband's ambition and his style, which meant that they did not talk much in intimate, personal terms. However, she had not thought that she could do very much about that.

Mr. G. used to get up very early to prepare for work. He would often travel. Only much later was she aware of the toll that took on their intimacy and sexual closeness and able to speak to him about it. After the children were older, he would take her with him on trips. She always went; it was regarded *by others* as a great honor for her and a source of enjoyment to visit exotic places where his office had clients or where he was invited to give some presentation or receive an honor.

For a time, probably because of the limits on his activity created by his illness, his availability and responsiveness to her and her help were comforting and seemed to lead to an improvement in their relationship. In some way they seemed to fit the classic pattern of the aging couple in which the man expects to be cared for at a later phase of his life, having fulfilled his earlier ambitions, and in which the wife returns to a caring and nurturing role because a commitment to a life of her own has not been solidly developed.

After a few months, the contrast between his current emotional availability and relative communicativeness and his previous style became apparent. They spent time talking over many shared past experiences, and she increasingly and openly described to him her feelings from the past, of which he had clearly been unaware. I encouraged her to do this. She felt as if her perspective sharpened and that feelings of which she had been aware in a fragmentary fashion coalesced.

Within the first few sessions an interesting additional issue emerged. Because the "main problem," Mr. G.'s illness, was quiescent, Mrs. G. started to talk about her older sister and, as she did so, became aware of a constellation she labeled a *paradox*. She felt that her feelings about her sister really were the kind that many people have about their mothers; the sister was domineering, perfectionistic, and always wanted things done right. She tended to pressure the patient. The sister had a daughter of her own who had had some emotional difficulties, but she seemed to be managing at the time. Mrs. G. contrasted her own children with her sister's. Her own children were married, and their marriages seemed relatively harmonious. The grandchildren were doing well, and there were considerable warmth and family loyalty and closeness. She had felt much closer to her daughter than to her son who had been more overtly successful in marriage and in achieving a higher standard of living, but there was a relatively comfortable relationship between Mrs. G. and her son as well. The son lived much closer than the daughter. Her son and his wife had a life-style that exhibited more permissiveness toward their children, less conventional patterns, and somewhat more radical ideas than did the life-style of her daughter's family. Mrs. G. felt a bit less comfortable with them and felt that he was not as communicative as her daughter. In part, she connected this with his identification with his father, and in part she felt it was related to a serious illness he had mastered successfully as a child but that seemed to make him reluctant to face any serious illness in a close family member.

In the therapy sessions, Mrs. G. returned to the topic of her sister and gradually realized how angry she was at her and how resentful she had been at some of the pressures. For years Mrs. G. had felt she was "being pushed around." For example, at one point while she was in therapy there was a large family party that she and her sister were giving jointly. She had wanted to participate by cooking some of the dishes, arranging for the flowers, and taking care of other details. Her sister agreed, but when Mrs. G. arrived to participate in her share of the activities, she found that her sister had already made all the arrangements. This made her very angry. She realized that in the past what she would have done would have been to find some excuse for her sister, rationalizing that her sister's perfectionism made it uncomfortable for her to give up control and permit anyone else to take part. However, this time, with encouragement, she decided that it really distressed her and made her feel angry and excluded. This was a chronic pattern in their relationship. She expressed these feelings to her sister, who was quite surprised. Mrs. G. then arranged for a luncheon with her sister during which she tried to communicate more fully how she had felt about these issues during the many years of their relationship. At the end of this meeting, Mrs. G. felt shaken and very tearful. She was frightened that she might have driven her sister away and blamed herself for alienating her. However, in reality, her sister was not put off and was reassuring to Mrs. G., acknowledging that she had strengths of her own, including the loyalty and success of her children. This problem was not resolved with one confrontation, needless to say, but Mrs. G. felt for the first time that she could be in a position of strength with her sister.

A change began in their relationship, in which Mrs. G. began to confront her sister about many such maneuvers. She gradually felt that her sister understood her better and regarded her more highly. She also found an unexpected ally in her brother-in-law who supported her in some decisions and family negotiations. One crisis involved some money that had been left to them jointly by their parents and for which they had to work out some disposition. Instead of accepting the plans that had been developed by her sister, Mrs. G. requested that they be renegotiated, and another solution was found more in keeping with her wishes.

Because of his illness, Mrs. G.'s husband spent much time at home. This resulted in greater interaction and communication between them. For about the first 6 months, the illness preoccupied them, but in addition, long-standing patterns of noncommunication made changes difficult. However, Mrs. G. began to describe to me and even to her husband in greater detail some of the stresses she had felt in the relationship. She felt that they had made decisions essentially on the basis of her husband's needs or the children's needs but never on her needs.

Mrs. G. had been aware of having a streak of stubbornness and a temper and had on occasion snapped at him or at someone else publicly. Sometimes, these outbursts seemed unpredictable, and afterward she felt very embarrassed. One such incident provided a good example for dynamic understanding of this pattern. Her husband had been honored by a group of people who had worked with him and to whom he was very devoted, as they were to him, and a dinner was planned for him. At the same time, a public ceremony was planned at another civic function where he was to speak and to receive an award. The award and the speech carried much prestige. Mrs. G. felt that the dinner the small group had planned was very genuine and personal, much more so than the more public occasion. They worked out an arrangement whereby it was possible for them to attend both events. At the gathering preceding the civic honor, a member of the smaller group was talking with her and her husband when someone came up and diverted them with some detail about the larger ceremony. Her husband was distracted, and she found herself snapping at him to pay attention to the man who had started the conversation. She sensed this was rude, could not understand what was going on, and felt that she had embarrassed everyone concerned. When we discussed it, she pieced together an understanding of the incident as a symbolic competition between feelings that were genuine and personal (that she valued highly and identified as representing such parts of his life as his family, the children, her own feelings, and, in general, relationships and feelings) and the ambition, competitiveness, prestige, and success that was represented by the public civic ceremony. When he seemed to be more attentive to the latter, she not only felt he was insufficiently appreciative of the others but also as if it was a rebuff to the values for which she stood and that she felt he had long neglected. She tried to communicate this to him and felt that he did understand what she was saying. However, it was more important for her to begin to understand some of her perplexing outbursts and alliances than to convey this to him.

She had developed a transference response to me as someone who could bridge both worlds, who knew the world of her sister and her husband's affairs but was also sympathetic to her needs and in some way allied with her daughter. She nevertheless gave me warnings when she felt I was pushing too hard or she was not prepared to absorb what I had to say. I think that if I had not been linked to a professional community with which her husband was affiliated, I might not have been seen as an "insider," and there might have been more mistrust. At the same time, the facts that I was younger and in a field related to that of her daughter, and that we met in an office that was at my home diminished the formality of the relationship.

My countertransference feelings were certainly affected by the status and accomplishments of her family and her husband. However, I was soon enormously impressed by her capacity for honesty, insight, and change. It seemed to me unusual that someone her age would be able to negotiate a major change in her relationship with her sister and to become expressive toward the man with whom she had lived lifelong in relative silence. I then realized my own stereotypes about age and psychic rigidity.

Certainly the roles of Mrs. G. and her husband had changed; he was no longer the tower of strength; *he needed her.* She felt some power resulting from his dependency and also some anxiety because he was no longer as strong a figure for her to depend on. This seems characteristic of the changes described for older couples even without illness (Troll & Turner, 1979), where the husband begins to look for care from his wife whereas she wants communication, warmth, love, and/or sex.

Through the years, Mrs. G. had maintained some contact with her college friends, and where possible she now resumed some of these connections with an eye to the future when she might be alone. Despite my encouraging her to fill her life with some activities, she found it difficult to return to the volunteer jobs because so many changes had occurred in those organizations that she no longer felt she belonged.

Other issues emerged. One incident involved some unexplained anger she felt toward her daughter. She could not understand it but felt very irritable with her and could hardly speak with her on the telephone when she called. Because we were meeting infrequently at that period, many events took place between the meetings, but she used our meeting time extremely well to explore the interactions that had led to the strain. They appeared to involve a competitive struggle between two of her grandchildren. One of them had become aware of some dependent feelings toward her parents and had made demands on them that Mrs. G. resented. They were able to resolve this, and she developed some insight into some of their past difficulties.

Following a trip to another city, she recalled some earlier travels. One year in particular had been a miserable one. Her husband had been asked to help with setting up a new business office in what was supposed to be a lovely area. However, no one had consulted her about the house that was obtained for them, and it turned out to be poorly suited for comfortable living, although it was well located with respect to her husband's work. She had never felt that she could have a say in those arrangements. When another trip was proposed shortly after this topic arose, she insisted that either she would stay home or, if they went together, she would take part in activities that interested her.

Communication with her husband continued to improve, and her feeling was that something had shifted in his values as he spent more time with her and at home. She felt also that the importance of his relationships with his children, grandchildren, and her had also increased. However, there was some recurrence of the old style. Once, when he was feeling physically weak, Mr. G. was asked to appear at a civic banquet as a speaker; she realized this meant much to him, and she worked very hard to make it possible. It took considerable planning. In the enthusiasm of the moment following the occasion, he invited a number of people to go home with them. She felt very irritated but responded and took care of the guests. Afterward, she was very angry with him for not being aware of how much effort the whole activity had cost her. She was freer to express her feelings in spite of the fact that he was ill.

In the face of her latent concern about the destructive potential of her aggressive feelings, Mr. G. also was undergoing some changes. He told her that he had never realized how much it had cost her to accompany him on trips, or how much effort she had expended to simply keep things going, or that she minded the strain. It had not occurred to him that she might have undeveloped and unexpressed wishes, expectations, and goals of her own, particularly because she characterized herself as unambitious, which seemed to imply that she was happy to be compliant. She did, indeed, behave in an accommodating, facilitating, and compliant manner but actually was a person with strong feelings about her own desires and reactions.

Mr. G.'s illness had remissions and relapses. A new lesion would be discovered and then he would respond to some form of treatment. Each time he maintained a certain level of well-being and enthusiasm. Once, however, she saw a look of anxiety in his eyes, and she was very shaken by this indication of vulnerability. It seemed to her that this was the beginning of the end. Outwardly, things had continued as they had before. The pace of traveling, community affairs, and talks diminished somewhat, although, as his health seemed to be failing more, honors continued to be bestowed on him. Because they were in town more consistently, she decided that she wanted to increase her psychotherapy visits. After almost a year and three quarters, she began to come almost weekly, a schedule that was interrupted by various events in their lives and in my schedule. She further consolidated her relationships with her children and their spouses, although not without some friction.

One important event was the celebration of her birthday. She had always valued her birthday, and it was sometimes overlooked in the family priorities. This time she said she really wanted the celebration to be as she wanted it, and the whole family gathered at a resort. It was a delightful occasion for her, particularly because she had been clear enough about her wishes to express them explicitly. Therefore plans could be made in advance, thus assuring their success.

After about the second year of Mrs. G.'s therapy, Mr. G.'s illness seemed to worsen. His status was not clear, and he was hospitalized for some further diagnostic work. He died suddenly about a week later. She missed several psychotherapy visits. She had handled all the arrangements and details appropriately, but she was upset about the events just preceding Mr. G.'s death. At the beginning of the diagnostic hospitalization, she had been angry with him because of his behavior; he had isolated himself from everyone, including her. She regretted her anger as she later realized that he had neither the strength nor the capacity to relate to anyone at that time. She had been with him when he died.

All in all, it had been enormously helpful for her to recognize the resentment of past years and to bring about a closer relationship before he died. She then had to mourn and afterwards to develop her own priorities. The first phase after her husband's death was one of coping. Therapy helped her to deal with the immediate demands and rearrangement of her daily patterns, adapting to the loss of previous routines, and responding to friends and condolences. It was not until she visited one of her children that she was able to respond with the full extent of her feelings of loss. When talking with her daughter about what kind of father her husband had been and becoming aware of the extent to which their grandchildren valued him, she realized that they knew he cared for them in spite of the relatively sparse communication.

She also responded in a particularly sensitive manner to sympathy letters that were addressed to her as an individual and that acknowledged her feelings or her needs and letters that referred to their marriage, rather than those that eulogized her husband's contributions and referred to his stature in the community. She was able to set limits that seemed appropriate as to how much she could tolerate at the time from contacts with relatives and friends, which she felt she could not have done previously. After several months of mourning, she began to want more contact with some of her husband's friends, and she explored and sought out those relationships that were meaningful to her. She also restored relationships with some of her old friends, many of whom were also widows. She began to think about moving from the house that she and her husband had shared, having always planned to simplify her living arrangements after he died. However, she realized that she was not yet ready to give up the house and for the time being resisted the pressure from family and friends to move, although she started to explore alternatives.

Mrs. G. was clearly a woman with considerable strengths, intellectual as well as emotional resources, sensitivity, warmth, and the capacity for insight. She had some obsessive-compulsive personality features, which meshed well with her husband's personality style. Because of social expectations and because of anxiety about her own ambition and aggression, she did not choose a life of competitive striving and achievement but was the model wife to an ambitious, successful, professional man and civic leader. The strains, however, became apparent and could have left her guilty and embittered.

She was unlikely to have sought psychiatric help because of her self-concept of being a strong person and her husband's devaluation of psychiatry if there had not been the stimulus of his illness and then consistent encouragement from a family member. In the course of the psychotherapy, which was initially designed to be a preparation for living alone and for adaptation to the loss of her husband, she made some important discoveries about herself, with genuine insights. These included reevaluating her relationship to her sister and gaining understanding of her relationships to her children and her husband. She was able to become more aware of her needs, more assertive, and in the process less given to previously occurring irrational outbursts of embarrassing and inappropriate anger. Although she had an appropriate depression at the loss of her husband, she also had support for recovery and finding priorities of her own that needed to be explored and developed further.

I found it unusual and remarkable for this amount of change to take place in the brief time we worked together. I had expected a more focused and limited response because of the nature of the problem and her age. It was impressive and gratifying to me as a therapist to have an expression of puzzlement change to one of illumination with the words, "Oh, I see what you mean," and then a reformulation that confirmed some clarification I had made. Mrs. G. also had an unusual capacity to pursue issues and to avoid simple rationalizations. She would be aware of contradictory feelings or of having some ideas and responses that seemed inconsistent with others, and she would explore them with energy and persistence until something was clarified and seemed to fit. This process resulted in changes in her mood and at times in her behavior. There were certainly effects on her day-to-day life. She developed new awareness of other people's motivations and of her meaning to her and to her husband. She was sensitive to ambition, conflict, and feelings of rejection and became clearer about both the assets and the problems of the adaptations she had made.

She has thought carefully and sensitively about where her ongoing supports might be and how to make them effective. She seemed prepared to encounter what lay before her, to approach feelings honestly, reassess her past feelings and judgments, assess her own needs, and try to arrange her life to meet them.

REFERENCE

Troll, L. E., & Turner, B. F. Sex differences in problems of aging. In E. S. Gomberg & V. Franks (Eds.), *Gender and disordered behavior*. New York: Brunner/Mazel, 1979.

13

When a Wife Dies

STANLEY H. CATH AND CLAIRE CATH

In keeping with the flexibility advocated by the senior author in psychoanalytic psychotherapy with the long lived (Cath, 1982), individual treatment of a 57-year-old man was converted to conjoint therapy with his wife and the therapist's wife. The shift was considered advisable for several reasons. From the patient's point of view, his therapist "had been through it with him before," by which he referred to the time when cancer had reappeared in his 56-year-old wife's second breast. Later, with the onset of her ominous back pains, he found his terrifyingly calm wife adamant about her choice of someone to consult, namely, *his* therapist. In their discussions, it became clear to him that through his 2 years of therapy, she had developed a "silent positive transference" based upon his sharing much of what he learned about his interactions with his families of origin and of generation. Reinforcing their decision to come together was the gratitude he and his wife felt for the therapist's clarifications and interpretations of the surgeon's verbal and nonverbal behavior, for example, turning his back to them as he talked, especially after her destiny had been sealed by the pathologist's report.

From the therapist's point of view, it seemed reasonable to agree to this appeal for conjoint work, but he felt he needed help and balance in an extremely emotional therapeutic task. It had been the case that his wife had been through a similar biopsy that turned out to be benign; she was more fortunate in that her surgeon, to be sure under less stress, had been equally benign. This common ground as well as the confusion patients feel in deciphering the strange ways some physicians deal with their own helplessness in the face of defeat had been shared with the

241

patient, and he in turn had shared this understanding with his wife. In retrospect, it is likely these earlier interactions set the stage for the conjoint therapeutic alliance in the presence of death that was to follow. Of equal if not greater significance, the initial therapist was overwhelmed by the unfairness of it all, not only to his patient but to the wife who had been reconstructed in the therapist's mind through her husband's mental representations as an unusually bright, considerate, self-possessed, and admirable woman. He recognized that he had developed a positive countertransference to both husband and wife but knew from past experiences that with couples this tended to have oedipal overtones. Thus, he suggested that a co-therapist might be helpful, especially if the wife might want some separate time of her own, which was an accurate anticipation. This form of conjoint treatment of a man and his wife by a man and his wife was considered consistently helpful by the couple, and it was particularly so to the initial psychotherapist dealing with the overwhelmingly complex countertransference race against therapeutic time engendered when death threatened to enter his patient's life.

THE INITIAL PHASE OF INDIVIDUAL PSYCHOTHERAPY

In the early 1800s, in Russia, a father died when his son was but 2 years of age. A few years later, his wife remarried, but the new stepfather refused to take her child. Put out to live with various aunts and uncles, the boy longed for a home and vowed that when he grew up no child of his would be without a father or be sent away. True to his word, he sired six children. Then, at the prime of his life, destiny decreed he abandon his children. Late getting home from the market on a Friday night, he stopped at sunset to pray at the side of the road. Three Cossacks on horseback spied the Jew praying. After teasing him unmercifully, they finally cut off his head. It is alleged his widow took to her bed, never to leave it again. The older children, including the father of my patient, replaced the mother in the home and the father in the fields, whereas the younger ones found jobs in nearby villages. As my patient Jack related this history of "father's raising himself," he emphasized the paradox that this man had seemed to him dependent and weak. His strength resided in the ability to arrange for stronger women, older sisters or a wife to serve him. More than a tragic family myth, this story of Jack's grandfather's death had been elaborated over the years into a justification for many of the feelings of angry deprivation and intense Jewish identity that smoldered beneath the surface of current familial relationships.

My first contact with Jack occurred in the late 1960s in a clinical setting, which was significant in terms of later transference implications. In his early 50s, he was the oldest of a group of psychiatric residents, all of whom were young enough to be his children. He readily revealed that after a series of anginal episodes he had given up a thriving, demanding family practice in a large eastern city to enter "the more relaxed field of psychiatry." Faced by the realities of a new, if not more taxing career, he was even more depressed. Unable to concentrate, he had fallen behind in his work, started to overeat, and gained weight. This was particularly alarming because both his father and brother had died of coronary attacks in their mid-50s. Although one EKG indicated a questionable myocardial occlusion, for him the death knell had rung. He fantasized that, like his grandfather, he would leave children without a father in the not too distant future.

Remembering a discussion of my paper on depletion anxiety in which the "midlife ego" is depicted as spending more and more time and energy monitoring age-specific psychophysiological changes in the body, he began to reflect upon his own postcoronary "hypertrophied sensor." Indeed, he realized how constantly he had been preoccupied with every physiological message of age that related organic change from within. In the second year of his residency, at the age of 54 and unable to concentrate or learn as quickly as he expected, he worried about early-onset dementia. These anxieties were alleviated by the suggestion that most of his psychic energy might be taken up with anticipating another dreaded catastrophe. My theory of depletion drain of energies seemed to be a more accurate acceptable assessment than his self-diagnosis of an endogenous depression and organic brain disease.

After his residency was over, at the age of 55, he asked for a consultation to consider psychotherapy. In our first interview, Jack explained that he was poorly prepared for the shift from a financially successful family practice of medicine to the field of psychiatry. Furthermore, explicating his isolation, old as well as new friends regarded him as radical, difficult to influence, and perhaps a bit too vocal in expressing his liberal views especially on sexuality. Several affairs with wives of colleagues had predated his coronary and career switch. These relations had not only complicated his life, but had added to the burning humiliation frequently verbalized by his tired and strained wife, Marsha. In contrast to his many grateful, admiring patients, in his mind she saw him as a despicable, hypocritical weakling, much as he had regarded his father. Following outbursts of rage at her attempts to reform him, he would become penitent, self-critical, and withdrawn for days. In his mind, he was passionate and political; she was disdainfully aloof and above it all. He considered her mainline ancestry and his Jewish ghetto backgrounds "one hundred and eighty degrees apart."

In this regard, although Jack knew that Marsha's manners, which so drew him to her when they first met, were still impeccable, he had come to regard them as supercilious attempts to manipulate him and the family. In part, he had always felt the children as well as himself were rebelling against these perfectionistic standards. In their arguments, she would remind him that her family considered their marriage unwise and beneath her dignity. Because of this narcissistic devaluation, gaining in-laws had not enhanced his self-respect. Like those of many couples in midlife, their marriage had become one of increasing complementary polarity. He was outspoken, crude but isolated; she was well mannered, sophisticated, and tactful enough to gather a circle of friends outside their relationship.

Disappointing Children

I gradually learned what Jack had meant by his "life collapsing." His history read like a crisis in slow motion. His oldest daughter, "molested" and impregnated by an older baby-sitter, had had an abortion 1 month prior to his first cardiac episode. Six months earlier, his son had received emergency room treatment for a drug overdose. The family's efforts to "talk him out of both soft and hard drugs" failed miserably. Overhearing some neighbors talking about "that doctor's son," Jack felt publicly humiliated. His younger daughter seemed "in the clear...too good to be true." But considerable apprehension about her was aroused when a teacher remarked, "Maybe still waters run deep."

Jack always felt that Marsha, in contrast to his Jewish mother, underestimated the seriousness of their childrens' difficulties. Their son's lack of interest in girls bothered Jack but not his wife. This, combined with indifference toward sports, made him suspect the worst: Was his son just passive or a homosexual? Had drugs seriously damaged his body or mind? In the parents' minds, the oldest daughter's boyfriend had seemed the "worst possible." In summary, Jack considered his body giving way to age, his marriage deteriorating, his son going nowhere if not homosexual, and his elder daughter a prostitute.

Jack's depression and anxiety about body–family integrity had retriggered some old anxiety about impotency. Partly because his physician had not encouraged him to resume sexual activity after his anginal episodes and partly because one of the attacks followed a night in which he and Marsha had fought prior to intercourse, sex, aggression, and angina were linked in his mind. Eventually, his intermittent impotency, combined with a lack of loving concern for his wife, led him to suspect that Marsha might look elsewhere for warmth and gratification.

Jack was rather nice looking, of medium build, if slightly obese, a superficially pleasant man with many assets. His brightness was complemented by a sharp wit. Always able to listen well enough to achieve well on examinations, he had become a concerned physician. But after serving in Korea, Jack found himself extremely unpopular because of his conservative views on the war in Vietnam. In one of their rare political role reversals, Marsha sympathized with the liberal antiwar protesters. Her friends regarded him as a "warnick." Several years had passed before Jack came to understand the deceits involved on both sides. Until he did, he suffered much social ostracism and humiliation. On one particular evening, he argued his case over some cocktails, went to the bathroom and returned to find that everyone, including his wife, had left for the theater without him.

Jack had returned from Korea to find a beautiful, little blond boy added to the family of wife and daughter. He recalled perambulating up and down neighborhood streets with pride swelling in his chest ("qvelling"), certain that the war had been worth the effort. During the early phases of his therapy, he related many stories reflecting his capacity to be altruistic, helpful, and a good citizen. He always had aimed at being the ideal family physician, feeling critical of any failure, lack of knowledge, or error in his judgment. Neither he nor any other physician knew enough. When his angina struck, he thought, "Time is running out...I will never be the perfect man...I might not even see my children get married or have grandchildren." With tears, Jack associated his cardiac episodes to the time his father first developed angina when Jack was in his junior year in high school. His father had died 6 months later, just prior to the economic crisis of 1929.

Catalyzed by the respect with which he regarded the doctor who had first relieved his father's pain, Jack converted his anguish into determination to become an ideal physician. Especially because her situation replicated the anger and rage he felt toward his father's desertion, Jack came to appreciate Marsha's anxiety about a sick man's moving to a new area and starting a new career. Although he had seemed insensitive to her apprehensions, now they caused him great inner pain. When I observed that he seemed more naturally to show his wife only the insensitive side and to conceal his concerns for her, a new phase of therapy ensued. After some time working on his defense of being the always competent physician, father, and husband, he was able to share these insights with her, alleviating some of her distress.

Resistance to Change

Facilitating this improvement was a spontaneous and unwitting intervention that had occurred during one of my teaching sessions. I had made a side comment on the difficulty some older people, including myself, have in changing familiar ground. As an example, I noted the striking contrast between the hawkish attitudes of the "command generation," mostly middle-aged or older men, and the dovish positions of the more youthful protesters. Using myself as an example, in regard to the Vietnam War,[1] I noted how the mature self may be enhanced by holding on to values appropriate in the past for much too long. I cited stories of Einstein's and Freud's resistances to changing their theories, but how with age each of them modulated their positions. He heard all this as empathic with his own position and later told me he had thought to himself that it would be unlikely that I would be overly critical of him. Jack then related both his perfectionistic, stubborn idealism, and his pessimism to his mother, and his militaristic stance to his father's vision that unless violent forces were controlled, people would be slaughtered and "worlds would collide."

There was one other piece of built-in transference; Jack knew of my interest in geriatric psychiatry. It happened that Jack's mother's last days coincided with the period prior to his anginal episode. Five years earlier, after Jack had "refused to take her in," his mother entered a nursing home. He described her as "a bitch," for one either did things her way

---

[1]This was described in the November 22, 1982 issue of *Newsweek* as "an uncertain war, fought for uncertain ends, and prolonged far beyond the hope of success."

or suffered her raging contempt. Accordingly, in time his father had become a virtual nonentity, who ensured his own safety by siding with her whenever she was unhappy with the children. This was an image he despised but feared that he had duplicated. There were some interesting oedipal counterpoints to this image of his mother as a destructive bitch who castrated men and the image of his father as a nonentity. During World War I, when Jack was about 4, his father, to everyone's surprise, enlisted in the service. Many evenings while his father was away, Jack's mother would take him into her bed. Some early memories or dreams, he was never sure which, contained the sound of footsteps climbing the stairs. He recalled his mother saying: "That's enough, you'll have to stop that." His associations led to the almost certain recollection that he might have been touching his mother's breast or some other part of her body. His further recollection of a scurried exit to his bedroom left him puzzled and frightened. This phase of maternal warmth and intimacy was abruptly terminated when his father returned after 3 years as a wounded veteran. Even though Jack never liked his father, he recalled feeling some compassion for his disability and an anxious sadness after his father's heart began to fail.

It was some time in therapy before these oedipal screen memories of a disabled father's returning from war to displace him were linked to Jack's sense of apocalyptic doom and his image of worlds' colliding. We learned that, to deny his sensed dependency and vulnerability, Jack had married a woman who needed him to break her dependency upon her domineering father. Together they formed a not-so-unconscious alliance in which he became "number 1," and others would not be allowed to intrude. Unfortunately, this came to include not only her family but their children as well. In the words of Jack's daughter, "We knew we were second class to Daddy...it didn't even help to be sick!"

Nourished by this marital alliance and considerable success in his work, certain of Jack's grandiose narcissistic and oedipal fantasies were realized. Soon he and his family were able to move to a nicer neighborhood, and by rubbing elbows with more successful people, he felt he closed the gap between himself and his wife's relatives. As a doctor, his status gave him considerable prestige. Still, he was sensitive to any criticism and was plagued by every, albeit intermittent, failure, especially with a cardiac or neoplastic patient. In family practice, it had seemed to him as if death was always lurking around the corner.

Marsha's Cancer

And then the bell tolled! Shortly after the birth of their youngest child, Marsha had an episode with cancer in one breast, leading to a mastectomy. From that time she became a volunteer, alerting others to the dangers of cancer. Four years prior to my initial consultation with Jack, she discovered a lump in the other breast. For a solid year, she said nothing about it to anyone. When it was found to be malignant, Jack was angrily grief stricken. In addition to having missed the reoccurrence, his professional pride was shattered. No longer could he maintain the ideal-ized image of the all-caring husband and all-knowing physician. Sens-ing that the emotional distance between them had led to both diminished physical contact and a subclinical depression (subintended suicide?) in his wife, and despite his scientific background, Jack shifted the blame intermittently between themselves and the gynecologist who had not "picked it up soon enough."

The anxious eventful months that followed, marked by the realiza-tion that Marsha had lacked the desire to preserve herself, contributed to the psychic overload that led to the shift in his career. The second bi-opsy report was remembered as the lowest point in their family life. To help his wife make the best possible decision and to recoup some self-esteem, Jack secluded himself in the library to read all he could on al-ternatives in the management of recurrent breast cancer. His practice suffered, not only because of his absorption in his wife's illness, but be-cause of a shift in hospital policy on admissions. When his wife chose another radical mastectomy, he supported her in every way he could, but he used the demands of a terminal case as an excuse not to be in the recovery room when she awoke. Somewhere deep inside, Jack remembered wishes that his wife would not awake, and rationalized them as his depressed concern lest she should have to go through the kind of terminal illness he had so often witnessed. On the other hand, he wished her to live no matter what followed, as he was terrified of be-ing without her steadying influence.

After the emergency was over, Jack immersed himself in restoring his practice and "lost track of time." Even before the operation, he had worried about whether or not he could perform sexually face-to-face with a nonbreasted woman, and, to be sure, it was difficult. Although he felt cheated, in psychotherapy he emphatically observed how she must have felt even more so.

I suggested that Jack's focus on and distancing from his wife's deformity was consistent with his need for perfection and that he probably had avoided grieving over the loss of it in her as well as in himself. Even his affairs may have served the same purpose. He responded with a long silence. Then his eyes filled with tears as he slowly revealed his sense that he had failed her, whereas she had stood by him through his anginal episodes. In the face of fantasies of finding another woman, one with two breasts, how could he maintain the image of himself as a perfect human being? In his revived grief, he asked the question voiced so often by those obsessives' realizing life is a terminal affair, "The right time to live and love is any time you're lucky to be healthy enough. We didn't seem able to do that...do many other couples?"

During his wife's convalescence, the family visited Jack's older sister's home. This happened to coincide with his nephew's acceptance to law school. He burned with the humiliation of the uncertainty of his son's finishing high school, and felt, in all likelihood, that he never would experience such "nachas." He associated to his youngest daughter's excelling in school as if she could make up to her parents for her sibling's failures. This effort was an open family secret. In retrospect, he regretted never having made more of this offering from her. I suggested that his inability to enjoy his wife and daughter's accomplishments might have had something to do with his intense envy of his father's delight in his sister. Jack recalled when he was so upset by his sister's nachas in her son that he became sick to his stomach and unable to eat. His rage seemed divided between her, himself, and his son. He wondered how his sister could be so cold and callous as to keep talking about her son's selecting dorms, and making the law review. In this regard, Jack recalled how much his own identity had been based on giving nachas to his parents. "I was the original nachas kid. What more could a nice Jewish family want, their son a doctor? I did what I was told, but what choice did I have?" Then, in comparing the relationship to his son, he began an exploration of the unusually vivid fear he had always had of his father.

> "In the old house where I grew up, my most vivid memory is still of the bathroom. Every day before my father went to work, especially when mother and father would fight, it would become my refuge. I would stay there for hours reading books on science or health. After the fight was over and he left, I would come out. If they fought at night, my father would sleep with her. It was like a Russian novel; I've read them all." Glancing at me humorously, he added, "Maybe I chose you as my psychiatrist be-

cause you referred to Dostoevski and Kafka. In family practice generally, I had kept away from psychology and psychiatrists."

He shuddered as he recalled the intensity of his father's rage. Then a vivid memory of his father's razor strap emerged. In the evening, exhausted by the day's work, his father often laid down to rest before supper. Unhappy "for her own reasons," Jack's mother would tattle to father about his son's misconduct. Flying into rage, either from the sofa or from behind a newspaper, his father would grab the strap from his own bathroom and chase his son into the children's bathroom. Usually escaping there and locking the door, Jack felt safe. He would read his favorite books for hours. His sister, whom his father favored, was never treated that way. Associating to his sister and the law school incident once again, it turned out that Jack's father had had many grievances. They included a lost law suit. "He couldn't afford a decent lawyer; maybe that's why he wanted me to go to law school." I asked if this connection might be at the root of his irritation on learning his nephew might fulfill his grandfather's dream.

After 2 years of biweekly psychotherapy, Jack's family relationships eased. At work he felt admired and respected once again. Appearing more mature than his younger colleagues, he had assumed the role of an older brother who took responsibility and displayed initiative. His children, no longer under pressure to fulfill his dreams, related to him more openly and affectionately, and his older daughter became seriously involved with a young man. Although both Jack and his wife loved this boy, their "living together" caused the mother much consternation. The son, still equivocating about his career, managed to return to school part-time, and the third child remained "a delight."

At this point, Jack's major complaint still focused on his disappointment in his wife, her aloofness, and lack of sexual response. His only serious depression occurred on the anniversary of his father's death. Exploration revealed he was not grieving over his father *per se* but over the revived issue of his inherited responsibility for his mother and her subsequent happiness or unhappiness as a widow. After living alone fairly well for 10 years, his mother had become progressively more demented. As is often the case, increasingly phobic about being alone, she made repeated requests to move into his home. Despite Marsha's willingness to establish a three-generation home, Jack adamantly refused. When the situation deteriorated badly, Jack placed his mother in a nursing home

against her will, whereupon she soon died. We now connected his aloofness in that situation with his devalued image of his aloof wife.

Jack had bragged to his wife of feeling a new independence through
therapy. On several occasions through the years of therapy, Marsha had
expressed interest in meeting me, implying she'd also like to tell her side
of the story. But Jack did not pick up her request for attention and a hearing until a pain in her back raised the question of recurrence of breast
cancer. While she was being worked up for metastases, he raised the issue of whether she could join him in couples therapy. Partly because I
had just lost a dear friend who smoked to metastic brain cancer, I tem-
porized and suggested we talk more about the wisdom and consequences of such a move.

A shattering conversation between husband and wife soon overcame
my temporizing. Despite his improvement, Marsha had confronted Jack
repeatedly with two great concerns. For if she were to judge on the basis of his tolerance for illness in the family and his "expelling" his mother
in the face of his wife's willingness to take her in, her future as a possibly sick, dependent older woman was grim indeed. If he had such faith
in Dr. Cath, she queried, "Wouldn't he be the one with whom to check
out my fears?...How do you justify your behavior with your
mother?...What did you learn in your therapy?" After Jack and I discussed his resistance to her presence as a threat both to his "I-know-
best" stance and to being "*numero uno*," Jack's overwhelming concern
for her by-now diagnosed metastatic cancer comingled with an increasing respect for his wife's courage and intuitive understanding brought
the four of us together.

Yes, there were four of us. As I explained to Jack, despite long years
in therapy with couples, a co-therapist not only ameliorated my concern
that I could not do justice to the needs of husband and wife, but a
woman, in this case my wife, would add a special viewpoint that might
enrich the process. Only in writing this down did I appreciate how much
the threat of Marsha's fatal illness had intensified my pain as well as my
race against therapeutic time. In general, this painful time sense probably inclines most therapists' countertransference with both patients and
families toward increased levels of empathic activity and toward reality.
I had long recognized in myself that the termination process often ac-
celerated the momentum of therapeutic action. In this last phase, when
the therapist should be seen as a more real person, the assumption has
been that this activity reflects a more resolved transference and better

reality testing. To be sure, therapy with middle-aged and older patients is more like working with adolescents and terminating patients, who are characteristically more active and interactive. But in this case, with terminal cancer, a special urgency difficult to elucidate but sensed by all concerned had adulterated and adumbrated both transference and countertransference.

THE PHASE OF CONJOINT THERAPY

In the first joint session, Jack and his wife, each for obviously different reasons, revealed haunting images of a lonely sick old age in which no one would care for them. Because of an impending bone scan, Marsha's insecurity took center stage, but, as noted before, it was couched in terms of her husband's seeming abandonment of his mother. Although our exact words are lost, we tried to diffuse the situation by observing that most middle-aged people are quite uncomfortable with the notion of inviting a parent "cascading into senility" to live in their home, especially during their children's adolescence. No one had the wisdom, even in retrospect, to know what might have been best. But probably Jack's intuition was correct because it was based upon the qualities of "the bond" he had experienced with his mother. Also, Marsha's judgment was equally correct because it was based on her experience with her mother who had died cerebrally intact. As we explored these historical antecedents, it seemed a three-generation home might well have been intolerable, exacting a price too great for everyone to pay.

It soon emerged that Marsha's concerns, inappropriate to Jack's reality with his mother, were quite appropriate to something in her own past. To reach this point, several clarification interventions were required. We had to differentiate two validities: first, Jack's experiences with and his mental representations of his mother; and second, his behavior in relation to his ailing wife in the present and the future. In one session, relieved of the burden of his projection upon her of the cold Wasp image, she observed:

> It's not just that you were hard on us and on her, but you were even harder on yourself. You insisted on your own guilty interpretation no matter what we said, so it would be natural for us to agree with you. It is true that I only know what I think I would have done had it been my mother, but I can't be sure even today. Now that you've let me in on what went

on between you and your mother in the past, I understand you had no choice.

To which he responded:

You don't hold it against me?...You don't hate me, or think I'm terrible? Didn't you wonder what I would do if it were you...if I put you away and let you die?

She then said:

Well, I had also thought what I would do if you had a stroke or died of a heart attack. We were not in a good position; I couldn't see how I could keep the house and raise the kids, and I had nightmares of the prospect of turning to my parents. I guess I have my limits with them as well as with you.

No longer able to retain the image of his wife as cool and unfeeling perfectionist, Jack burst into tears and among the four of us there was not a dry eye in the room.

It became clear that Marsha's feeling about family affiliation had indeed played a part in her object choice of a Jewish mate. She was determined to have warmer family relationships than her parents had had. Jack's refusal to give up the image of betrayal by his parents as well as his betraying them was sensed by her as a betrayal of her unconscious contract with an idealized Jewish family that she intuited would have healed her childhood wounds.

Jack went on to recall how he had recognized that whenever he fell away from the ideal image of a loving Jewish son (the successful doctor), he became depressed. Whenever he could not repair either his mother's "ancient wounds" or his wife's current ones, he felt defeated and worked harder away from home. Familiar with theories relating stress to cancer, Jack began to work through some of his guilt over Marsha's illness. In this regard, it has been found that most cancer patients adapt better than their spouses up to the very end, and Jack was no exception. But in these early interviews, we interpreted Jack's initial distancing of his wife and her illness as related to guilty fears he might do something wrong or not be able to protect her any more than he had his mother, which might add to his already considerable reservoir of regrets. After this phase, his irritability and tendency to distance and devalue Marsha almost disappeared.

With these themes as our major foci, Marsha became a very strong source of support to her husband, and he to her. Rather than remaining critical of his tendency to bury himself in his work, she conceded it might have been impossible for him to have done otherwise. And no longer feeling that need to prove that he would not abandon her, she began to change her position that he had abandoned his mother. After a series of radiation treatments her condition seemed stable. "The women" met several times alone, facilitating the emergence of a number of correlations. These included, much to Jack's surprise, a confession that watching him improve over 2 years had made Marsha feel envious and left out. To her, it had seemed he was more devoted to his therapist than he was to his family. This led to a discussion of Jack's old infidelities. Marsha had regarded me as similar to one of her husband's paramours, or even worse, like a "secret family." This had special implications, for, in his 30s, Jack had been shocked to learn that he had a secret half brother, a child his father had sired with another woman. Indeed, a secret family had been one of Jack's fantasies during one of his affairs. We all agreed that Jack's willingness to share his therapy might help undo this "secret" pattern.

It seems, in retrospect, that instructing older people to refrain from discussing therapy may be unwise. This advice was originally based on the fear of dilution of material, but, at least in the light of this case, such advice now seems superfluous and unnecessarily restrictive if not counterproductive.

Adolescent Associations

Further sessions focused on distancing mechanisms used either when anxious expectations of illness or death of significant others were fantasized or when they actually threatened. As is so often the case, our discussions of death were followed by associations to sex, birth, and rebirth. Issues arose about why they could not accept their daughter's living with her boyfriend. Would these youngsters ever marry? Would they ever become grandparents? Although both Jack and his wife inwardly approved of the idea of premarital sex, it rekindled frightening associations of their adolescence. They speculated on what it would have been like if they had had the opportunity to go through college living together. Marsha claimed innocently that she had not discovered how babies were made by then. Jack described his adolescent shock at learning the facts of life. "In my mind, it was impossible for my parents to have engaged in sex." Even four-letter words repelled him. In college, Jack was impotent in his first attempt at intercourse. His failure so confused and terrified him that he considered suicide and consulted a psychiatrist. Indeed, the years between his father's death and his attempt at intimacy had been lonely and seclusive, although studious and productive. It was shortly after this failure that he first met Marsha. Her seeming coolness facilitated a rapid platonic courtship and marriage.

In individual therapy, especially through the transference, we had learned that Jack offset feelings of impotent ineffectiveness by humiliating others with his sharp tongue, much as he had done with his less educated mother and family. We had also reconstructed that his sexual anxiety might have reflected the simultaneous arousal and inhibition experienced in his mother's bed during his father's absence. During conjoint therapy, in contrast to this ambivalent, seductive mother whose loving attachments waxed and waned and who betrayed him to his father, Marsha's steadiness and aloofness emerged in a new light. Although this strength was what Jack needed, we suspected he could not enjoy and respect it fully. Sharing this understanding helped Marsha gradually reevaluate and forgive Jack for his seeming rejection of the best part of herself and his seeming abandonment of his mother. But even in this setting of new understanding, Jack described himself as "the kind of a person who never forgave." Indeed, from his wife's point of view, Jack had transferred much of his distrust and unforgiveness onto his children. Then, unable to tolerate their resentments, he would try to talk them out of the same suspicious recalcitrance that plagued him. We suggested he feared they would ultimately distance themselves from him and hate him as he had hated his parents. It emerged that discipline would often be preceded by "I know you will hate me for this."

The words *hate* and *rage* became strikingly associated with *heart* and *attack*. Jack now connected these associations with the Jewish calendar, as he usually became particularly morose and irritable just before Jewish holidays. Furthermore, his wife observed that at times it seemed he had bullied his children in exactly the same way that he had been treated in the ghetto. A surprising series of associations revealed a latent pride in having survived the ghetto, in his heritage, and in having been raised as "an ethical honest Jew." Jack's son's drug addiction and his daughter's sexual behavior reflected poorly on this image of the ideal courageous Jewish physician. With tears in his eyes, he asked Marsha if she minded this secret pride in his background—the memories of his mother's greeting the Sabbath bride in the ritual of lighting candles, and so forth.

On further reflection, we all agreed this seemed an important nucleus around which some of Jack's earliest, best, and warmest memories of his mother were consolidated. Indeed, they had had to be walled off and repressed, and this was the first time in their marriage that he had shared this secret pride with his wife. It had been an unconscious part of himself and his past that had been kept from her that had contributed to and reinforced his defense of devaluating both pasts. Then he recalled it was only after his father's death that he began to ridicule his heritage and its rituals, as if he had to distance himself from the man and his Jewishness. Then after his heart attack, he began to wish secretly that he had married a Jewish woman who might reinstate some of these rituals and their associated nostalgia. Still he did not want his children "to be so Jewish as to be bound to my nachas formula...[that] they would be intellectual and independent enough not to have to make peace at any price...a form of cowardice characteristic of Jews." Jack considered these dynamics related both to his choice of a Christian wife and to his adamant militarism. He had supported the Israeli efforts at recognition because "it was time for the worm to turn."

In the past, Jack had described his very young son's behavior during his first heart attack as lacking feeling or appropriate concern. The therapist observed that often children are not able to respond to the implications of such events "in an adult mode until adolescence"; that his expectations were not of a young boy but of an older, wiser, and more empathic person of more advanced age or possibly of an idealized parent. Could his ancient guilt about his lack of concern for "the wounded warrior" and his aging dementing mother be at the root of some of this overcriticism of his son? Now in conjoint therapy, Marsha was able to contribute a different view of these events. She related how truly upset her son had been about his father's ill health and told us how he tried to be "a stoic soldier."

Jack's misreading led us to a reinquiry into his own response when his father had fallen ill. He felt safe enough to recall how he had failed to show any emotion then or earlier, when his father returned from war. In all probability, we reconstructed, his father may have reproached him, possibly "never forgave" him, and made him feel guilty much as Jack had done with his own son. Then he linked his gloom-and-doom pes-

simism to fear he would not be prepared for, or respond appropriately
to, sudden disasters. As a family physician, this had been a constant burden. Almost as much as his heart attack, it had been another motivat-
ing factor in his change of career. Jack confessed that in a distorted way
his heart attack had been welcome. It reduced the potential for dying a
more horrible death, either of cancer or the chronic degeneration of organic brain disease. With either condition, he might end up in a nursing home like his mother. We raised the possibility that he also might
have felt relief not to have to burden his family and be as disappointed
in their lack of manifest concern as others had seemingly been with him.
Then his "Aha!" revealed a sense of enlightenment. "How could the
nachas kid do this to his mother?" He had always been surprised if not
angered that others did not feel as much guilt and obligation or try as
hard as he did to please.

In response, Marsha wondered if he realized that his sense of ob-
ligatory trying did not come through when she was worried about the
impact upon the family should her cancer prove inoperable and her illness protracted. Because she had never felt sure of Jack, she had taken
comfort in teaching the children to grow up on their own, not to be
spoiled as she had been, and to be "model soldiers." In her opinion,
the question was still valid. At what point would he be unable to tolerate her and put her in a nursing home to die alone? As if resonating with
the countertransference of both therapists, Marsha asked all of us, "Can
I count on your compassion?" Then we learned from Jack how the family joke, "Look at Daddy crying," pained him; he cried whenever he
watched sad television or movies. And Marsha's fostering the "model-
soldier" stance in the children had been infuriating because it reinforced
the tendency to conceal sensitivity and overconcern. But Marsha remembered shortly after her first mastectomy, sometime after her daughter's
pregnancy and the exposure of the son's drug problem, that Jack had
become even more tyrannical. It was his empathic response to movies
in contrast to such family crises that made the family see him in exactly
the same way as he saw them; namely, lacking in compassionte concern.
He noted sadly, indeed, that this was true and that he had shown more
emotion when the cat died than at his mother's funeral. Ironically
enough, shortly after her abortion, their elder daughter began to work
in a nursing home. There her need to nurture had been rewarded by constant appreciation and love from both staff and residents. Reflecting on
this, her father noted, "Isn't it strange? She's doing something I feel I

should have done. I could never take care of old people comfortably before. Maybe one can learn from one's children." This theme of lack of compassion for weakness, illness, aging, and death led to a discussion of the family's difficulties in openly grieving over real or sensed losses. This behavior, the ease with which they all were able to express feelings of loss over displaced or vicarious characters on television, was interpreted as concealing how very much they needed and depended on each other. It probably explained why Jack was so hard on both his wife and children: She represented the side of himself that would like to have been a cool, dispassionate soldier; the children represented the side that was hungry for love, approval, and deep connection.

Complex Countertransference

To repeat, even though the senior author had worked with geriatric and terminal cases for years, he sensed that his countertransference was more complex than usual. Very real and repeated clinical experiences had led to a core residue of resentment related to the shortcomings of a physician's empathic resonance with chronic or dying patients. Parenthetically, two decades of his life had been spent, only partially successfully, in trying to include courses on aging, dying, and death in his medical school's curriculum. Finding his own ideals sorely challenged by this physician's responses to his mother's dementia and Marsha's cancer revived certain aspects of his positive and negative oedipus complex. With empathy split between patient and family, sensing the race against therapeutic time, he enlisted a co-therapist with whom to reflect on these issues and to dilute the tension both during and after sessions.

After 2 years of individual psychotherapy and 1 year of conjoint therapy, in Jack's words, "We are in a different place and mood." Radiation and chemotherapy had held Marsha's lesions in check. As new and deeper levels of family connectedness were reached, Jack's self-esteem was raised, and he was no longer irritable, depressed, or overly concerned about his cardiac status. Once he passed the age at which his father had died, his fear that he would suffer an early cardiac death diminished even more. Lifelong feelings of being used had been analyzed as a "paranoid" defense against a sense of worthlessness as well as a distorted wish to use and hold onto others. No longer as ashamed of himself or his children and more comfortable with his wife, he seemed better able to work without offending his peers, supervisors, or friends.

His daughter started psychotherapy, but his son remained adamantly opposed to any intrusion into his personal life. When his wife felt reasonably confident that "the new Jack" would be able and willing to support her if she suffered a relapse, therapy was interrupted. For the next 2½ "good years," Marsha's breast cancer remained dormant.

But then their fears and ours became a nightmare. A new and even more virulent form of cancer from other female organs threatened to terminate Marsha's life within 6 months. Both returned for therapy. Jack preferred individual time in which, sobbing unabashedly, he could rail against the incredibly unfair fate he had dreaded most. Marsha, taken up with an exhausting course of experimental chemotherapy and radiation treatments, came infrequently, mostly for conjoint sessions. It was striking to all of us how she maintained her dignity, composure, and independence until the very end. Typically, she took concern for her husband and children as a point of departure. The realization that cancer seemed to run in the female members of Marsha's family was a great burden. As a couple, they decided to do everything they had postponed for one reason or another. We encouraged this race against sensed deprivation, for in work with dying patients we had learned not to offer the customary cautions or euphemisms, with one exception. It is true, we preferred over several sessions, that all of us live owing one ultimate debt to life, namely our death. We all await meanwhile the failure of some one or more of our tissues, organs or systems; this is a vulnerability in all probability related not to heredity *per se* but to genetics. According to the latest theories, of which we shared what we knew, cancer probably results from a failure in immunocompetence, of which one of many factors might be familial. It seems we all co-exist with pathogenic viruses and "viroids" from birth to death. What diminishes our resistance to their taking over of cells is not clear. But once a fatal diagnosis is known, as long as one is not incapacitated or in pain, a choice must be made, either to live until one is dead or to die before the cessation of life.

Marsha's Death

We all knew what Marsha's choice would be, and she disappointed no one. The children and family rallied around to take excursions into the country and a few local weekends away. But as her strength ebbed over the next few months, her unconsolable eyes began to stare into space reminding all of us of our conjoint helplessness.

Soon home visits were made to spare her energy. As she toured the house reminiscing about mementos, she allowed herself to cry and express some of the bitterness of it all. The visit and the reminiscences stimulated a series of thoughts ending with what it felt like to imagine another woman enjoying her house, paintings, and husband. But one of her last gifts to Jack was the wish he would not spend the rest of his life alone. Marsha's last months were bedridden with many philosophical excursions into why people had to die like this. Somehow, she and Jack clung to these weeks as precious times, for in them she found the answer to her question. Indeed, in her horrible time Jack not only had compassion, but nursed, cleaned, and comforted her in the most distasteful of circumstances. One day he stood at the foot of her bed watching her sleep, thinking sadly of how she looked like a child and a skeleton at the same time. She called to him and died in his arms.

When the funeral was over, individual therapy resumed. As was his wont, Jack found comfort in intensifying his work. He seemed cried-out for the most part, but intermittent hours were spent grieving over his past lack of appreciation for Marsha. His children's distance bothered him most because they avoided coming home, although they phoned reasonably often. In his dreams, he spoke to Marsha and accused her of desertion and heartlessness, associating the reproach not only to her death but to the old theme of his children's seeming lack of concern. Only now it seemed true. Not so parenthetically, Marsha appeared in two dreams of the senior author.

Then Jack met Louise at a dinner at the home of old friends. The next few months were focused on his devaluation of the potentials of the new relationship, his fear of loving and losing someone again, and the strange paradox of how much like Marsha, Louise was. But the most vigorous opposition came from the children, who voiced their incredulity that anyone could take their mother's place plus "it was all too soon." To the therapist, Louise was what the doctor ordered, for Jack blossomed like a teenager, regaining the vitality and joy thought lost forever. In part out of guilt, in part in truth, Jack agreed with those who felt no one would ever compare with Marsha, but to his credit he persisted in trying to overcome the temptation of "living with the dead out of a sense of loyalty." Almost a year after Marsha'a death, Jack married Louise and began a new chapter of his life.

Two years later Jack returned for therapy. The next few months were focused on the difficulties attendant upon his children's adamant unwillingness to accept a step-mother. With the pregnancy of his by-now-married but still cooly distant daughter, he felt certain he would never be allowed to be a grandfather to the child. Once again, as pessimism threatened to overwhelm him, he catalogued all his sins as a father. He was reminded of his tendency to judge prematurely by superficial characteristics mirroring his own, as he had with Marsha. When his grandchild was born, so was a refueling grandparenthood (Cath, 1982). Soon he, but not his second wife, was warmly welcomed into a newly formed family. Within a short time Jack was ready to end therapy once again. In the termination hour he was ecstatic, fully enjoying the role of a loving grandfather. In his opinion, his daughter and son-in-law saw him in a different light when they saw the love he "poured over the baby." He said: "What I have to remember is to put myself in the other person's place, and I will be all right...You taught me that...You've been a smashing success...I've not been an easy patient." To which I responded: "No, it hasn't always been easy, but it has been worth-while." "Well" he laughed, "you can't say I'm a fast worker...it took over 60 years to get to this point."

Soberly he added:

> I wish she could have been here with me, and I wish my son could have seen the way I handled the baby. The biggest mistake we made was the unconscious pact that I would be number one. I know the children resented it. With my grandchild I can show my children that it's not true—not any more. You know somehow I even feel maternal, as if I have to take Marsha's role too. I just love holding the baby and talking to it. I wish my son and my new wife could share this joy. They must feel left out. My son seems to choose to be left out. He always lagged behind his sister like a shadow. Could he still feel that way? I guess I'm ready to try to make friends with him on his terms, on any terms, and not to criticize him...if he could share our joy. Do you think I'm ready?

CONCLUSIONS

In psychotherapy with older people racing against time, the therapist is sorely challenged by his or her knowledge that failure in any organ or organ system may be brought about by circumstances far beyond his or her control. Unknown genetic determinants, the effects of stress upon immunocompetence, and the complex interactions within the family all interdigitate to summate in what is commonly called human destiny. Countertransference may be contaminated by the therapist's anxiety that all therapy may soon be in vain.

REFERENCES

Cath, S. H. Some dynamics of middle and later years. *Smith College Studies in Social Work,* 1963, *33*(2), 97–126.
Cath, S. H. Vicissitudes of grandfatherhood: A miracle of revitalization? In S. H. Cath, A. Gurwitt, & J. M. Ross (Eds.), *Father and child: Developmental and clinical perspectives.* Boston: Little, Brown, 1982.
Cath, S. H. Psychoanalysis in old age. *Journal of the American Psychoanalytic Association,* submitted for publication.

14

The Ant and the Grasshopper in Later Life

AGING IN RELATION TO WORK AND GRATIFICATION

Ralph J. Kahana

This chapter deals with aging in relation to work and gratification, and with the aims and results of psychoanalytic psychotherapy. Contrasting cases of two men are described, one severely limited in his ability to work by symptoms and inhibitions, the other a lifelong overworker. The first case illustrates some special features of therapy with older persons. The second is an unusual example of long-term, potentially "interminable" treatment beginning at midlife, with one of the goals conceived as preparation for old age.

As therapists, we have been fascinated with and challenged by the wide variety of life-styles encountered, any of which may prove adaptive or maladaptive in later life. We expect the consistency of personality structure and life-style that we call *character* to persist and be reflected in corresponding life experiences; yet we often discover that a style that worked well early in life has not proved effective later on. Sometimes the converse is true when previously maladaptive behavior becomes more successful with advancing age. We learn to value fairness and wishfully anticipate that effort and sacrifice will be rewarded. Yet life is often unjust. The hardworking ant of Aesop's fable does not always fare better in the long run than the improvident grasshopper.

Another version of this paper was presented at a scientific meeting of the Boston Society for Gerontologic Psychiatry and has appeared in *The Journal of Geriatric Psychiatry*, 1983, 16, 7–32, under the title "A Miserable Old Age—What Can Therapy Do?"

There is a deeper inequity in the life cycle. Libidinal, ego, and psychosocial development follow the principle of epigenesis (Erikson, 1939) in which each stage is built upon a sequence of earlier stages. At every step, adaptability is a function of the successful unfolding and surmounting of the preceding ones. The relation between earlier and later life is often in accord with the biblical adage: "Unto everyone that hath shall be given." Richly endowed and well enjoyed childhood and youth appear to guarantee a successful and gratifying adulthood and old age. And it follows that unsatisfactory early life foredooms unsatisfactory aging. This was exemplified in a memorable way by Max Beerbohm (1872–1956), a British writer, caricaturist, and drama critic.

THE GIFT OR THE MISERY OF OLD AGE

Beerbohm was educated at Oxford University and made a reputation while still an undergraduate as a witty, polished essayist. His essays, parodies, short stories, and a novel, written mainly from the 1890s through World War I were modest in number but of high quality. His caricatures of political, literary, and artistic figures of this time, including Queen Victoria, Lord Balfour, Ibsen, Shaw, Henry James, Oscar Wilde, Yeats, Kipling, and many others, are among the finest ever created. He married in his late 30s, and before the age of 40 he withdrew to the Italian Riviera where he spent over half of his long life, becoming an object of literary and social pilgrimages, like Bernard Berenson and W. Somerset Maugham. From his 50s on, his artistic output diminished and he lived in semiretirement. Small, slight, easily fatigued, thoughtful, and kind, he retained the elegant manner and dress of the Edwardian era. A noted conversationalist, his charm in his later years was enhanced by a persistent childlike gaze, irreverent humor, a joy in playing elaborate, benign, practical jokes, and pleasure in food and in receiving and unwrapping gifts (Cecil, 1964).

At the age of 63 he accepted an invitation by the British Broadcasting Corporation (BBC) to give a talk on "revisiting London" (Beerbohm, 1958a). He approached it with his usual meticulous care, and it was a triumph. Other radio talks followed, including one about his childhood enthusiasm for statesmen that was entitled "A Small Boy Seeing Giants." He stressed the fact that he was on the verge of old age, elderly and anachronistic, an elegant Rip Van Winkle who preferred the old days. We should observe that being "past his prime" came naturally to him. Oscar Wilde, who died when Beerbohm was still in his 20s, said that "the Gods have bestowed on Max the gift of eternal old age" (Beerbohm, 1958b). In 1939, Beerbohm was honored with knighthood. During World War II he returned to Britain where, at age 70, he did a number of further broadcasts on the BBC.

One of his biographers (Behrman, 1960) wrote that it was odd that one of the least popular writers of the world should have become, next to Winston Churchill, the most popular broadcaster in England during the most critical moment of its history. In January of 1942, while London was blacked out and a vast number of its inhabitants were sleeping in the underground and in shelters, and the fires lit by incendiary bombs furnished the only illumination, Sir Max treated his listeners to the program called "Music Halls of My Youth." He delivered it when it was well past his own bedtime. In a soft, courteous, quavering, elderly voice, he said he assumed that most of his listeners who were up and doing would "know little of the subject on which I am going to dilate with senile garrulity." After talking about a number of performers, he ended with a few words to his listeners on how he had come to squander his youth drinking in the words and music of these vanished ghosts.

> Perhaps you will blame me for having spent so much of my time in music halls, so frivolously, when I should have been sticking to my books, burning the midnight oil, and compassing the larger latitude. But I am impenitent. I am inclined to think, indeed I have always thought, that a young man who desires to know all that in all ages and in all lands has been thought by the best minds, and wishes to make a synthesis of all those thoughts for the future benefit of mankind, is laying up for himself a very miserable old age.

Beerbohm expresses the lesson of epigenesis. In this instance, to put it simplistically, "If you don't have fun when you are young, you won't when you are old." This is an especial danger for the very old who live in their memories, drawing upon the past for gratification. His observations remind us that Aesop's moral "It is thrifty to prepare today for the wants of tomorrow" should be qualified by the Biblical adage "Man doth not live by bread alone."

Before proceeding to the history and treatment of the underworker and the overworker, our allegorical grasshopper and ant, a brief orientation toward psychoanalytic or dynamic psychotherapy is in order.

Much of this concerns psychotherapy at all ages, but the applications and special features seen with older patients are emphasized.

PSYCHOTHERAPY AND GERIATRIC PSYCHOTHERAPY

It is usually simpler to diagnose psychopathology than it is to plan and carry out psychotherapy. We categorize psychological maladaptations roughly as taking a limited number of forms, such as neuroses, character disorders and psychoses, or depressions, stress reactions, interpersonal difficulties, and so on. In contrast, the possibility of helping an individual usually depends upon a number of factors and circumstances in his or her personality, life experience, physical health, family, and community as well as the therapist's skill, experience, personality, and theoretical orientation. With so many variables we find a range of possible therapeutic goals and approaches. The goal of therapy may be to relieve suffering, to allow normal functioning, or to prevent future problems. The aims or strategies and methods of treatment include support, adaptive intervention, and character change. Supportive methods involve identifying and mitigating stresses and assisting or modifying the patient's caretaking environment in order to halt regression and relieve distress. Adaptive intervention seeks to promote adaptive strengths in order to reinstate the best level of functioning that the patient has attained hitherto. Character (structural) change represents a further development and integration of drive derivatives, ego and superego functions, the self, and other components of personality through conflict resolution (Kahana, 1979). Just as each of us has in his or her personality an admixture of the entire book of psychological normality and pathology, every therapy utilizes all of these methods in some degree.

Often the principal method of choice is not apparent until after a trial of therapy during which the diagnosis and the patient's potential for improvement have become better established. Depending upon the method selected, the schedule of treatment will range from a consultation, to time-limited or brief therapy (as in crisis intervention), to open-ended psychotherapy at set intervals from three times weekly to monthly, to psychoanalysis four or five times a week. Follow-up may be ad lib or prescribed. In making this choice with a patient of any age, we consider the acuteness and severity of the disturbance, his or her tolerance of tension and regression, reality testing, adaptive capacity, motivation for treatment and ability to use insight, and the quality of the patient's personal relationships. All of these determine the possibility of consolidating a working or therapeutic alliance, including a manageable or interpretable transference. With older patients especially, we pay particular attention to their tolerance of tension and regression and to their family and other social environment as a source of support or stress.

There is a tendency to favor shorter forms of therapy for older people or even to neglect psychotherapy entirely. This downplaying of therapy occurs for a number of reasons. Sometimes the choice is dictated by realistic considerations, such as the vulnerability to stress of a significant group of the aging and elderly, that may limit treatment to crisis intervention. Another reason for this tendency is historical, as in the case of the older person who grew up in an era when dynamic psychotherapy was not widely available and never learned to accept it as potentially helpful. Finally, the reason may be irrational, for example, the ageistic prejudice of caretakers against investing therapeutic time and effort in people with a "limited future." Countering this trend among the public and the healing professions is increasing interest in geriatric psychotherapy and experience with the whole range of treatment methods, including psychoanalysis (Sandler, 1978).

Irrational emotional responses in the form of transference and countertransference are intrinsic elements in the therapeutic process. The patient's unconscious tendency to transfer onto the therapist expectations and feelings held toward important figures in his or her past provides the alert therapist with valuable information and the possibility of responding helpfully. The therapist's countertransference, the impulse to repeat with the patient his or her own early patterns of relationship, provides him or her with essential information and therapeutic opportunity when he or she is aware of the fact and meaning of his or her feelings and is in control of his or her actual responses. Basic problems in all discussions of these elements are the limits of acceptable disclosure and the large amount of detailed information (e.g., personal history, free associations, context) necessary to do justice to the subject. It is easier to deal with transference and countertransference at a general level than to discuss it in the individual case.

In general form, many transference–countertransference paradigms encountered with older patients are well known. For example, preconscious attitudes often correspond to the parent-child relationship. The older patient may react like a parent or grandparent to the younger therapist, and the therapist may respond like a child or grandchild. Frequently, though more surprisingly, a younger therapist may be cast in the parental role. Unconscious oedipal conflicts are, of course, universal and may be centrally important in a given case. Character attitudes (hysterical, obsessional, dependent, masochistic, narcissistic, paranoid, schizoid) enter the therapeutic relationship from both participants, and these tend to be accentuated in older people. Social roles play a part in the form of culturally influenced patient behavior and stereotyped attitudes of healers, such as "bedside manners" (Bibring & Kahana, 1968).

Clinical writings have much more to say about the personal lives of patients than of therapists, if only because it is less difficult to protect the privacy of the former. Regarding the emotions of therapists, again it is easier to generalize. It is in the nature of psychodynamic factors that they function antithetically, in opposite ways at different times. For example, the same ego defense can serve as an adaptive tool or as a resistance to constructive change. Thus, the factors that establish and enhance the therapist's interest and skill in working with older people can also give rise to countertransferences. These may include positive early relationships with older persons, for example, grandparents, and identifications with family members, traditions, and teachers involved in caring for the elderly. The geriatric therapist may be optimally patient and accepting toward the slower reactions of older persons and have empathy for the narcissistic injuries to which the aging are prone. His or her life experiences may include observing or actually undergoing some of the major stresses of aging such as disabling physical illnesses and object losses. Yet, under certain circumstances, positive motivation can hypertrophy into excessive therapeutic ambition, objectivity can be lost, and identification and empathy regress to introjection and oversensitivity. The residue of ambivalence in the most favorably negotiated life experiences may become activated. Any or all of these might precipitate countertransference in its many forms.

THE UNDERWORKER AND THE OVERWORKER

Two men will be described, both of whom suffered from depression and anxiety, but with differences in character and contrasting life styles. Each entered treatment skeptical about what therapy could accomplish. The first, an elderly bachelor, had never been able to achieve independence from his family. In an ironic, joking, self-depreciating, and imprecise way, he said: "I have no problem with retirement because I have never worked." Despite these limitations, he had pursued certain interests, and when he was not acutely depressed he had a capacity for fun.

The second man was sole owner of a small manufacturing business. He worked long days and on Saturdays, brought work home on evenings and Sundays, and rarely took even a brief vacation. He monitored every step in the creation of his manufactured product, advertised it and dealt with potential buyers, hired and trained employees, served as complaint department and troubleshooter, and invented new products and processes. His independence had been achieved out of necessity, very early and painfully. He had married and had a child. Despite his talents and achievements, he experienced little esteem and enjoyment.

These men were not optimum candidates for expressive, insight-centered treatment. Although they had never been psychotic and did not show the pervasive anger evinced by many who suffer borderline pathology, their lifelong conflicts, expressed in character formation, had preoedipal roots and narcissistic components. Their understanding of their own motives, relationships, and life patterns was limited and selective. Nevertheless, in these patients, the trial of treatment led to a shift of aim from support and mitigation of stress to adaptive intervention in the first case and to a degree of character change in the second. It usually requires intensified treatment to effect such shifts. In these instances, treatment was extended over time, but the sessions were scheduled only once every 2 to 4 weeks. The question arises about the extent of conflict resolution and repair of early traumas and deficits that is possible under these circumstances. Will there be relinquishment of infantile omnipotence, acceptance of realistic limitations, establishment of narcissistic balance, sublimation of primitive drive derivatives, and age-appropriate maturation?

The Lonely "Grasshopper"

A bachelor of 71, Mr. K., was referred to me by a psychiatrist who treated a young relative of his. The relative had described him as sitting in his apartment, depressed, afraid to go out, and reluctant to have any visitors. Two current contributing causes of the patient's depression and isolation were apparent. His younger brother by 6 years and only sibling, to whom he felt closely attached, had recently entered a nursing home because of an advanced state of chronic illness. The patient had been further isolated by the closing of an artists' club that he had attended regularly.

His father had died of a myocardial infarction when the patient was 11. His mother, the dominating influence in his life, had died at 90, 10 years before I met him. The patient had not been able to move away from his mother until his early 40s, and then only to an apartment in the same building, and with the help of a year of psychotherapy. His room at his mother's had been taken by one of her brothers. This unmarried uncle had had an adventuresome youth. In his later years, after retiring from work, he became depressed, began to drink, and finally committed suicide by jumping from the window of his sister's apartment.

The patient had been partly deaf for 30 years. Around the time of his mother's death, he was found to be mildly diabetic. Recently, he had developed angina pectoris. Mr. K. managed his diabetes without insulin by carefully monitoring his diet and took his heart medicine as prescribed. In contrast to his conscientious attention to his medical care, he declared with a mixture of defiance and guilt that he was a heavy cigarette smoker. And he confessed, with anxious overstatement, that he drank too much at times.

Mr. K.'s declaration that he had never worked was not literally true, but he had been supported throughout his life by a family business founded by his mother that was continued by his brother.

The patient looked his age. He was of medium short stature; he presented a neat figure, with thinning hair, a lined, square-shaped, yellowed face, complete with eye glasses and hearing aid. He wore an old tweed jacket, shirt and tie, dark pants, and black loafers. When not depressed, he often sported a conspicuously large button in his lapel bearing a cheerful adage or greeting, for example, "Merry Christmas." He carried one or more books or newspapers or magazine articles to show or give me as well as a pocket full of photographs and a wallet stuffed with news clippings.[1] In the waiting room, he deliberately put away his cigarette and entered my office ready with stories or jokes. He

---

[1] I have reported this use of mementos as a form of communication in the case of another single, potentially isolated older person (Kahana, 1967). The books, articles, programs, photographs, and letters brought to the therapist are not only aids to reminiscence and communication but serve as symbols of past objects and experiences akin to transitional objects.

even played harmless practical jokes, such as with a dollar bill on an elastic string. He was a friendly one-ring circus.

The patient remembered almost nothing of his early childhood, dating his recollections to his brother's birth. A photograph at age 4 showed him dressed up by his mother in a Buster Brown suit and haircut—a cute but baby, sissy outfit. His brother had insisted on wearing long pants and got his own way, whereas the patient was still unhappily dressed in shorts.

The mother had come to Boston from Europe in her 20s. The patient believes that she was basically timid, but she presented a facade of aggressiveness, particularly in her work. She was very antagonistic toward men. While the patient sat frozen with embarrassment and apprehension, she fought with waiters in restaurants and salesmen in stores. The patient attributes to this his long-standing fears of dining out and of shopping. His mother was obsessed with determination that he should not know about sex. When a girl fixed her stocking in public, his mother praised him for looking the other way. His concept and experience of sex became sadomasochistic: Men fooled and used women; boys conducted gang rapes of girls; female prostitutes performed without feeling. He was always afraid of women and never married.

Mr. K.'s fears dated to age 11 when his father died. His father was quiet and nice but away all day at work in his small manufacturing business. "We didn't see much of him. Sometimes mother would tell him that I had been bad, and he would hit me lightly with his strap. I didn't blame him." His father had little organized social life. He never belonged to lodges or clubs and was overweight and smoked. When he fell in the street with a heart attack at age 39, his wife received a telephone call that he had been taken to the morgue. Before the father died, the maternal grandmother, in her 90s, lived with them. In her last years she had a leg fracture and a psychosis.

The patient's mother started her business after the father's death. The patient recalls long, dragging hours when he and his brother awaited her return from work. There were frequent changes of apartments in tough, rundown sections of the city. Some children on the street had guns, and hoodlums "nearly murdered" the patient. He was determined to encourage his brother to find suitable friends and become free of this environment.

In his teens, the patient began to pursue two related interests, one, in an art form in which he possessed modest skill, and the other in amateur photography, recording people and events. He collected memorabilia, posters, programs, and catalogues, and his own photographs of the professional artists with whom he became acquainted over the years.

After finishing high school, Mr. K. started preprofessional training but could not keep up with the work. During his 20s, the years of the great economic depression, he served briefly in the National Guard, and then opened a small, secondhand book shop that was more a hobby than a financial success. He still had many books from that venture and would bring some to his therapy hours.

A psychiatrist who visited the bookstore became his friend and, later, was instrumental in the referral for psychotherapy. Of the year of psychotherapy in his early 40s, he said:

> Emotionally, I was an infant then and took my first steps. I had moved out of mother's apartment and begun a relationship with a girl of 18. Our sexual experience was satisfying, and she wanted to marry. But we had little in common in terms of interests and backgrounds. She was always on the go, and I wanted a quiet life. My family was opposed to the whole thing.

In spite of the gain in autonomy, he remained pessimistic, regarding himself as hopelessly messed up. "I would have needed 10 years of treatment for minor improvement."

I prescribed a tricyclic antidepressant medication and referred him to a newly opened, nearby senior day center. The young woman director visited him in his apartment and facilitated his entry into the center. His misgivings abated, as he found himself valued for his interests and humor, a scarce man in a situation with a preponderance of older women. He was really engaged by the attractive younger women on the staff—arts and recreation instructors and college student volunteer workers. Mr. K. reported sleeping better in a week and showed improved mood after 3 weeks. In therapy he spoke of his fears, especially that his brother would die and then he would drink and commit suicide like his uncle. He hinted at sexual urges that threatened his self-esteem.

At the end of 2 months, the patient shifted his dependence to the center. His visits to his brother in the nursing home became less traumatic, and he told of fantasizing that his mother was still alive in her apartment downstairs. Two dreams, reported after 5 months, expressed positive transference and easing of depression. The first dream was of his therapist's smiling in a group of doctors, and he associated it with a party given by his psychiatrist friend 35 years before. In the second dream, he was standing on a shelf of sand overlooking a beach and, suddenly, he was afraid that he would fall hundreds of feet to his death. He climbed down and discovered that the shelf was only a few inches above the beach.

These dreams are akin to many reported by children; they are almost undisguised wish fulfillments. They followed daydreams that his mother was alive and had not left him. In the first dream, his good, supportive friend, the psychiatrist, had returned in the person of the therapist. In the second dream, he had gained reassurance against suicide, which was depicted as falling to his death. The dreams not only indicated that the amelioration of his mood had been sustained but suggested that this improvement had extended deeper into unconscious levels revealed during sleep when ego controls are relaxed. The dreams were not distorted or accompanied by the shock of surprise or defensively disavowed, as we might see in a breakthrough of unconscious material. I commented that they expressed his better mood and good feeling about me. This was an affirmation and clarification of emerging preconscious thoughts and feelings rather than a true interpretation of unconscious content. It was possible to avoid confrontation, which might have provoked the negativistic insistence on "no improvement" or even on worsening, which is so common among people emerging from depression. I did not remark upon his dependence on me, which I welcomed as positive transference, not resistance, at that time.

It is my impression that these dreams were consistent with the childlike aspects of the patient's personality rather than indicative of any general characteristic of the dreams of older persons. In therapy, I respond to dreams of later life as I do to those of younger people, in the context of the therapeutic process and with consideration of the individual's character structure. This is in accord with the observation that the aging collectively represent the entire spectrum of personality and life experience. Freud's basic discoveries about dreams, including the dream as a window into the unconscious, the importance of wish fulfillment, the significance of memories of the preceding day or two, and the role of symbolism and the dream work, are applicable at any age. From the physiological side, studies show that REM sleep, the principal dream time, is not reduced appreciably in the nondemented aged (Regestein, 1980).

By the 6th or 7th month of therapy, the patient reported occasional ventures into the community, for example, excursions with a group from the center and attending concerts with a friend or staff member. He gave illustrated talks on art history at the center. I learned that some of his memorabilia, which he had given away to an artists' society, had been included in an exhibition in the city. He took photographs of the center, its members, staff, and activities. When he lunched there, he made a point of contributing beyond the subsidized cost of the meal.

In therapy, Mr. K. spoke more explicitly of his sexual interest in younger women and his fear of being a dirty old man in the eyes of others. I distinguished between fantasy and action, observing that his actual behavior with these women is like that of a fond relative. His unconscious response was to tell me about the play *The Elephant Man* that is based upon the account by the British surgeon, Sir Frederick Treves (1853–1923), of his discovery and humane treatment of Joseph Merrick (1862–1890), a 21-year-old man who was monstrously deformed by neurofibromatosis and exhibited as a sideshow freak. The patient brought me a copy of Ashley Montagu's book *The Elephant Man: A Study of Human Dignity* (1971). I interpreted to the patient that (unconsciously) he saw himself as the Elephant Man, an outcast, set apart and doomed, not by grotesque physical deformity and illness, but by shame over what he felt to be his personal failure, immaturity, and, above all, his "dirty" sexual wishes. In his wishes, he placed me in the idealized position of Treves, the noble doctor who rescued the Elephant Man, recognized his intelligence and sensibility, and restored his dignity in his remaining days. In reality, I *had* affirmed his dignity and his right to the enjoyment and privacy of his sexual fantasies.

In Treves' original essay, written over 30 years after the events, Merrick was said to have been "basely deserted" and abandoned by his mother to the workhouse when he was quite small. Treves thought that Merrick's memory of his mother as "very beautiful" was a comforting romantic fiction. Later research indicates that his mother was loving and caring (Howell & Ford, 1980). She died of pneumonia when he was 10 3/4 years old. After his father's remarriage, 1 1/2 years later, the increasingly lame and ugly boy found himself in competition with stepbrothers and stepsisters. Eventually, he became an outcast and was unemployable. He ran away to his father's warmhearted younger brother, until poverty forced him to enter the workhouse at age 16. He remained there for 6 years in grinding, regimented penury before escaping to the sideshow, where his exhibitors treated him with concern after their own fashion.

We did not pursue the further implications of the Elephant Man's story for my patient's early relationships with his mother and younger brother. In Mr. K.'s previous therapy, he had concluded sadly that his mother was not aware of the harmful effects upon him of her attitudes toward men and sexual life. He tended to regard his resigned hostility to her as a settled issue. Similarly, he defended his reactive protecting disposition toward his brother that had replaced his early ambivalence. Much later in treatment he brought a review of a book, *Mother Love: Myth and Reality*. The author believed that the majority of infants in a sample of mainly middle-class families in prerevolutionary Paris had been sent to wet-nurse in the country or simply abandoned by their parents, that is, "mother love is a gift, not a given."

By the time of my first summer vacation, 10 months after starting therapy, the patient had sustained his improved mood and increased level of activity. When I returned, Mr. K. told me with pleasure that he had been chosen as one of the 350 "Grand Bostonians" to receive municipal honors in celebration of the city's 350th anniversary. The center and his neighborhood had nominated him in recognition of his contribution to art history. He showed me the program listing his name and a copy of the certificate.

During that fall he appeared more animated, expressed anger at public officials who cheat and steal, and reminisced about Boston in the 1920s. He complained of lonely evenings but was unable to have his apartment refurbished and set in the order he regarded as requisite for visitors. In late fall, a respiratory infection led to pneumonia and diabetic ketosis. During his hospitalization, a niece straightened up his apartment, but his resistance to having visitors remained. While he convalesced at home, the center called him daily, serving as his telephone "lifeline." His illness interrupted therapy for 6 weeks.

Mr. K. reappeared in my office thin and cheerful, carrying a review of Jean Strouse's (1980) biography of Alice James—another talented, nervous invalid. In similar fashion, from time to time, he brought in other literary works or journalist's articles that dramatized and illuminated his own conflicts as the Elephant Man had done. These writings and his jokes, maxims, observations, and occasional reported dreams seemed to express three overlapping themes: sexual concerns, fears of madness, violence, and suicide, and the childlike versus the mature aspects of his character.

In a collection of short stories by Alberto Moravia the patient found one expressing the legitimate sexual needs of an older man. He brought in an issue of a national magazine, with the founder of psychoanalysis on the cover. The magazine sensationalized a recent book purporting to uncover an affair between Freud and his sister-in-law Minna; thus Freud was another dirty old man. He discussed the filmscript of the classical motion picture *M* of 1931 (Lang, 1968) that told the tale of a man who seduces and murders little girls. The forces of good and evil fight for the man's soul as he is pursued by the police, citizens, and the criminal underworld.

On one occasion, the patient began to speak of Vincent Van Gogh and his brother Theo, identifying himself with the artist who was supported by his brother (the only one who believed in him), suffered mental illness, and committed suicide. Many newspaper pieces about old people being assaulted and robbed served as vehicles of his aggression and rationalization of his phobias. However, he did observe that a number of older women at the center went out in the community carefully, without the intensity of fear that he experienced, that is, fear can be worse than reality.

The more childlike aspect of his personality was often expressed in his jokes. Like a doctor or professor, he would put a degree after his name, choosing the letters LSD, for "low sodium diet." "Pediatricians earn as little per visit as psychiatrists: It's hard to ask a baby for $50." Jokes and witticisms also served to cloak or express his mature observations: "I tried counting sheep to get to sleep, but it was no use. I'm an old goat, and my attention wandered." "There is a lady at the center who attends all funerals: The deceased cannot object." He quoted, "Youth is an act of nature; age is a work of art." The President was a special target of his humor. He handed me a packet of ketchup, saying "I've brought some Reagan vegetables." He also kept me posted on the amount of Mr. Reagan's earnings and pension from the State of California. Franklin Roosevelt's social legislation, he said, "passed without the aid of jelly beans."

Although Mr. K. tended to play down his own insight and maturity, it did come through; for example, the recognition that his joking had a defensive function, protecting his self-esteem. He shared with me one of his clippings, a thoughtful piece of art criticism in the field of his interest and made insightful and considerate comments about past and current acquaintances.

Shortly after the second summer interruption, the patient had the following dream, which was reported in September:

I had a fight with a big, broad-shouldered man. I was angry and hit at him.
I was awakened by falling out of bed and striking my lip [on a piece of fur-
niture]. It wasn't you; it was a bigger man.

I assured him that it was, indeed, me, and we discussed his need to defend against feeling deserted and angry. At this time, we discontinued
the antidepressant medication; subsequently, he felt better without it.

There are certainly many questions regarding his treatment. Can his
phobias be moderated further? How much change in character has occurred or is possible? Is he less grandiose? Is he better protected against
object loss, for example, the death of his brother? Might he have been
helped as much with less effort by an early decision to see him only at
monthly or bimonthly intervals in order to monitor the medication? Can
treatment ever be terminated? Should the frequency of therapy hours be
reduced progressively as suggested by Wayne (1953)? Some answers will
be ventured later, where they can be compared with similar issues in the
second case.

The Overworking "Ant"

The second patient, Mr. L., a married man of 65, was 38 when I first
saw him. At that time, he complained of anxiety and depression which
had reached the proportions of a panic. The youngest of four children
and now the sole survivor, he had a brother 6 years older who practiced
a profession; a sister 1 year older, who was unmarried and self-
supporting; and another brother, Tom, 3 years older, who had been a
partner in their small manufacturing business.

Two years before we met, Tom had committed suicide while
depressed, after spending the previous 2 years in and out of a mental
hospital. The patient had been immobilized with shock and grief for
several days after his brother's suicide. A psychiatrist had helped him
through the most acute affliction, but he remained "on a roller coaster"
of depression and remission. Subsequently, he saw another psychiatrist
who put him on a mild tranquilizer and a mild stimulant, which he had
used ever since. Mr. L. did not feel that these two therapists had understood his distress; perhaps he had not explained things well enough. But
he said, "there is no magic"—indicating his disappointed wish for a
magical cure.

The patient's wife was 4 years younger than he. Like her husband, she was vulnerable to anxiety and depression but was talented and worked very hard in a field in which she had held positions of leadership. When I first saw Mr. L., 27 years ago, he and his wife had been married for 6 years and had a 3 1/2-year-old son. His wife gave birth to a daughter about 4 months after therapy began.

The patient's earliest recollections were palpable screen memories, manifestly suggestive of fantasies. The first, at age 3, was of nursing at his mother's side. According to another memory, which was merged with a doubtful family myth, the cause of his mother's death, when the patient was 4 years old, was "some female disease" that had been the result of an unsuccessful attempt to produce an abortion while carrying him. His father, a tailor, had to place the three younger children in a large institutional home. For the patient and his sister this placement was preceded by a period in a foster home. A memory of being caught at age 6 in sexual exploration with two other children was associated with a recollection of becoming ill with whooping cough that turned into pneumonia and led to an ambulance ride from the foster home to a hospital.

His brother Tom was his protector in the large institutional home. Mr. L. recalled Tom as a leader who surpassed him in schoolwork, basketball, music, and dancing. Of the food in the home, he said that all meals afterward in life were an improvement. The patient had contracted head lice at age 10 and fought valiantly but unsuccessfully to avoid the shame of having his head shaved. He related these experiences to his persistent feelings of insecurity and inferiority, fear of poverty, and shyness in groups. Nevertheless, the atmosphere was humane; there was a rude but enjoyable summer camp; and the children were taught marketable skills. His and Tom's later business was an outgrowth of this training. Leaving the home meant leaving friends and Mr. L. made no others until he went to college. The home, at age 12, was the last place in which he felt that he belonged.

When the patient was 12, his father married a woman in her late 30s and the family was reunited. His stepmother had a 13-year-old daughter from a previous marriage. Neither the patient nor his siblings got along well with the stepmother whom they felt to be domineering and unfairly partial to her own child. With their father, she opposed his having a paper route and going to college. Mr. L. qualified these reproaches, saying that perhaps he blamed her too much; after all, she did bring the family together. His complaints against his father were less mitigated. His father did not talk with him, did not give him school lunch money, did not see that he was prepared for his Bar Mitzvah, did not come to his graduations or teach him to drive. He regarded his father as a self-depreciating failure.

The patient went to work early, providing his own clothing at age 15. Despite his parents' opposition, he attended and graduated from a state university, supporting himself with two or three jobs after classes. Mr. L. joined the ROTC and enjoyed sports, believing that he had "guts" then. He blamed himself now, however, for fearfully expecting disasters. He continued to reproach himself for his inability to get into an Ivy League college and for his failure to pass an examination that would have given him a government position as a factory inspector.

During World War II, the patient was a noncombatant instructor in the army air force, and he had an initial, brief experience of clinical depression. After the war, he and Tom started their manufacturing business; they had conducted it for several years when Tom's severe depression began.

Two Periods of Treatment

There were two distinct periods of treatment with me. The initial segment was psychodynamic psychotherapy of a depressed adult beginning in his late 30s. In the first 6 years, comprising almost half of the total hours, we met weekly, ending with his discharge as improved. Mr. L. returned after a year, following his father's death, and the treatment became an "interminable" follow-up. The second, much longer portion, evolved into a process of sustained support, assistance of maturation, and very gradual working through of narcissistic conflicts, with preparation for aging in mind.

The patient's grief over Tom's death was a major issue in the initial 2 1/2 years of therapy. After that, he spoke of his brother around the anniversary of the death, and his feelings were revived notably on two other occasions. The first occasion, 4 years after beginning treatment and 6 years after the bereavement, occurred when he began to consider merging his business with that of an older man as partner. The second was his father's death 9 years, almost to the day, after his brother died. I will pass over the therapy of his grief—which followed a familiar pattern. Eventually, for example, he could recall with intense guilt the deeper death wish to have his brother out of the way. In an introjective identification with Tom, the patient feared that he, too, would end as a suicide. In time, with the fading of grief, guilt appeared to be replaced by a masochistic fear of success.

We met weekly during the first 4 years of treatment and then monthly, with more frequent sessions during crises. Transference issues were most notable in the first 2 1/2 years. The patient had seen each of the two previous psychiatrists for about six interviews, and it is not surprising that the first harbinger of transference appeared in the 6th hour when he confessed to feeling envious of young, successful men. This feeling, which was now directed at me, resurfaced at 6 months. Mr. L. thought that my work was easier than his own because he was under constant pressure to develop new ideas, processes, and products. At that point, he also indicated greater trust, feeling that I was the one person with whom he could venture to talk about himself. In time, he came to speak of envying my youth (then), my success (his idealization), my (imagined) Ivy League background, my ability to understand and to help verbalize his feelings, and even my vacations.

Resistance in treatment also appeared quite early; it appeared initially as the fear that confronting certain feelings might lead to some sort of breakdown. After a few months, this became modified into a concern that he might appear "dumb" or "crazy" to me, and I would look down on him as weak or worthless. He was particularly afraid that I might react with excessive alarm or rejection to his occasional thoughts of suicide.

Mr. L.'s feelings of anger were expressed initially toward the psychiatrists who had not saved Tom. Then he recognized that he was angry at me as a component of his envy and feared my retaliation. Eventually, we connected this with his anger at his father for having been a poor provider and a poor model of an adult man. An element of competition with me began to appear, and in time he became aware of many strong competitive urges directed at other people as well. An indication of positive, dependent transference came in the 4th month, when a week's interruption of therapy led to intensification of depression that was followed, after my return, by the first definite improvement in mood. Near the end of a year, Mr. L. spoke of having to suppress positive feelings toward me lest they be interpreted as weakness or currying favor. In time, he was able to voice the wish that his son might become a physician.

We were able to explore his fears of poverty, "breakdown," and suicide, his fears of "experts," of the rich and powerful, and of being criticized or criticizing others and thus courting rejection. He felt humiliated by small failures or temporary setbacks. When, for a time, he enlarged his business through a merger, his partner's bragging and perfectionism further injured the patient's self-esteem. Gradually, we uncovered his underlying grandiose self-expectations and perfectionism, which lay behind this oversensitivity and contributed to the tendency to overwork.

Tenacious feelings of guilt that were associated with unconscious fantasies of being responsible for his mother's and brother's deaths were present as were feelings of shame and guilt that were related to persistent adolescent sexual fantasies involving his stepmother and stepsister. As a consequence of this guilt, Mr. L. did not feel that he deserved to succeed in life. The pattern of overworking was anchored in insecurity and self-punishment as atonement for guilt feelings; it was ego syntonic, requiring repeated interpretation to enable him to recognize and approach it as a problem to be corrected. In a patient with this type of depressive or masochistic character structure, it is not easy to distinguish immediately between stresses and gains because of the "negative therapeutic reaction." In this reaction, gains experienced as improvements or successes are felt unconsciously to be undeserved; that is, they evoke guilt. Conversely, setbacks and failures relieve guilt. Because reassessment of one's life is itself potentially a gain, both as a positive experience and as a means of enhancing adaptation, the person with a depressive character may resist this aspect of psychotherapy.

The patient's principal current stresses were experienced in his business. He fluctuated between depression when orders were slack and anxiety when production deadlines were near. Turnovers and incompetence of personnel were his bane. Four-and-one-half years after we started, he experienced another kind of major stress when the sudden appearance of a melanoma required immediate removal of one eye. Mr. L. and his wife were more concerned about each other's reaction than about themselves. The surgery was successful, and he handled it in a sensible and emotionally appropriate fashion. This favorable reaction to surgery and handicap had both rational and unconscious determinants. Unconsciously, the operation and defect represented a punishment, thus assuaging guilt. At the same time, he was realistically encouraged by the evident improvement in his overall functioning brought about by therapy. Tangible indication of this improvement had occurred a few months before the operation when he was finally able to buy a house for his family. Within a year, sustained improvement led to stopping therapy by mutual consent.

Return to Treatment

The patient's return to treatment, 7 years after we first met, was precipitated by his father's death. This loss, like the deaths of his stepmother, mother-in-law, sister, a sister-in-law, and oldest brother during the following 16 years, mobilized memories and feelings, and promoted reassessment of the meaning and impact of old relationships. These losses aroused the wish to improve his life, enjoy some leisure, and know more about the world of art. The deaths of his father and siblings all occurred near Labor Day, coinciding with the anniversary of Tom's suicide and thus awakening echoes of that grief. Not all of the stressful losses that he experienced were by death. One of the worst brief recurrences of acute depression followed his son's departure for college.

A major problem in the business, illustrating his slow rate of change, concerned a foreman he had employed for many years. This man, whom the patient regarded as indispensable—the only employee who could be relied upon to run the production line—was bigoted and paranoid. With innuendo and menacing actions, he made life intolerable for any worker who was not white, conservatively dressed, and beardless. Several years went by before the patient even mentioned the problem, and it took another 9 years before he could stop placating the foreman and let him go. Within a year or two, the shop underwent a renaissance; everyone relaxed, beards bloomed, and colors glowed; production went on. Almost 20 years after we first met, there was a lasting upturn in business with the acquisition of an extremely active and successful outside salesman who brought in a stream of orders.

With the purchase of a house, the patient began to become rooted. He and his wife gave parties occasionally for friends and neighbors, including some young academics and business people. From time to time Mr. L. mentioned playing golf on a weekend. His children pulled him into cross country skiing. The couple bought a half-interest in a country cottage. As his 60th birthday approached, Mr. L. began to consider the possibility of retirement in the future. Two years later, he spoke thoughtfully of his eventual, normal death, with practical concern for the security of his family.

In both courses of therapy, some of the most ordinary parent–child experiences introduced an element of pleasure into his existence. During the first interval, while on a dutiful visit to relatives, Mr. L. took his 5-year-old son to see the Statue of Liberty, and he felt, momentarily, like a happy boy again. Taking the son fishing aroused self-reproach: "I should do more for the boy.'' The patient, however, also became aware that he was not repeating with his son the neglect that he had experienced at the hands of his father. He could even admit that he enjoyed himself with the children.

The children's development promoted reworking of his own formative experiences. His son's masturbation at age 4 revived painful memories of being punished for sex play. When his daughter, at age three, announced that she was a boy and gave herself a boy's name, he responded in a more relaxed, accepting way and with some amusement. Awareness of his son's oedipal attachment led to screen memories of his mother. His children's perceived shyness promoted discussion of his own social timidity. During the second phase of therapy their generally healthy development gave him assurance. Mr. L. could accept their adolescent ventures with an expectable level of concern. These included his son's February vacation trip to Sarasota with collegemates (the boy acquired body lice), his son's beard, habit of smoking pot, and living with the girl he eventually married. He also accepted his daughter's departure for college and dropping out for a semester.

In the psychotherapy, there was repeated clarification, reassessment, and some working through of feelings and conflicts that were related to the sources of his symptoms. Among these anxieties and disturbing emotions were his fears of poverty, weakness, rejection, criticism, and suicide, his feelings of envy, anger, and competition, and his manifest low self-esteem and underlying grandiosity. Mr. L. came to recognize the chronicity of his depression and how it affected every aspect of his life. He also rediscovered past pleasures: He had been a good sailor at camp and had enjoyed some of his Army experience. Much work was done on his self-boundaries, for example, acknowledging his differences from Tom or seeing that many concerns about his son were *self*-concerns.

In the course of our discussions, he could reevaluate experiences that had remained as the residues of trauma, for example, the painful disappointment when he had not succeeded in becoming a government factory inspector. In his mind, this had stamped him as a failure. Late in therapy, when his business was prospering, the patient and I could enjoy the analogy to the fictitious tale of the illiterate, underpaid shammes or beadle of an impoverished village synagogue: One day the board of directors discovered this man's illiteracy and fired him as unqualified for the position. He was forced to go out into the world of business and, after many years, became a millionaire. An acquaintance, upon hearing this story, was amazed at his achievement in the face of such limitations and exclaimed: "Imagine what (more) you would have been today if only you had been able to read and write!" The millionaire replied, "I know what I would have been—the village shammes."

Again, in the case of Mr. L., questions arise concerning the type of treatment and the outcome. It is my impression that few cases are reported of treatments considered to be interminable, and those comprise mainly psychoses and psychotic character disorders. Therapists may regard such cases as failures of treatment or the intrusive substitution of a quasi-parental relationship for a therapeutic one. In this instance, the overriding consideration was the patient's initial vulnerability, his limited tolerance of therapeutic regression, and his persistent need for support based on severe traumatization in childhood. There were in all about 480 treatment hours, the time equivalent of 2 1/2 years of psychoanalysis. Therapy was vis-à-vis. Transference was interpreted when I believed it constituted a resistance, or as it expressed developmental fixation or progress. For the most part it was mildly positive. Extratransference clarification and interpretation played a significant role. I interviewed Mr. L.'s wife with him on several occasions during his depressive crises.

Overall, the patient was helped with his acute depression and showed a gradual capacity for better resolution of narcissistic and oedipal conflicts. He matured in ways appropriate to the life cycle, with consideration of aging, possible retirement, and natural death. There was partial amelioration of his overwork tendency and growth of the capacity to enjoy life.

WORK AND RECREATION

Mark Twain said it best:

> Work consists of whatever a body is *obliged* to do, and play consists of whatever a body is not obliged to do. (*The Adventures of Tom Sawyer*)

However, the common contrast of work and recreation is only a rough approximation of experience. Work is certainly forced upon us by necessity. It attaches us to reality, especially to the human community, but it also serves for the gratification of all kinds of drives (Freud, 1930). Optimally, it has many rewarding aspects, including permitting sublimated discharge of aggression, serving as a major source of self-esteem, and providing social status. It affords the pleasures of mastery, craftsmanship, and creativity; it gains us a measure of independence and the means of recreation; and it provides a necessary counterpart to more purely pleasurable activities. And it satisfies our superego. The overworker epitomized the pathology of work that is without pleasure. Moreover, he tended to turn his recreation into work, for example, renovating his summer cottage.

Both men, the underworker and the overworker, came from hardworking families, had experienced the great economic depression of the 1930s, and regarded working as the symbol and the reality of security. Both valued the work ethic. The underworker valued it explicitly and consciously, believing himself to be a failure by that stringent standard. The overworker valued it implicitly and unconsciously, and he lived by it. Both had major impairments in the ability to work effectively. This is more obvious in the underworker who never established his independence fully and who lived hedged in by phobias. Although the overworker was productive and innovative, his work lacked gratification and suffered by virtue of his difficulty in delegating responsibility. At times, worsening depression interfered with his effectiveness. Both men had suffered early and severe psychological traumas that left them with vulnerable self-esteem. Each acted as though his survival were almost constantly at stake. The underworker preserved himself by his phobic avoidance, rarely leaving his apartment for the "dangerous" streets. The overworker behaved as if his continued existence was predicated upon uninterrupted work.

CONTRASTING AIMS OF TREATMENT

Except at the very start of treatment, when both patients were severely depressed, requiring immediate attention and evaluation of suicide risk, the aim of psychotherapy differed significantly in these two cases. This followed from differences in personality that were apparent from the beginning. The underworker, Mr. K., had more impairment of ego functions, particularly executive functions, was fixated upon shame, had more limited and superficial personal relationships despite a much wider circle of acquaintances, and was generally more immature and dependent, with an appealing childlike manner. He was more likely to assume that he would be cared for, as he had been by his mother. The overworker, Mr. L., in contrast, had more intact ego functions, suffered from guilt (expressed in a masochistic-depressive character structure), and was a counterdependent do-it-yourselfer. He had a richer network

of family and social relationships and, later on, his children's development offered him many "second chances" to become more mature and
flexible.

The underworker was seen in old age, when he had begun to show
early signs of debilitation, which became evident later when he had
pneumonia.[2] Because of debilitation and lessened resilience, it is more
typical for older people to enter treatment at a point of crisis than it is
for younger ones. Good experience with therapy earlier in life and the
encouragement of family members who have themselves benefited from
psychotherapy help to motivate and sustain treatment, as they did in this
case despite Mr. K.'s initial misgivings. Because his crisis had come on
slowly, and it was an effort for him to leave his apartment for the office
visits, we decided, after the initial evaluation, to meet every second
week. Another point of decision for the therapist came at the end of 2
months. At that time, the patient was less depressed, able to satisfy some
of his needs for care, stimulation, and affirmation of self-esteem at the
senior center, and had become more objective in his relationship with
his brother. Although Mr. K. did not indicate any wish to stop, one
might have considered meeting less frequently to monitor his antidepressant medication while remaining available for any recurrent crisis.

My decision to continue was based upon the following: Mr. K.'s improvement was recent, and his commitment to therapy still tentative. If
we met infrequently, he might not call in time before he was in a more
serious state of depression, or he might lose confidence in the treatment.
His painful dependence upon his brother was not sufficiently alleviated,
and he was in a process of mourning in anticipation of his brother's
eventual death. I was not sure that he would continue to resolve this dependence and grief with only the minimum of support. On the positive
side, I thought that he had potential for a higher level of improvement.
Despite the phobias, he had a social life built around an interest in art
and books. His art history activities represented a sublimation and a link
to younger generations, and his humor was an adaptive asset, which was
attractive to people. In therapy, he did not repeat himself in a stagnant

---

[2]The debilitated or frail aged are the small group who, toward the end of life, show the
limiting effects of chronic and multiple physical illnesses, diminished functional reserve
of various organ systems, constriction of activities, increased realistic dependence on others,
depletion of self-esteem and satisfactions (with more reliance upon the memories of past
gratifications), and the armoring of defenses against painful affects induced by accumulat-
ing losses of significant people. (Kahana, 1979)

fashion; instead, he enlarged upon his interests and tried to engage me and address my apparent or presumed interests in psychoanalysis, literature, local history, and current events.

This positive attitude and a degree of objectivity about his problems indicated that further development of a limited working alliance was possible. All of this suggested that the aim in therapy of adaptive intervention might be more appropriate than the limited one of support. On the other hand, to go beyond adaptive intervention would require a greater degree of self-awareness and tolerance of tension than he possessed. Mr. K.'s inability to achieve autonomy and his long history of symptoms weighed against the goal of deeper character change.

This cautiously favorable estimate of the patient's potential was borne out by his beginning, spontaneously, to bring in anxieties and feelings of shame. He continued to work on these and on the fears of insanity and aggression, narcissistic needs, and his self-depreciating tendency. Continuation of therapy enabled me to answer some of my early questions about him. For example, when I first heard that he had given away much of his art history collection and was giving away his books, old postcards, and other acquisitions (he offered some of these to me), I wondered to myself whether he was making plans to die or was expressing a need to be given to. In time, I concluded that this had represented mainly a certain generosity of spirit, which had been evident previously in his early determination to protect and save his younger brother. The same admixture of altruism (sublimation) and reaction formation was manifested in his encouragement of artists.

The leading transferences were compulsive and narcissistic, and to a lesser extent masochistic. Positive feelings predominated. "Good" compulsive attitudes, reminiscent of a latency child, were evinced in the way he consciously worked on problems. Negativism and passive aggression were less evident unless, for example, he felt pressured to confront his phobic anxiety. Mr. K. tended to idealize the therapist and to seek out affirmation of his own worth. A psychoanalyst was a fellow member of the avant garde and, masochistically, a fellow sufferer from the attitudes of the vulgar. Masochism was also expressed in self-deprecating humor, with the expectation that the therapist would join in the laughter. I tried to be aware of these attitudes in order not to accept them unquestioningly or overreact against them. Overacceptance promoted the illusion that all was going well, until this gave way to a frustrated feeling in me of getting nowhere. Overreaction against these transferences took the form of impatience and irritation with the self-deprecation and the urge to become too active or even aggressive.

What was the outcome of treatment? The phobias persist, but they have been moderated to the extent that he takes more frequent outings, arranging to go with companions or staying overnight in a familiar, safe environment. His narcissistic balance is restored as seen in a sustained improvement of mood. He is less ashamed of his sexual wishes and less afraid of his aggressive impulses. This is evidence of a degree of conflict resolution. Significantly, he can reveal more openly his mature interests and artistic judgments, the more sublimated and fully developed side of his character. Abatement of the unconscious grandiosity is evident in his acceptance of limitations and in more reasonable self-expectations. Beyond this, there is little further repair of early traumas and deficits, which were mainly the influence of his parents (both actual and in his unconscious fantasies), that he has long regarded with resignation. It is my impression that he has a better prospect of mourning and successfully surviving his brother's death. He is more separate and objective in this relationship, and he can use therapeutic support when and if he experiences that loss. At the time of this report, the question of terminability of therapy is undecided. He has not indicated a wish for reduction or interruption of treatment.

The second patient, Mr. L., the overworker, began therapy at midlife. Although ostensibly he had settled his occupational and marital choices some years before, he felt trapped rather than fulfilled in his existence. Symptoms of midlife crisis, such as restlessness in his career and marriage and an upsurge of narcissistic entitlements, were overshadowed by long-standing impairments of autonomy and self-esteem and by acute despair following his brother Tom's suicide. It took several years to mitigate this depressive emergency. During this period, the aims of treatment were to facilitate mourning for his brother, to help him rebound from other then-current traumatic experiences, and, to a limited extent, to clarify his masochistic-depressive reactions, such as turning hostility upon himself. After 6 years it appeared that the general aim of adaptive intervention had been achieved. He functioned as well as he ever had. In addition to his wife's continuing help, he had gained the support of an older man as business partner, who was a symbolic substitute for Tom.

When Mr. L. returned to psychotherapy after his father's death and had once again mastered his grief and regression, it was clear that he needed some form of continued treatment. There were two reasonable choices. We could stop then and resume when further crises arose, or we could continue regularly, attempting to modify his character structure. Left on his own he would endure moderate anxiety and depression, and this equilibrium would be interrupted by episodes of more severe and alarming regression. Thus far in therapy, Mr. L. had changed slowly but definitely, employing his assets of intelligence, a degree of self-awareness, motivation, positive transference and ability to tolerate painful affects. He continued to be involved, willy-nilly, in a variety of human relationships that held promise of stimulating him to further constructive change. Accordingly, we decided to go on, choosing monthly intervals as an efficient pace. Over the long run the criteria of progress, reflecting structural changes, were indices of maturation.

It is not a simple task to describe the course or effects of maturation in an individual case because it is not simply a matter of the easing or disappearance of symptoms. Favorable change in psychic structure does not mean transformation to a different type of character. The general rule still holds that, as we grow older, we become more like ourselves, or, in the French saying, "The more things change, the more they remain the same." At 65, the overworker would still react with envy in the transference or respond to an improvement in guilty fashion. But, in contrast to similar feelings at age 38, he quickly showed evidence of objectivity and self-awareness and saw the repetitiveness and exaggeration in his behavior, even its humorous aspect. Although Mr. L. retained the general tendencies of his masochistic-depressive character structure, he showed greater appreciation of his own accomplishments vis-à-vis those of others, increased acceptance of realistic ideals, and relatively more sense of responsibility as against self-sacrifice.

The perspective of maturation is that of the life cycle. To be mature is to have undergone natural growth and development with potential capabilities realized. The watchwords of psychological maturity are "appropriate," "realistic," "assimilated," "differentiated," "neutralized," and "flexible." Mature behavior is appropriate to the person's age and life cycle stage. It presupposes good reality testing and is based upon well-assimilated life experiences. Assimilated experiences, feelings, and meanings are integrated, cumulative, and are available to memory. They serve as guides to participation in new events. Differentiation refers to the capacity to recognize more precisely the meanings and determinants of events and the differences between them, including nuances, shad-

ings, and ambiguities. Neutralized psychic responses make differentiation possible. They are characterized by thoughtful, planned behavior
rather than impulsive action. Being flexible means being able to be appropriately grown up or childlike, self-concerned or attuned to the needs
of others, and able to change one's course or viewpoint when it is indicated.

In Mr. L.'s life, as it focused in therapy, he addressed major life cycle tasks: parenting, making a contribution to work and to the culture,
the reworking of narcissistic conflicts in preparation for losses, illnesses,
and other narcissistic stresses of old age, and the anticipation of lessened
activity and more leisure. Improvement in reality testing was seen in the
correction of projection onto others of self-expectations. Assimilation of
experience was marked by gradual working through of conflicts and anxieties and the gaining of perspective on his life. Differentiation was apparent in the enrichment of his perceptions of others, especially his children. Evidences of neutralization were increased thoughtfulness, less
need to prove his worth through overwork, and better narcissistic balance. Flexibility was reflected in his enjoyment of recreation.

With the underworker, compulsive and narcissistic transferences had
predominated. In contrast, the overworker developed early ambivalent
transferences of envy, idealization, and trust, which shifted later to competition and positive identification. These transferences could be clarified for the patient without encountering major resistance. They were
not in a form or of an intensity to provoke unsettling countertransferences. On the other hand Mr. L.'s masochistic-depressive style and slow
rate of change aroused countertransference feelings of helplessness and
impatience and doubts about the value of my efforts. Sometimes my attempts to confront him, as with his masochistic behavior toward the
bigoted foreman, acquired a sadistic coloring. This had to be recognized,
understood, acknowledged to the patient, and controlled. The spacing
of interviews tended to dilute the intensity of such transference-
countertransference struggles.

SUMMARY

"If you don't have fun when you are young, you won't when you
are old." This lesson of epigenesis is highlighted briefly as expressed in
the life and writings of Sir Max Beerbohm, the British writer, critic, and
caricaturist. The psychopathology of work and play is explored as seen

in the psychotherapy of two men. Both suffered depression, in part on the basis of early narcissistic injuries. The first, treated in old age, had never been able to hold an independent job or maintain an autonomous existence; yet he had preserved his childhood capacity for enjoyment. The second, seen from midlife to the threshhold of old age, an unusual example of long-term "interminable" therapy, was an overworker who had not been able to achieve inner security, self-esteem, or pleasure. General strategies or aims of dynamic psychotherapy have been outlined, particularly as applied with older patients. Common transferences and countertransferences with this group have been described. The aims of support, adaptive intervention or structural change, the individual transference manifestations, the use of clarification and interpretation, and the handling of dreams have been discussed as they applied in the two cases. Maturation, preparation for old age, and the restitution of narcissistic balance have been considered in relation to outcome of treatment.

References

Beerbohm, M. *Mainly on the air.* New York: Knopf, 1958. (a)

Beerbohm, M. *Max's nineties.* Introduction by Osbert Lancaster. New York: J. B. Lippincott, 1958. (b)

Behrman, S. N. *Portrait of Max.* New York: Random House, 1960.

Bibring, G. L., & Kahana, R. J. *Lectures in medical psychology.* New York: International Universities Press, 1968.

Cecil, D. *Max: A biography.* Boston: Houghton Mifflin, 1964.

Erikson, E. H. Observations on Sioux education. *Journal of Psychology,* 1939, *7,* 101–156.

Freud, S. Civilization and its discontents. In J. Strachey (Ed. and Trans.), *Standard edition* (21:59). London: Hogarth Press, 1930.

Howell, M., & Ford, P. *The true history of the elephant man.* London: Allison & Busby, 1980.

Kahana, R. J. Medical management, psychotherapy and aging. *Journal of Geriatric Psychiatry,* 1967, *1,* 78–89.

Kahana, R. J. Strategies of dynamic psychotherapy with the wide range of older individuals. *Journal of Geriatric Psychiatry,* 1979, *12,* 71–100.

Lang, F. *"M.": A film by Fritz Lang.* (Translation and Introduction by Nicholas Garnham, Classic Film Scripts.) New York: Simon & Schuster, 1968.

Montagu, A. *The elephant man: A study in human dignity.* New York: Outerbridge and Dienstfrey, 1971.

Regestein, Q. R. Sleep and insomnia in the elderly. *Journal of Geriatric Psychiatry,* 1980, *13,* 153–171.

Sandler, A. M. Problems in the psychoanalysis of an aging narcissistic patient. *Journal of Geriatric Psychiatry,* 1978, *11,* 5–36.

Strouse, J. *Alice James: A biography.* Boston: Houghton Mifflin, 1980.

Wayne, G. J. Modified psychoanalytic therapy in senescence. *Psychoanalytic Review,* 1953, *40,* 99–116.

15

Being Sick and Facing Eighty
OBSERVATIONS OF AN AGING THERAPIST

MARTIN GROTJAHN

I do not mind being 77, but to be 80 soon is a different matter. I have doubts that I will live that long because I am sick and definitely handicapped. Death, however, remains unconceivable for me as being nothing—totally nothing, a black hole in the universe.

ON BEING SICK

I have been sick—kidney stones, gallstones, appendicitis—but sickness came and left my life, and I continued more or less as before.

This, my last sickness, is different. It stays with me, and I have to live with it. It is here to stay with me, and in time to come it will win.

For all my life I looked forward to growing old with great expectation. In my fantasy, it seemed I would become wise, slightly detached from the worries of this world, beyond desire and temptation, without frustration, and therefore without anger, rage, and fits of temper. Finally, I would be without guilt, without obligations and duties. I just would be alive. That would be true freedom; freedom from inner drive; freedom from outer temptation or threat. I thought as an old man I would finally be what I was supposed to be: I myself and Free.

I assume that I had reached maturity by now and had reached a time in my growth where I could deal reasonably well with inner and outer reality. The assignment of my age is now to achieve wisdom, which is the ability to deal with the unavoidable reality of death. That seems to be the last assignment—and it seems to escape my reach. So far as I am concerned, old age seems to be combined with a certain amount of physical deterioration and illness, but the mind should and could grow some more if given a little time longer. If I could express my wish in that matter, I would say I need one more year—or two.

Facing 80

Facing 80 in 1984, I probably have to realize that I am already old—to my surprise. I don't really feel it. I do feel sick at times.

I started to work with the aged, individually and in groups a long time ago, in 1936. I became a consultant for gerontology in two universities—but I never felt old. Other people around me got old, but I did not. I could walk as well and as far as always. I never noticed whether the road went up the mountain or came down.

I could think and work out clinical experience as well as ever or better than before. I became 60, 65, and even 70, not feeling much change. This is remarkable for me because I always have been and still am my favorite patient and constantly under self-observation. I think I stand in good and constant communication with my unconscious. My self awareness had become my trusted working tool for understanding patients and myself. When I could understand myself, I could understand others. When I was in a resistance, every patient seemed to follow me, and work slowed down and even stopped.

Never have I felt the need to consult any therapist after my training analysis 50 years ago. Since then, I always felt I could take care of myself and of us, meaning besides myself, also my wife and my son. As I took care of them, they took care of me.

My marriage continued where my analysis left off. It was not necessarily in the form of a dialogue but mostly in the form of a continued self-analysis. I analyzed myself as if I were my own favorite patient, and I analyzed my patients as if they were myself—more or less.

Anyhow, feeling young or old, I decided to work less when I became 75. I wanted to have more time for contemplation, more time for doing nothing. I tried to do more of nothing. I tried not to follow any ambitions left in me from former times, but there was always another essay to write, another lecture to give, another book to think about, and another city to visit.

My son Michael, who sometimes seems to have learned already what I still have to learn, asked me: "Did you ever sit down and do nothing?" That did it—I started to do more of nothing.

Sudden Illness

Then suddenly it happened. I got an "asthma" attack, which I never had experienced in my life. I was not especially surprised or alarmed. I had been allergic to dust, especially when the wind blew from the desert. I reacted sometimes with severe vasomotoric rhinitis. I had often wondered why I did not have asthma because my brother and sister suffered with it.

That night I could not sleep, and an indescribable terror overpowered me. I felt I was being annihilated and destroyed. I was facing absolute stark, timeless, and formless nothingness. Ernst Simmel told me once that he did not mind dying so much as being dead. I felt beyond dying. I know death fear, but this time death was already in me; it stopped my breathing and stopped my heart.

I lived through that night, or, rather, my wife lived me through. She did not do anything; she just was there with me, and I was not alone. We waited for death or for the morning, whichever might come first. I told her about this anxiety. In the morning we went to my doctor. In his office I already regretted having come. I felt better and did not feel I had the right to bother him. The "asthma" was almost gone; if there ever was a man with "imagined health," it was me.

My doctor was not fooled: He was shocked. One look at my electrocardiogram showed a total left bundle branch block that had not been there on previous occasions. My doctor suspected that I was having a coronary occlusion right then and there. He also knew me well enough not to tell me. I probably would have walked away, not believing him. So he called an ambulance first, and when I saw those men with the litter and the oxygen, he told me, and I didn't see any way to protest against hospitalization. I went to the intensive care unit, in the ambulance, with sirens blaring, and with my wife in hot pursuit of us, desperately trying to keep up with the ambulance.

I still did not feel old: I did not even feel sick. I felt annoyed about the whole circus performance.

Angina!

I needed a second, much more serious congestive heart failure to realize that something was seriously wrong with my heart. That did it: At first I felt sick, then old. I had angina pectoris attacks, spells of dyspnea, later palpitations, and most of all, overpowering, humiliating anxiety attacks, which I considered most inappropriate for a psychiatrist. The typical angina pain developed only a few weeks later.

It was a panic without visual images, far beyond any words. It was a certainty of impending death. Only the kind face of my wife would reassure me (and nitroglycerin of course relieved me promptly). The fact that my son appeared —he is, like my wife, also a physician—gave me courage and hope as well as it showed me that other people took my condition seriously. So I was not only hysterical, I was sick!

A slow recovery followed: As long as I live within my restrictions of most limited walking and a strict low-sodium diet, I live quite in comfort but now definitely like an old man. I do not work anymore, and I walk little. Peculiarly enough, I feel all right about it. All of a sudden, 50 years of work in psychiatry, psychoanalysis, and group therapy seems to be enough. Now I have no more worries about patients, no more guilt that I don't understand somebody well enough, no more bad conscience that I do not know how to help them more. I feel free from the guilt that goes with our work: The feeling of never being as good as one ought to be to help somebody. Let other people worry now. I am through with work and worry: I am a free man.

I sit in the sun watching the falling leaves slowly sail across the waters of the swimming pool. I think, dream, draw, sit. I feel almost free of this world of reality. This fall, this Southern California "winter" seems more beautiful than I have ever seen it.

Whoever would have told me that I would be quietly happy just sitting here, reading a little, writing a little, and mostly enjoying life in a quiet and modest way, I would, of course, not have believed. That a walk across the street to the corner of the park would satisfy me more than a long walk when only 2 years ago I thought a 4-hour walk was just not enough—that surprises me.

I have time now. I do not know how much time is left for me to live, but I am in no hurry: I am in no hurry to get anywhere, not even to the end of time. That can wait. When that time comes, I will try to accept it. I have no illusions; it will not be easy.

Right now I live in the moment, and I want to sit here a little while longer, quietly, and hoping not to sit in anybody's way.

I always thought old age is an achievement in itself. I now know better: To get sick and to live on, *that* is an achievement.

How to Face the Nothingness of Being Dead

When I was born, the old and wise woman from the neighborhood came to foretell my future. She listened to the screams of my rage and said: "He will love the yellow of eggs, but he will learn nothing." My mother loved the poetry of these words, and I have heard them often.

I did not do badly in the almost 80 years of my life. I even learned how to live a little from the people who did not know and came to me to learn. But now I am stuck again. I am not ready to die, not ready to say goodbye to this life. I am not ready to say goodbye to myself. That seems to be the worst: to say goodbye to myself. Through all the years, I have built myself, and in that way I am a self-made man or a "self-found" one.

I know dying is unpleasant, but to be dead is *Nothing*. I like that even less. Sure, I am a narcissist. Who in our profession is not? I think of all the investment I have made in myself: the analysis, endless training, the continued self-analysis, the drive to understand, to give insight, and the wealth of knowledge accumulated in a lifetime. All this I should give up?

Fifty-five years of marriage were built with care, study, insight, learning, and patience, and grew to ever deepening love. I am a most impatient person of genuine bad temper, but I worked on myself: I tried to deepen my insight, to become a better therapist and a better person. And finally, all should turn to ashes? Just because my heart does not want to do its part anymore? One does not need to be a narcissist to find that unacceptable. To say goodbye to myself and vanish into nothingness? Well, it shall be done. Nobody claimed it would be easy.

I would not want to live my life all over again. I would not want to go to a Prussian school again—to worry about being loved—or not. I am equally certain that I would only accept the offer to live a much longer life, in relative health. I would so much like to see "who wins" or what happens next.

Deaths of Friends

How come so many of my friends accepted death as a matter of course? It may be just that, that death may happen to me too: I hope it will not be tonight and not tomorrow either.

My friend James got angry, very angry; he knew that scotch and a tranquilizer took the edge off his rage. And when there was no more rage in the course of a long night, there was no more James either.

My friend Byron did not want to die, but he was obsessed by the idea that he did not need to be in pain. So he took sedation, ever heavier sedation, until he felt no pain anymore. He finally felt nothing, not even himself, and so he was dead.

Maria wanted to die before her arms became paralyzed. She had a degeneration of her spinal cord. And so she took a heavy overdose of sedation, made love as she had planned, said goodbye to herself and was gone.

I knew a murderer for whom to kill was the ultimate fulfillment, an indescribable lust. When he was told he would have to die and was made ready for execution, he turned to me and wanted to know whether he would hear his blood rushing out of his neck? That, he knew, would be the moment of greatest lust. I did not know the answer, but I did not interfere with his lustful hope.

My friend George could not die and wanted me to help him. I told him as long as he needed help to die, he was not ready, and I would be on the side of life. When he would be ready, he would not need me and would die. He heard me and even understood me, and he died that night.

The poor little rich girl, Juliana, suffered and suffered, fought, and suffered some more. She had no illusion and finally followed her husband silently, obediently, submissively, into the unavoidable nothing.

If I think that millions of people will greet the sun tomorrow morning and I may not, I get mad. Well, I am old. I had a good and full life. I tried my best, and I should be ready to leave, or at least I should be able to learn how to accept the end and wait quietly. I loved and was loved and that I shall not take with me? Then I will not go!

I still love the yellow of eggs, and I do not learn my last lesson. I live quietly; it is now a life of moderation and meditation, but I live. It is the nothingness I fear. I remember the nothingness of narcosis, and I know there is nothing to remember; there is no suffering and no boredom; there is not even a feeling for nothingness. It will not be terrible: It will be nothing.

DREAMS OF DEATH

Last night I dreamt about my father, who had been my mother when I was a child. He died 51 years ago. He did not say anything in my dream; he never did talk much. Silence was his answer, and silence is frequently a symbol of death in dreams.

Dreams of death are often beautiful. It always has struck me as sad that when people finally have beautiful dreams, they are dreams of death. In these dreams, people dream about beautiful castles, which represent the houses of the parents, frequently of the dead parents. I dream frequently of the university in the City of God, the city of learning for me. In these dreams I have the vague feeling I don't belong there, or I do not find my room, or my room has been given away to other people. When I dream about beautiful landscapes, fountains, and streams, I associate immediately with fantasies about the marvelous life hereafter, in which I seem to believe only in my dreams.

How banal and naive death symbols may be even in the dreams of a person as complex and supposedly sophisticated as an aging therapist! They are dreams of traveling: To ride the train from here to hereafter; the slow emptying of the train, meaning the departure of so many friends; collecting books and notes, symbolizing all my knowledge I want to take along and can't; jumping out of the train over a deep and dangerous looking trench; being in that part of Berlin where my father died many years ago.

A Dream of My Own

The following dream was dreamt in the night after a visit to my physician, who was as pleased with my state of health as I was.

> I was riding in a train, going from a suburb of Berlin (the city of my birth) to the terminal in a dilapidated part of Berlin. I was aware that the train got slowly empty of people. I had made myself comfortable, unpacked several books, many papers, notes, pens and pencils, and writing paper. I realized that I would have to leave the train at the next stop. I had increasing anxiety to get my belongings together, stuffing them in several briefcases, looking back whether I left anything. The train stopped, the door opened, and there was a deep, bottomless trench—or empty space— between the train and the station platform. I thought that other people got out there, and so would I. I stepped back and then ran with full speed to the door. I made a gigantic jump, landing with all my stuff "on the other side."
>
> I realized it was late when I left the station. I could not walk to visit my father, wanted to take a taxi, but there were none. There were only a few horse-drawn carriages, as I remember them in Berlin from the time before the war back in 1914. They did not stop when I tried to flag them down. So I woke up highly annoyed.

A patient of mine succeeded in visiting me while I was in the intensive care unit of the hospital. (I do not remember his visit.) A year later, when he visited me at home, he told me a "most banal" dream. He saw an airplane overhead. Suddenly it took a nose dive, could not pull out of it, and crashed into a tree. "Just like that tree in front of your window." The pilot got out of the plane as if nothing had happened to him. When the man started to tell the dream, he was not aware of its meaning; when he, however, mentioned the tree in front of my window, the meaning became clear to him.

I have learned how to wait, and I too have learned how to be silent. When my time comes, I hope it will not be up to me to accept it or not. There will be no choice, I hope, no alternative, not even an acceptance. There will be nothing. Come to think of it, that is what my father finally meant I should do: I should do nothing and quietly enjoy my existence as long as it lasts.

LOVE IN A MARRIAGE OF FIFTY-FIVE YEARS

We—that is, my wife and I—have known and loved each other for a long time. It was 57 years ago that we met for the first time, and we have been married for almost that long (55 years). We never regretted our love, even if it was not always easy. The greatest conflict between us was always that I am never, and my wife is always, worried. I don't want to worry because it diminishes my hope and confidence in the future. My wife must worry because, she says, "I am not happy if I have nothing to worry about."

People often ask us: How did you manage to live together for such a long time, in this time of divorce? My wife feels embarrassed by this question. She does not think our marriage was an endurance test she won.

It seems to me that people do not "solve" problems or conflicts—not even in psychoanalysis. People live out of them—or away from them—they don't really forget them. As they go through a new phase of their lives, new conflicts arise, and the old ones become less important. A long psychotherapy is sometimes justified because, in such situations, a therapist tries to keep his or her patient going long enough until he or she has grown and turns to new periods in his or her life, leaving old conflicts behind.

Of course, it helped that our marriage was blessed by good luck—

for which I give my wife full credit—and I take some credit myself. It is one thing to be lucky; it is of equal importance to be ready for it, to use it, and to go on from there to the next stroke of good luck. The first chance to escape is always the best; the first chance to success will never return.

We have not lived our lives together without grief, unhappiness, even despair. But the peculiar fact remains that all these tough times have brought us closer together. I once asked her: How would you live without me? And she answered with that calm smile of the ageless woman, ''After you have gone, I will follow you soon. Don't worry.''

Sex in Old Age

When I read about the joy of sex in old age, I have to laugh. It amuses me to guess the researcher's age and experience, according to his claims. When an old man talks to young or younger would-be sexologists, he rarely tells the truth. Old men are as unreliable as informants as boys in puberty showing off. And old women talk about other people's sexuality but never, or very rarely, about their own. What old people know and what they say to each other, if they have the courage to face the facts of old age is quite different from what they told the researcher or wrote as answers in his or her questionnaire.

Sex in old age—and with that I mean age closer to the 80s than to the 70s—seems to be split in pregenital indulgences and, I feel tempted to say, ''postgenital'' or ''postambivalent'' feelings in the form of tender love, which is mostly asexual love. It is nevertheless true love, as it is deep and of everlasting strength.

Old people love less and mean it more. Old people have intercourse less often after a couple of coronaries, or when taking diuretics, but they feel deeply, nevertheless.

This is a great lesson old people could teach the younger generation. There is nothing to regret or to envy in the younger ones. To love and to feel loved in old age anticipates that the old ones I am talking about have not become lonely, frustrated, bitter, and despaired.

The enjoyment of looking remains strong and alive in old age. A young and pretty nurse in an intensive care unit is sent by the gods and is appreciated as that. When she combines her attractiveness with good humor—and that includes tolerance and kindliness—everybody will be happier for it in a quiet way.

Sex cannot be repressed nor can it be sublimated. It certainly can be controlled or disciplined. Sex has to be enjoyed. But sexuality may certainly become less important in later years. Then, tenderness in love and friendship can grow like never before. I feel it in relationship to my son and my friends—the few ones who are still around—but most of all I feel it in my relationship with my wife Etelka. I also feel it from her. (She is almost as old as I am.) Her name means for me the strange one—the one who came from the dark into the light—the ageless, the understanding one. She always had a kind of superior attitude toward me, which I tried to change for many years and later accepted. It is that kind of benevolent superiority that experienced and mature women develop most frequently when they have been mothers. They then identify with the Mother and begin to feel that men identify forever with the Son.

When our son left us to start his own family, Etelka changed her attitude toward me somewhat. She no longer treated me as the older of two, but I had become now the only one. I remained still, definitely, one to be taken care of. I once asked her: "What would you do if I would grow up overnight?" She only smiled and left the question unanswered. To have felt the nearness of death together was a binding, loving experience, even if I do not recommend it for that purpose.

To feel the nearness of death had done something else to me: It has taught me how to cry, how to feel tears welling up in my eyes. I have often wondered why I never could cry—neither on the death of my father, my brother, my mother, my sister, nor anybody else. Tears of homesickness seemed ridiculous to me.

When I came home from the hospital, I had become old. Etelka smiled at me and said: "I have adopted you."

It is this kind of tender love I needed and to which I tried to respond in kind. To have that kind of love makes us both happy. Life becomes worth living all over again when such tenderness is the final renewal.

My story would be incomplete if I did not mention my son, who has become my friend in these times of sickness. He saw me when I was closer to death than to life in the intensive care unit. It seems that to feel the nearness of death washes away all aspects of ambivalence in old and in young. With a different intensity, this is also true in my feelings to my friend who was with me and still is.

I hope when my time comes to say goodbye to this world and to myself and when I sink into nothingness, I will have enough presence of mind left to say my last words. I would like to say once more and for the last time to my wife: "I love you."

16

Issues and Strategies for Psychotherapy and Psychoanalysis in the Second Half of Life

ROBERT A. NEMIROFF AND CALVIN A. COLARUSSO

In this concluding chapter, we shall delineate some clinical issues crucial to the psychotherapist or psychoanalyst trying to work effectively with middle-aged and elderly patients.

DEVELOPMENTAL FOCUS

We are impressed again and again by the usefulness and power of the developmental or life-cycle orientation in the day-to-day clinical setting. Incorporation of this approach can significantly improve the therapist's understanding of the purpose, process, and results of his or her work. Quoting from the Conference on Psychoanalytic Education and Research report of 1974:

> The implications of the developmental orientation for clinical work stem from the view of individual human development as a continuous and life-long process. One important part of this longitudinal view is the conceptualization of mental illness not in the medical model of disease entities affecting a fully developed organ system, but in the model of functional disturbances which not

303

only impair the current functioning of the individual but impede the development of still-evolving psychic structure and function in one or more of its lines
or aspects. By placing mental illness within the broader context of the ongoing process of development we emphasize that the aim of treatment is to enable development to proceed in all of its dimensions. This viewpoint keeps in
the foreground the awareness that one is treating a person, not an illness.
(p. 14)

The report spelled out additional advantages to viewing the individual
as still developing:

The longitudinal view of the patient as still developing has a further advantage. It focuses on the formation of psychic structure *in process* and under-
scores the contiguity of normal and pathologic outcomes. Psychopathology
is thus understood in terms of psychogenetic and psychodynamic deviations
from normal development and the route of reversibility in treatment is highlighted. *We treat not syndromes but developmentally arrested human beings, who
have through their own defensive activity participated in the formation of their pathology and must in the same way participate in its undoing.* [italics added] (pp. 14–15)

The implications of these formulations for the therapist are profound.
First, a patient *of any age* is understood to be in the midst of dynamic
change, as is amply demonstrated by all 10 of the clinical cases and the
many vignettes in the preceding chapters. Through interactions with
their therapists, all these patients, ranging in age from 40 to 80, were able
to grow and develop. We believe that the key to their successful treatments lay in the ability of their therapists to focus on the current, phase-
specific adult developmental tasks as well as the residue from earlier experiences and conflicts. This point is misunderstood by some of our colleagues as suggesting a superficial attention to the "here and now of
adult experience" exclusively. Not so. We reiterate that the developmental psychotherapist takes *both* childhood and adult experience into account. The therapeutic tasks focuses on three goals: (1) defining the relationship between infantile experience and adult symptomatology; (2)
elaborating the effects of the infantile experience on all subsequent developmental tasks, from childhood through adulthood; and (3) focusing
on the reengagement of the adult developmental process.

The developmental approach has considerable utility in the diagnostic process. In addition to a DSM III assessment and psychodynamic conflict formulation, the clinician is urged to make a *developmental* diagnosis based on a thorough history and assessment of his or her patient's
developmental arrests. As we described in Chapter 3, the concept of *arrest*, which has proved very useful to child analysts, is too rarely applied
in work with adults. Through fixation or regression, progression along

a developmental line may be halted at any point along the life course. In addition to the childhood past, attention must be paid the adult past (Colarusso & Nemiroff, 1979, 1981; Shane, 1977). Employing the concept of developmental arrest, noting where fixation has occurred in the life cycle, and formulating the patient's current, phase-specific developmental tasks allow the therapist to add considerable specificity to his or her diagnosis. This is helpful not only in being able to formulate goals but in initial communications to patients as to why therapy is indicated and what needs to be worked on during it. The approach was first suggested by Erikson's (1959) life cycle model that elaborated the impact of the various stages of development on patients of different age ranges. Most recently, work by Gould (1978), Levinson, Darrow, Klein, Levinson, & McKee (1978), and Vaillant (1977) has further delineated stages of adult growth and change. Levinson *et al.* (1978) schematized a longitudinal life structure with alternating periods of transition and stability, a particularly pertinent construction. It is striking how many of the patients described here first came for help during transitional periods in their lives. Being able to locate his or her patient on the life cycle clarifies the therapist's conceptualization, and he or she is able to describe to the patient the phenomena of the particular period, a maneuver that can immediately strengthen the therapeutic alliance. Subsequently, working on phase-specific problems keeps the treatment on course; indeed, in brief psychodynamic therapy, resolution of the phase-specific transitional task may be the main goal.

Levinson *et al.*'s (1978) description of the midlife transition (ages 40–45) is particularly illustrative of the nature of transitional phenomena in general. The state of mind of an individual at such times involves false starts, emotional turmoil, and despair. "Every genuine reappraisal must be agonizing, because it challenges the assumptions, illusions, and vested interests on which the existing structure is based" (p. 108). The Levinson group goes on to say:

> Every life structure necessarily gives high priority to certain aspects of the self and neglects or minimizes other aspects.... In the Midlife transition these neglected parts of the self urgently seek expression. A man experiences them as "other voices in other rooms" (in Truman Capote's evocative phrase). Internal voices that have been muted for years now clamor to be heard. At times they are heard as a vague whispering, the content unclear but the tone indicating grief over lost opportunities, outrage over betrayal by others, or guilt over betrayal by oneself. At other times they come through as a thunderous roar, the content all too clear, stating names and times and places and

demanding that something be done to right the balance. A man hears the voice of an identity prematurely rejected; of a love lost or not pursued; of a valued interest or relationship give up in acquiescence to parental or other authority; of an internal figure who wants to be an athlete or nomad or artist, to marry for love or remain a bachelor, to get rich, enter the clergy or live a sensual carefree life—possibilities set aside earlier to become what he is now. *During the midlife transition he must learn to listen more attentively to these voices and decide consciously what part he will give them in his life.* [italics added] (Levinson *et al.*, 1978, p. 200)

The developmental focus not only highlights transitional phenomena, it attends to the possibilities for arrest around phase-specific adult developmental tasks, giving considerably specificity and relevance to the therapy. Arrest in the face of such tasks is often expressed indirectly as patients experience the pressures unique to the second half of life; the more the therapist understands about special adult developmental concerns, the more informed and comprehensive his or her approach can be. In Chapter 2, we included King's (1980) excellent summary of some of the main sources of anxiety and concern during the second half of the life cycle (see p. 32). Keeping those in mind has improved our own ability to appreciate the specifically adult difficulties encountered by our patients.

In many of the cases included in this book, the therapists obviously paid particular attention to the issues cited by King. Miller's contribution describing the development of intimacy at age 50 (Chapter 7) is a very good example. Mr. K., a 50-year-old bachelor, came to analysis because of a desire to achieve heterosexual intimacy and an urgent feeling that time was running out. In the background was the fact that his mother was dying of cancer. An important juncture came when his mother died and the patient tried to deny the significance of her death. Sensitive to the midlife developmental tasks of mastering time limitation and death anxiety, Miller persistently confronted him with his denial and encouraged an exploration of its meaning and the need for the defense. The patient expressed his unconscious feelings of loss and hostility in the transference by leaving to go on vacations. Eventually Miller was able to interpret those feelings toward the mother (analyst) and connect them with his patient's lifelong inhibitions toward women of his own age. When Mr. K. started to date, his unconscious fear and hostility emerged again and was worked through.

With regard to the view that only supportive treatment is indicated for the older patient and, conversely, the exploratory treatment is always countraindicated in the face of advanced years, we note that all the cases in *The Race Against Time* attest to the fallaciousness of those too-prevalent suppositions. This was patently so in Notman's moving case (Chapter 12). There, a 68-year-old woman was referred for supportive therapy to prepare for the loss of her husband and living alone. With an open-ended view of development, however, Notman was able to help her make important discoveries about herself. She achieved profound insight about her relationships with her older sister, her children, and her husband and was able to become more assertive and more aware of her own needs, in the process becoming less given to irrational outbursts of embarrassing and inappropriate anger. Our own experience and that of our collaborators reported here attests to the human capacity to use a therapeutic relationship beneficially for growth and suggests that there is waste, if not danger, in an assumption that older patients are not capable of in-depth self-exploration and change.

THE BODY IMAGE

Awareness of and preoccupation with changes in the body in the second half of life are universal phenomena, inadequately conceptualized in the psychoanalytic literature, despite the fact that Freud (1915) placed great emphasis on the influence of the body in early mental development, especially the concepts of the erogenous zones, those circumscribed areas of heightened bodily sensation that are partially responsible for mental development in infancy and early childhood. Similarly, integration of mind and body is dealt with extensively in the psychoanalytic theory of adolescence. The profound biological upheaval of puberty renders much existing mental organization inadequate and requires a reworking of psychic structure, with basic alterations in the mental apparatus. A number of years are necessary to integrate the changes and again achieve a balanced relationship between mind and body.

Yet, for the adult years, a much longer span, we have no defined theory of mind–body relationship until the occurrence of the climacteric (Benedek & Maranon, 1954). Even Erikson (1959), who refers to bodily zones and modes through adolescence, speaks of adulthood only in such abstract terms as intimacy, generativity, and stagnation. In our clinical experience bodily changes start to play an important role in the psychological reactions of men and women as early as age 35. These include small changes in strength and endurance, slightly perceptible changes in skin and muscle tone, some decreases in energy and vigor, mild hearing or vision loss and slower reaction time, loss or graying of hair, or minor change in sexual interest, with occasional impotence. These small bodily changes are reacted to by many people in midlife with considerable anxiety because they symbolize time running out and stir feelings of anxiety about death. These issues are important for both men and women but may be particularly poignant for women in our youth-oriented culture. Middle-aged men are frequently still seen as attractive and sexual, whereas prevailing sociocultural views equate female sexual desirability with a youthful body. Simone De Beauvoir (1974) put the difference starkly:

> Whereas man grows old gradually, woman is suddenly deprived of her femininity; she is still relatively young when she loses the erotic attractiveness and the fertility which, in the view of society and in her own, provide the justification of her existence and her opportunity for happiness. With no future, she still has about one-half of her adult life to live. (p. 640)

In the course of midlife development, there is a normative conflict between wishes to deny the aging process and acceptance of the loss of a youthful body (Colarusso & Nemiroff, 1981). The resolution of this conflict leads to a reshaping of the body image and a more realistic appraisal of the middle-aged body, resulting in a heightened sense of appreciation of the pleasures the body can continue to provide if cared for properly through appropriate activities. However, as mentioned previously, many people react to the changes of aging as a narcissistic injury (Cath, 1962) that in some may result in pathological regression. In a number of ways this regression takes the form of a search for a new body. We have worked with middle-aged patients who suddenly feel an urgent "need" for inappropriate forms of plastic surgery, whereas others leave spouses in search of young mates who have the "hard body feel" and will be their "fountain of youth." Another, more pathological form of regression stimulated by changes in the adult body can be the sudden emergence, for the first time, of perversions. Although earlier fixations exist in such individuals, we have found that specifically adult factors, namely, change in midlife bodily appearance and sexual functioning, can act as powerful sources of narcissistic injury, triggering regression and perverse behavior.

In patients who narcissistically overreact to bodily aging, the normal mourning for their young adult bodies seems to be short-circuited; instead of the resolution of a normative developmental conflict, they attempt a magical repair of body image through surgery or by attempting to fuse with or borrow another person's younger body. In *Adult Development*

(Colarusso & Nemiroff, 1981), we summarized these responses to the narcissistic injury involved in bodily changes during adulthood:

1. *Repairing the body:* actual attempts at repair including plastic surgery, dyeing hair, makeup, exercise, and diet.
2. *Finding a new body:* the search for a new body or parts of a new body through hetero- or homosexual relationships.
3. *Substituting for the body:* adult toys and hobbies such as bigger and better boats, houses, cars, and so on which are used symbolically to compensate for and repair the changes in the body. (Colarusso & Nemiroff, p. 89)

Because adult patients are so deeply influenced by the body, it is incumbent on the therapist to continually assess the patient's thoughts and feelings about physical appearance, function, and aging. Such attitudes may be repeatedly avoided because of the narcissistic injury involved and may not be brought into the treatment unless the therapist is aware of the powerful resistances against them. Active exploration is often indicated, particularly when there is a question of possible organic disease. Appropriate therapeutic intervention may include referral and consultation with medical specialists and evaluation of the results with the patient. Neglect of the adult body in treatment may grow out of the *therapist's* need to avoid the issue. Because therapy is usually done by people in their 30s, 40s, and beyond, therapist and patient are often trying to master the same feelings about bodily decline. The following is a case illustration of a middle-aged women's denial of her physical problems and the necessary interventions by her therapist.

A woman of 38 avoided seeing a cardiologist despite the presence of symptoms (occasional missed beats and an arrhythmia) because of her strong belief that the symptoms were psychological. She did indeed have a cardiac neurosis, based in part on the death of her mother from a heart attack and a serious operation of her own, both at about age 10. She subsequently developed an anxious preoccupation with bodily functioning and a profound fear of physicians. After the establishment of a therapeutic alliance and an extended period of work on the cardiac neurosis, the patient was able, at the therapist's suggestion, to see a cardiologist. The confirmation of definite but controllable organic disease led to a marked increase in cardiac anxiety and major reworking of the infantile factors in the cardiac neurosis, including her rage at her parents (and in the transference, the therapist) for subjecting her to the operation (and to the adult cardiac evaluation).

Many of the patients discussed in this book were preoccupied in a major way with bodily changes and their aging bodies. In the Caths' poignant case (Chapter 13), after suffering a suspected coronary occlusion, Jack, the 54-year-old physician, felt that his death knell had rung, and he was obsessed with his own postcoronary "hypertropied sensor." Both therapist and patient were able to clarify how constantly the latter had been preoccupied with every physiological message of age-related organic change from within. In the second year of residency training, the patient was unable to concentrate or learn as quickly as he expected and suspected early-onset dementia. Cath (1962), who first wrote a paper in which the "midlife ego" is depicted as spending more and more time and energy monitoring age specific psycho-physiological changes in the body, interpreted to this patient that his problems of concentrating and learning were not a manifestation of organic brain disease but that the patient's energies were being depleted by his anticipating some dreaded bodily catastrophe. Again, after the patient's wife developed breast cancer, Cath's sensitivity to the importance of the body in adult life and issues of loss and narcissistic injury was manifested when he agreed to conjoint sessions with the patient, his wife, and his own wife as cotherapist, to discuss, sort out, and clarify the terrifying death sentence of malignancy. The Caths (Chapter 13) describe the confusion patients feel in deciphering the strange ways some physicians deal with their own helplessness in the face of medical defeat. In this case, the surgeon turned his back to the couple as he talked, especially after her destiny had been sealed by the pathologist's report.

Similarly, in Levinson's case (Chapter 9), the patient first came for treatment when she was 62 and was able after years of depression and isolation to finally reestablish contact with her children after nearly 30 years of estrangement. Development was resumed once she was able to function as a mother and progress to her new role as a grandmother. Central in this case was Levinson's ability to work flexibly with Mrs. A.'s multitude of somatic ills, some of which were real and some of which were imagined. Initially, she presented as a markedly obese, 220-pound woman, who was alcohol dependent with many physical complaints. So much of the therapeutic work revolved around real and imagined concerns about physical well-being that Levinson had to work then in close collaboration with the other physicians involved in Mrs. A.'s care. He needed a detailed understanding of the reality of her physical problems (and that reality was constantly changing) in order to help the patient understand and accept the limitations involved. It was also necessary to differentiate for the patient and himself the organic aspects of her condition from those that were primarily psychogenic. Levinson states,

> Like all older patients, Mrs. A. had to integrate a rapidly changing body image with powerful feelings from the past about physical appearance and well-being; in this patient, her physical beauty and slimness were central cornerstones of her self-esteem for most of her life. (p. 187)

As in the Caths' case (Chapter 13), it was crucial that the therapist serve as an ally and translator, bridging the gap between the recommendations of the medical and surgical specialists and her understanding and acceptance of their treatment. These parameters did not interfere with therapeutic progress in this case but cemented the therapeutic alliance and facilitated aspects of maternal and paternal transference. As the patient felt cared for in the therapy, she was better able to care for herself (physically and psychologically) and was able to progress developmentally and achieve new growth.

Probably the ultimate in the absolute centrality and importance of bodily well-being and body image in adulthood is expressed by one of Barbara Myerhoff's "old ladies" in her study of growing old in Venice, California (Myerhoff, 1978):

> Every morning I wake up in pain. I wiggle my toes. Good. They still obey. I open my eyes. Good. I can see. Everything hurts but I get dressed. I walk down to the ocean. Good. It's still there. Now my day can start. About tomorrow I never know. After all, I'm 89. I can't live forever. (p. 20)

SEXUAL MYTHS

Sexuality in later life has given rise to much myth and misunderstanding, despite the ready availability of scientific information. Similar to cultural taboos about infantile sexuality before Freud's great discoveries, sex is thought to be something older people are finished with (biologically) or should be finished with (psychologically). Berezin (1969) traces the origin of the myth that old age is a sexless era, or if it is not it should be, to the timelessness of oedipal feelings. "The oedipal child fiercely clings to his convictions that his parents do not indulge in sexual activity" (p. 132). Berezin tells the story of Sam Levinson, the comedian, who once said,

> When I first found out how babies were born, I couldn't believe it! To think that my mother and father would do such a thing!...My father—maybe, but my mother—*never*! (p. 132)

For Berezin (1969), a consequence of this attitude is that older people adopt a negative view of their own sexual desires, fantasies, and feelings. Thus, the myth of the sexless older years held by young people and the culture in general becomes a self-fulfilling prophecy when they themselves reach old age. Older patients who find they have strong sexual desires are overwhelmed with guilt and shame and feel that they are oversexed. This clinical observation has been made by a number of investigators, including Berezin (1969), Bowman (1963), English and Pearson (1955), Kleegman (1959), Rubin (1965), and Wolff (1957). Thus, it is most important for therapists working with patients in the second half of life to confront their own stereotypes and biases about sexuality in later life, to see if they are interfering with their work and to become as knowledgeable as possible about the scientific evidence in this area.

Weinberg (1969) has concisely reviewed some of the scientific data in this area. The overall conclusion supported by all studies to date is that, when health, opportunity, and partners are available, the elderly can and do enjoy sexual activity (intercourse, masturbation, and fantasies) well into old age. For example Kinsey, Pomeroy, and Martin (1948), studied 126 males and 56 females of 60 years or more and found for most males that the rate of decline in sexual activity in old age did not exceed the rate of decline in their previous decades. The oldest person who was still active was an 88-year-old man married to a 90-year-old woman. The point is that an individual's later life sexual activity is consistent with his or her characteristic lifelong sexual patterns. Newman and Nichols (1960) conducted a large study of 250 persons ranging from 60 to 93; of the 149 who were still married, 54% indicated that they were still sexually active. Only the 75-and-older group showed a significantly lower level of sexual activity. Of 101 single, divorced, or widowed subjects, only 7 reported sexual activity. Freeman (1961) studied 74 men whose ages averaged 71. Seventy-five percent indicated that they still had sexual desire, and 55% indicated a sexual activity, the frequency of which ranged from three or more occasions per week to once every 2 months or less often.

In *Adult Development* (Colarusso & Nemiroff, 1981), we discussed a number of sexual myths related to aging: (1) that the menopausal syndrome is caused solely by estrogen deficiency; (2) that postmenopausal women cannot enjoy sex because of the physiological and psychological effects of estrogen withdrawal; and (3) that a decrease in testosterone levels is responsible for the decline in sexual functioning in older men.

As to the first myth, our review of the evidence indicated that the menopausal syndrome cannot be attributed to estrogen depletion alone, except for those symptoms with a clear somatic basis, namely, the hot flashes of vasomotor instability. It was our hypothesis that many menopausal symptoms may be psychologically based, occurring in women with an exaggerated response to phase-specific developmental events such as loss of fertility, aging of the body, and loss of the mothering function. We feel the implications for treatment are significant. Diagnosis and treatment should be based on a combined psychobiological approach that assumes that the reasons for the occurrence of the symptoms are more complex than simple hormone loss and that treatment must do more than replace the hormone loss. A combination of dynamic psychotherapy and hormone replacement is probably indicated in most cases.

In the minds of many is the myth that elderly women gradually become asexual, primarily because of the physical and psychological changes produced by diminished estrogen production. It is assumed that there is a direct relationship between aging, specifically hormone depletion, and the loss of sexual interest and ability. Masters and Johnson's (1966) work bears directly on this issue. Their research showed definite changes in the sexual organs of older women attributable to diminished estrogen production but that could not be correlated with sexual capacity or performance. To quote them:

> Thus the simple fact remains that if the opportunity for regularity of coital exposure is created or maintained, the elderly woman suffering from all of the vaginal stigmatas of sex-steroid starvation still will retain a far higher capacity for sexual performance than her female counterpart who does not have similar coital opportunities. (pp. 241–242)

It is clear that the therapist who treats the elderly woman as a dried-up, asexual "prune" will be perpetrating a long-standing, harmful myth and may be doing his or her patient a disservice by ignoring such vital factors as sexual attitudes, physical health, and the availability of sexual partners.

The last myth we investigated was that a decrease in testosterone levels is responsible for the decline in sexual functioning in older men. We reviewed a number of studies that demonstrated a lack of any clear-cut evidence for a significant decrease in testosterone production with age and uncertainty about the relationship between testosterone levels and sexual functioning. These studies cast doubt upon a simple biological etiology for any decline in male sexual function with age (Harman, 1978, 1979; Sachar, Halpern, Rosenfelt, Gallagher, & Hellman, 1973). Similarily, there is considerable doubt about a correlation between the

314 CHAPTER 16

so-called "male menopause" and symptoms of impotence with direct biological changes. Masters and Johnson (1966) comment on the problems of secondary impotence:

> The fear of performance reflecting cultural stigmas directed toward erective inadequacy was that associated with problems of secondary impotence. These fears were expressed, under interrogation, by every male study subject beyond forty years of age, irrespective of reported levels of formal education. Regardless of whether the individual male study subject had ever experienced an instance of erective difficulty, the probability that secondary impotence was associated directly with the aging process was vocalized constantly. The fallacy that secondary impotence is to be expected as the male ages is probably more firmly entrenched in our culture than any other misapprehension. . . . In most instances, secondary impotence is a reversible process for all men regardless of age, unless there is a background of specific trauma. (pp. 203–204)

As with the studies regarding estrogen depletion in women, therapists will do a disservice by assuming that their male patients' complaints of decreased sexual interest or impotence is automatically the result of lower testosterone levels. Sexual anxieties, regardless of the patient's age, are complex problems that need to be explored both biologically and psychologically in an open-ended, nonsimplistic fashion devoid of sexual myths.

Because older patients have the potential for a full and active sexual life, we should not be surprised that their sexuality would be manifest in the psychotherapeutic situation. Gitelson (1965) describes very successful psychoanalytic psychotherapy with a depressed, inhibited 66-year-old woman who developed a passionate erotic transference as her treatment developed. Through fantasies, dreams, and associations, she experienced erotic thoughts and sensations about her analyst, her former analyst of 20 years ago, her dead husband, and a co-worker in her current life. Eventually, the patient recognized that these thoughts and feelings were about a man whom she had met and fallen in love with when she was 17. She and Gitelson discovered how she had unconsciously yearned for this man all her life and how her feelings of guilt, masochism, and depression were in part unconscious punishments for her erotic feelings that she was now experiencing fully via the transference for the first time at 66. At the conclusion of her treatment, her depression had lifted, she felt less masochistic, and her inhibitions to participating more fully in family, social, and community life were markedly improved.

In the case material in this book, Crusey's beautifully described case of short-term psychodynamic psychotherapy with a 62-year-old man (Chapter 8) illustrates many of the issues discussed in this section. The patient was referred to Crusey after he had suffered a myocardial infarction and was under considerable emotional stress. His stresses were related to the fact that he was both carrying out full-time responsibilities as an executive and caring at home for his wife of 38 years, who had 2 years prior to his infarction suffered a stroke that left her paralyzed. His doctor had recommended that she be placed in a convalescent center, which raised many conflictual feelings for the patient.

As treatment began with Mr. D., there were immediate manifestations of a sexual transference to Crusey, who was some 30 years younger than he. These feelings started to be acted out through an affair with a younger divorced nurse. Because of the immediacy of this reaction, Crusey needed to explore the possible connections to herself, courageously pursuing the psychodynamic exploration and resisting the temptation only to support or try to manipulate the older patient's environment. However, this was not without trepidation, as Crusey realized that some of her countertransference reactions to Mr. D. were of an oedipal grandparent type. As she states,

> My concern was how to engender respect and develop a therapeutic alliance with a patient who approached each session as a date, particularly a patient who was old enough to be my grandfather. (p. 165)

Also,

> I was listening to a man close to my grandfather's age, who had a responsible, authoritative position in a major firm and was discussing difficulties of an infantile nature. How timelessly intact the unconscious has remained! (p. 157)

When Dr. Crusey was able to sort out these feelings, she was in a position to acknowledge the therapeutic legitimacy of discussing the patient's sexual feelings for her. The correctness of her intervention was borne out by the patient's producing a patently Oedipal dream about his parents and himself:

> I was on the back porch with my mother who was shampooing my hair. She promised to give me some strawberries if I didn't fuss too much while she washed my hair. We had just finished when my father walked in and started yelling at my mother for giving me the last of the strawberries. She was supposed to save them. (p. 157)

This triangular oedipal dream and the associations to the dream opened the door to a considerable amount of repressed genetic material that was very germane to Mr. D.'s lifelong sexual conflicts and defenses. This case illustrates how older patients develop erotic transference toward their therapists, regardless of age, theirs or their therapist's, just as younger patients do. These transferences, again, just as with young patients, are based on the powerful imprinting of the primary objects, namely, the mother and father of the nuclear family. Crusey's appreciation for the "timelessness of the unconscious" is very apt here. Another important paradigm emerges in the case of Mr. D., that of the multigenerational transference, which we discuss in more detail in the next section of the chapter. The patient developed a variety of generational transferences toward the therapist. As Crusey describes:

> In the many transference postures of our therapeutic relationship, I was the domineering mother, the seductive lover, and the unborn daughter. Mr. D.'s age uniquely impacted on the treatment in each of these situations. As the domineering mother, I needed to juxtapose Mr. D.'s feelings about being a good little boy with his very real adult circumstances and accomplishments. Similarly, it was important that I respect the healthy sexual drives of a 62-year-old man while simultaneously understanding the adolescent oedipal impulses as his seductive lover. Finally, the transference relationship of the unborn daughter provided Mr. D. with the opportunity to care for and mourn the loss of the opportunity for his own child while we maintained the boundaries of our therapeutic relationship. (p. 165)

The effectiveness of therapeutic work in this case was directly related to Crusey's ability to accept and work nondefensively with the undiminished intrapsychic sexuality of her older patient as it developed in the transference relationship. As a result of his psychodynamic psychotherapy, Mr. D. was able to establish a new and healthier homeostasis, reexperience and revive long dormant erotic feelings, dramatically confront the realistic limitations of his age, and attempt to accept his losses.

Finally, Weinberg (1969) raises a very important issue about the sexuality of the aged, stating that the aged have lost their cultural erotic value and appeal and seem to pass to the sidelines. Although older people may not have the opportunity for direct sexual expression, they still need sublimated or alternative forms of human contact. Weinberg writes sensitively:

> If old people are invisible, they are also untouchable. No one seems to want to touch the older person. Very few seek physical contact with them. Yet what seems to be instinctual and acquired needs for contactual relationships are sought by all living organisms. We are all too ready to touch and even caress and pat the young and the cat or the dog, but not the aged. Our physi-

cal encounters with them are perfunctory, with no warmth or conviction behind them. Theirs is a psychobiological hunger that usually remains ungratified. If sensory organs of the skin of the old become dull, as they so often do, it is as if this were in response to an anticipated deprivation. There is no need to feel, if feelings are to be denied. It is an unspoken grievance that needs to be redressed. (p. 213)

TRANSFERENCE AND COUNTERTRANSFERENCE

Transference and countertransference in the second half of life are complex phenomena, requiring that the analyst understand his or her patient in an adult developmental context. This complexity is particularly well illustrated by three issues: (1) the relationship between the adult past and the infantile neurosis; (2) multigenerational or reversed transference; and (3) specific countertransference patterns in treating older patients.

Relationship between the Adult Past and the Infantile Neurosis

In Chapter 4, we suggested that transference phenomena in adulthood, in addition to being new editions or elaborations of infantile experience are also expressions of new experiences and conflicts from those developmental stages beyond childhood and the continuation of central developmental themes (although in altered form) from childhood to adulthood. All three factors are represented in the present by psychic structure that is vastly different from that which existed in childhood, and is still undergoing continuous change and refinement, regardless of the age of the patient. In such a framework, the adult past as well as the childhood past is understood to be an important source of transference (Shane, 1977). Further, transference phenomena are recognized as simultaneous expressions of current midlife or late adulthood developmental conflicts *and* recapitulations of the infantile past. We find our views very much in agreement with those of Cohler (1980) who stated in an important paper on adult development psychology and reconstruction in psychoanalysis:

Consideration of the impact of psychological development across the life cycle on the experience of remembering the past shows that is impossible to consider an objective past apart from developmentally determined views of this past which emerge successively during childhood, adolescence, young adulthood, and middle and old age. The fantasies which emerge during the oedipal phase are but prototypes of such developmentally determined fantasies which are associated with each of the phases of development across the life cycle. Review of findings from empirical research on the memorial process at middle age, and of the reminiscence process of life review in old age, suggests that there are also fantasies distinctive to phases of development. (pp. 174–175)

We suggest that the relationship between the infantile neurosis and subsequent experiences may be divided into three steps:

1. Developmental experience during the preoedipal and oedipal phases predisposes the individual to the possibility of an adult neurosis. During the oedipal phase, for the first time, sexual and aggressive impulses are expressed primarily through the framework of triangular object relationships. Because of the combination of drive expression and ego development that occurs then, the psychic apparatus is capable of responding with neurotic symptom formation in response to conflict, namely, the infantile neurosis.

2. Subsequent developmental phases, both in childhood and adulthood, participate as well. When the infantile neurosis is not resolved, the neurotic pattern may continue unabated from the oedipal stage onward, traceable through each later phase of development where it is elaborated by new experiences; or the neurotic patterns may disappear, only to be precipitated by later events.

3. The adult presentation of the neurosis is the result of the infantile predisposition, subsequent elaboration, and current developmental experience. All of these are condensed into the symptom picture forged by the psychic apparatus of the present. In a sense, the adult mind rewrites the experience from childhood, shaping its presentation in the adult transference. Thus, all three aspects (organization and predisposition, subsequent elaboration, and adult presentation) are important to an understanding of the transference and the determination of technique. Coltrera (1979) has expressed a similar developmental view of transference. He states:

> The transference neurosis is very much developmentally determined, its character and focus changing throughout the life cycle according to phase-specific developmental and conflict resolutions and their subsequent internalizations. (p. 189)

These conceptualizations lead us to suggest that, technically, it is not enough to help the patient gradually see the relationship between the infantile and adult neurosis, that is, the oedipal and preoedipal reconstructions. That is but one step in the therapeutic process. It is necessary for patient and analyst to detail the elaboration of the neurosis in adolescence and adulthood, relating it to significant life events, and to describe the neurotic interference with normal adolescent and adult developmental tasks. Then, as described by Shane (1977), the patient should apply the insights and freedom gained in analysis to his or her present and future development. As with the child analytic patient, he or she should be able to return to the mainstream of development relatively free from the powerful skewing effect of the neurosis. Cohler (1980), expressing the developmental view, succinctly describes an important goal for the analyst:

> There are a number of developmentally salient conflicts which are called forth at particular transition points across the life cycle and which have the effect of reorganizing the personal biography in ways which were not possible earlier in the life cycle. The task is to understand this process and the means by which a consistent personal history has been created as a result of these transformations. Increased awareness of this process is among the most effective means of fostering the capacity for self-observation and for increased neutralization which Kris (1956) views as an important goal of psycho-analysis. (p. 187)

Multigenerational Transferences

The therapist who works with older patients is the object of powerful transference feelings from *all* stages of the life cycle. This experience increases the complexity of the therapeutic task, requiring a considerable degree of empathy, a developmental understanding of transference, and much flexibility. In Chapter 11, Hildebrand, discussing some of the complexities of the multigenerational transferences of his intriguing case presentations, suggests that

> we need to be prepared to embody both early and adult figures in the patient's life in order to help revalue and rework the past in the conventional way. On the other hand, much more than with younger patients, we have to become the embodiment of the ideal child or children whom the patient needs as the guarantors of his or her immortality and thus the future. (p. 218)

This later point we might call *reversed transference* because it reverses the usual paradigm of analysand experiencing the analyst as a parental authority figure but rather experiences the analyst as a much younger individual. In most of the case reports presented here, the multigenerational transference experience was encountered. We can best illustrate this phenomenon by reviewing some examples.

In Levinson's case (Chapter 9) of the 62-year-old woman who finally was able to accept her roles as mother and grandmother, there were a number of striking examples of multigenerational transferences. Initially, the transference was one of the therapist as the all-knowing, good father who could protect and dominate. As the therapy progressed, within the transference, Levinson became her "lost child, young, naive, and experienced, learning about the world from a wise, loving mother/grandmother" (p. 183). Mrs. A. was now transferring feelings and wishes from her adult past about her experiences as a mother and her as-yet unrealized maternal ego ideal. A son or daughter transference (reversed transference) is not a variation or a replacement for the traditional versions of transference; it exists side by side in older patients with the more traditional forms of transference.

The shifting generational transference was well illustrated in Cohen's work with an 80-year-old woman (Chapter 10). The patient, a childless widow who sought psychiatric treatment for the first time at 80 because of the death of a close friend and increasing feelings of loneliness, quickly developed a transference relationship with Cohen. In fairly rapid shifts throughout the therapy, Cohen was seen as a son, a lover, or a father. Particularly striking was the development of the erotic transference in this 80-year-old woman. Cohen vividly describes the shift in the transference from being a son to being a lover:

> As therapy progressed, the transference changed. She started to talk more about her relationships with men and took noticeably more care in her appearance around me. In one of our sessions, she brought in a framed 9-by-12-inch photograph of her in her 20s that was designed to stand on a table. I was sitting behind a desk, and she beside the desk on that occasion. While talking about the photography, she placed it on the desk in such a manner that it partially blocked my view of her. *It seemed that she was trying to get me to see her physically as a younger woman.* [italics added] (p. 199–200)

Hiatt (1971) studied the transference-countertransference problems in the dynamic outpatient psychotherapy of 19 patients ranging in age from 60 to 84 and followed them for a 15-year period, both during therapy and after termination. He describes myriad transference patterns, which we have called *multigenerational transferences*. His cases demonstrated that patients over 60 have accrued many more key figures in their histories than younger patients. For example,

> A spouse may occupy a greater span of years than a parental figure, and children, who may be all that remain of the patient's family constellation, tend to alter the transference seen in psychotherapy. In the "replaying of the cho-

rus'' of those growing older, the therapist should try to uncover the ''infantile neurosis''; however, other significant figures than the patient's parents
may have an impact on the transference which the patient reflects with his
physician. (p. 593)

Hiatt (1971) has ordered the multigenerational transferences into four
useful categories.

(a) *Parental transference.* The patient reacts to the therapist as a parental authority, forming a parent–child relationship. In many instances, the
older patient because of dependency needs endows the therapist with
omnipotent powers and transfers to the therapist a ''godlike'' trust, similar to the hero worship.

(b) *Peer or sibling transference.* In therapy, the patient may put the
therapist in the role of a deceased spouse, a confidant, a close colleague,
or not unusually a younger or older sibling. According to Hiatt (1971),

This group looked to the therapist to confirm ego reality, help with decision
making, and to share experiences of an interpersonal nature involving other
members of the family. It may be somewhat startling to the therapist to have
his age ignored and be transformed into a most trusted symbol of the patient's
spouse, business associate, or roommate. (p. 594)

(c) *Son, son-in-law, grandson transference.* This ''reversed transference
reaction'' is quite common in working with older patients. In this situation, the patient may consider himself or herself the superior or the
teacher of the therapist and the therapist the pupil, strongly denying dependency feelings.

(d) *Sexual transference.* In Hiatt's cases, the transference reaction was
similar to those seen in much younger hysterical girls. These patients,
at advanced ages, were still struggling with unresolved oedipal feelings.

Specific Countertransference Patterns in Treating Older Patients

All the typical countertransference responses that therapists have toward younger patients are experienced with individuals in middle and
late adulthood. However, there are others that are more directly related
to the older patient's age and position on the life course. First and foremost is the therapist's reaction to his or her own aging. Therapy is done
for the most part by individuals either entering middle age or well into
middle age or older. In our experience, the issues involving their own
aging process, that is, bodily changes, significant losses, appreciation of
life's limitations, and death anxiety, are difficult to confront. Further,
those therapists practicing dynamic psychotherapy or psychoanalysis face

their aging without the benefit of therapy or analysis because, for the most part, they have had their treatment experiences in earlier training years and, as a rule, are reluctant to again enter a treatment process unless a specific crisis is upon them. There have been many examples of countertransferences reported in the cases presented in this book. Hassler, for example (Chapter 6), is most open and forthright in discussing his own countertransference and how it interacted with the patient's transference.

Mr. B., an intelligent, articulate architect sought analysis after a year of depression, self-doubt, and intermittent resentment toward his adolescent daughter. The onset of depression coincided with her entering puberty. In a far-reaching and successful analysis, Hassler and his patient were able to explore and resolve many issues. Very valuable in this case presentation is Hassler's description of his own countertransference reactions to his patient's aging and mourning the loss of his youth. In reviewing the process of the case, specifically around the 40th birthday, Hassler noted that he ignored many of the patient's references to aging and then did not explore the patient's obviously ambivalent feelings about the birthday party or its significance to the patient. Most striking, in the analyst's denial of the aging process, was his omitting to inquire about the detail of "the halftime" in a nodal dream at that time. In retrospect, Hassler associated his denial to his own hoped-to-be-forgotten birthday coming up in the next month. In his candid assessment of the case, Hassler states,

> Although Mr. B. adapted rather well to the realities of turning 40 and was able to move toward a successful termination in analysis, there might have been yet further gain in his perspective on the adult challenges and meaningful pleasure he faced if the analyst had wondered on any number of occasions about the significance of the aging process. (p. 114)

Thus, in the treatment of the patient in the second half of life, it would be well not only to be sensitive to the patient's associations to aging, direct and indirect, but also for the analyst rigorously and continually to question himself or herself about the ways in which his or her own feelings about aging (or the denial of same) are playing a part in the treatment. Hassler sums up these issues well:

> For both the middle-aged (or older) analyst and his or her patient, thoughts and feelings about the finiteness of time and personal death, although disguised, are rarely absent. Both partners in the analytic process deny on various levels the clinical and developmental significance of this objective time

> frame. This is complicated by the immersion in a transference–
> countertransference relationship where the nontime frame of reference of
> childhood often prevails as part of a technical procedure that is not defined
> by time parameters. Perhaps an increased understanding of adult develop-
> mental processes will provide a conceptual bridge between these different time
> references. (p. 115)

As we discussed earlier in this chapter, the therapist who does not understand the power of the sexual life of older patients may be dismayed by both the patient's sexuality and his or her own sexual response to the patient. This may be due to unresolved oedipal feelings about parental sexuality. The countertransferences have their sources from both childhood, which are related to the infantile neurosis, and adulthood, which are related to oedipal triumph and guilt over aging or dead parents (Colarusso & Nemiroff, 1979). For example, an analyst's initial responses to the erotic transference of a 70-year-old woman were shock at the intensity of the patient's sexual feelings and surprise when he became aroused in response. Self-analysis led to the awareness of considerable curiosity about such a sexual encounter, and he traced his countertransference to fantasies related to infantile sexual desires for his mother.

Because of physical and/or emotional vulnerability and isolation, the older patient may wish to be dependent on the analyst. Because of the patient's age, relative nearness to death, and realistic difficulties, the analyst may respond inappropriately by becoming either unduly supportive or controlling. His or her countertransference response may be based on infantile wishes to control and dominate the formerly all-powerful oedipal or preoedipal parent, who is now a helpless captive in the transference–countertransference bond. Countertransference responses may also be related to later stages of the analyst's development, expressions of unresolved conflict from adolescence through middle adulthood that are based on his or her experiences with his or her own parents as they aged and perhaps eventually died.

Although not strictly a countertransference response, close attention should be paid by the analyst to his emotional reaction to interactions with his own parents in the present because they may be approximately the same age as his patients and dealing also with the developmental tasks of late adulthood. Hiatt (1971) points out how many clinicians agree that it is quite important for therapists to have a clear understanding of their relationships with their own parents and grandparents before treating other people's parents. Unexplored countertransference reactions stemming from a therapist's own parents may lead to oversolicitiousness, idealization, and unrealistic expectations of strength or subtle deprecations, competitive feelings, and pity. "Sometimes the therapist feels that the older patient should be obeyed, feared, or praised—strong remnants of his own childhood" (p. 597).

A final example of countertransference in work with older patients involves sibling issues. As mentioned, not only do older patients develop strong sexual and aggressive transferences toward the analyst, but a strong son or daughter transference should be expected as well. Often, the analyst is seen as the ideal, caring child, respectful of, and attentive to, the loving parent. Wishes in the analyst to be the favorite or only child readily complement the patient's desires to treat him or her so, leading to a mutually gratifying interaction within the analysis rather than analytic understanding. The analyst may also enjoy "favorite child" status in his or her mind by making comparisons between himself or herself and the patient's grown children, who may be approximately his or her age. In the countertransference, his caring, involved attitude could be seen by him as superior to the more realistically ambivalent, less involved response of the actual child. In the event of serious illness or other disruption in the patient's life, the analyst may meet and interact with the patient's children, thus encountering a real situation in which those feelings could be acted out.

Hiatt (1971) has categorized specific countertransference reactions on the part of therapists as follows:

1. *An omnipotent or unrealistic hope.* An example of this countertransference is the therapist's denying the realistic infirmities of his or her patients, imputing more strength to them than exists, and denying his or her own fears of death.

2. *The feeding of one's narcissism and gaining personal gratification.* Because of the tendencies of the older patient to hold his or her therapist in awe and consider him or her omnipotent, the therapist must carefully guard against playing an omnipotent "godlike" role for his or her own narcissistic gratification.

3. *An unreasonable anger and desire to avoid work with the older patient.* Older patients (like younger ones) can be quite manipulative and demanding. With regression that is associated with aging, oral, aggressive, overly dependent behavior can provoke countertransference responses of anger and withdrawal.

4. *The feeling of pity and sorrow for a person at the end of life.* Therapists may overidentify with the accumulated misfortunes of older patients,

thereby not providing them with the necessary professional empathy and realistic assessments of their possibilities.

LIMITED OBJECT TIES, TERMINATION, AND DEATH

It is appropriate that we conclude with some impressions of the unique issues of termination of therapy with the older patient. The transference neurosis emerges, in part, because of the intense relationship between patient and therapist. The therapist is predictably there, and if the patient is in analysis, the analyst is there, day after day, week after week, available to the patient within analytic limits. For young patients, the tie to the therapist, as intimate as it may be, is usually only one of several significant relationships. The patient remains deeply involved with a spouse or lover, children, friends, and relatives. Such is not always the case with an older patient. The spouse may be dead; children, even when attentive, may be separated by distance. Stanley Cath (1965, p. 40) feels that "the maintenance of meaningful object relationships may truly be said to be the principal psychic task of the later years." When the older person has a limited number of significant object ties, the analytic relationship is all the more important, and the emergence and course of the transference are strongly affected. Positive transference themes may become intense earlier in the analysis; the patient may be more reluctant than usual to give them up because the gratification obtained may fill a void of loneliness. Negative transference may be more difficult to analyze because of the patient's reluctance to jeopardize the valuable relationship. This difficulty in resolving the transference also complicates termination. Symbolically, the continuation of therapy represents the continuation of life itself, whereas termination involves the real loss of a sustaining object tie and may signify death. This tendency to use the analyst as a real object in an exaggerated way is not, however, characteristic of all older persons; many have rich and varied relationships and can tolerate the deprivation required by the analytic situation.

Kahana's most insightful comparison of the therapies of two very different elderly men (Chapter 14) bears on some of the issues raised previously in regard to termination. Specifically, in dealing with the issue of terminating the "ant's" treatment, Kahana had to take into account the patient's lifelong vulnerability, limited tolerence of therapeutic regression, and persistent need for support based on severe traumatization in childhood. For these reasons, particularly considering the patient's age, he conceived of the treatment in an appropriate, nondefensive way, as an interminable one. However, although support was important, Kahana was also able to interpret transference at significant points in the treatment. Grotjahn (Chapter 15) also points out that we should not be afraid to offer our patients interminable therapies by saying,

> It seems to me that people do not "solve" problems or conflicts—not even in psychoanalysis. People live out of them—or away from them—they don't really forget them. As they go through a new phase in their lives, new conflicts arise, and the old ones become less important. A long psychotherapy is sometimes justified because in such situations a therapist tries to keep his or her patient going long enough until he or she has grown and turns to new periods in life, leaving old conflicts behind. (p. 300)

Kahana expresses well the goals and results of his sensitive and patient long-term therapy with his older patient:

> Overall, he was helped with his acute depression and showed a gradual capacity for better resolution of narcissistic and oedipal conflicts. He matured in ways appropriate to the life cycle, with consideration of aging, possible retirement, and natural death. There was partial amelioration of his overwork tendency and growth of the capacity to enjoy life. (p. 284)

Termination in therapy is frequently associated with dying and death anxiety. Of course this is an issue we all must face; Freud was fond of quoting Goethe's famous saying, "Each man owes nature a death." Therapy in the second half of life can be extremely useful in, first, confronting our mortality, examining our own specific fantasies and anxieties concerning what death will be like for us, and placing dying in the perspective of our total life. Lifton (1979) has brought attention to the contemporary awareness of death and the human need for a sense of continuity. In Lifton's opinion, Americans have awakened to the importance of death and anxiety about death, but "more elusive has been the psychological relationship between the phenomena of death and the flow of life." Lifton has applied his ideas to the life cycle and specifically to adulthood.

An integration, or balance of immediate fulfillment and ultimate connectedness, grows from the adult's capacity to be aware of death without being incapacited by anxiety about it. The image of death, what Erikson calls "an ego chill," a shudder attending the awareness of our possible nonexistence, is for the most part suppressed in American culture during young adulthood. However, Lifton and many other researchers, including ourselves, find that sometime during the late 30s and early 40s thoughts of one's own death persistently intrude into consciousness. Tasks are carried out in a "race against time" with a sense of "now or never." This urgency may peak during the midlife transition, but we feel an important point is that in one form or another, conscious for some and unconscious for others, the anxiety about death pervades much of the second half of life, particularly at key transition points.

Grotjahn's moving and courageous description of his own illness and his self-analysis (Chapter 15) is an inspiration for all of us. He vividly describes his aging process and the period of time when he became seriously ill and attempted to deny it. On the night of a serious attack of dyspnea, secondary to his as yet undiagnosed coronary heart attacks he faced his death anxiety:

> I could not sleep, and an indescribable terror overpowered me. I felt I was being annihilated and destroyed. I was facing stark, timeless, formless nothingness.... I thought it was embarrassing and shameful for a psychiatrist to feel anxiety. (p. 295)

Later on, having more attacks now secondary to congestive heart failure and angina pain Grotjahn says that "it was a panic without visual images, far beyond any words—a certainty of impending death. Only the kind face of my wife would reassure me" (p. 296). Grotjahn tells us that he was always "his best patient," and with his considerable powers of introspection, he tries to enjoy the time he has left, still trying to comprehend what his own death or "nothingness" will be like.

> I have time now. I do not know how much time is left for me to live, but I am in no hurry. I am in no hurry to get anywhere, not even to the end of time. That can wait. When that time comes, I will try to accept it. I have no illusions; it will not be easy. Right now, I live in the moment, and I want to sit here a little while longer, quietly, and hoping not to sit in anybody's way. I always thought old age is an achievement in itself. I now know better: To get sick and to live on, that is an achievement. (p. 296)

Grotjahn's "race against time" is over; he is content to stop running, to introspect, and to feel cohesive and together with his loved ones and the world. However, like many of the patients described in this book, in both therapy and life, growth and development, new insight, and self-realization seem to be a never-ending process.

REFERENCES

Benedek, T., & Maranon, G. The climacteric. In A. M. Karch (Ed.), *Men: The variety and meaning of the sexual experience.* New York: Dell, 1954.

Berezin, M. A. Sex and old age: A review of the literature. *Journal of Geriatric Psychiatry,* 1969, 2, 131–149.

De Beauvoir, S. *The second sex.* New York: Vintage Books, 1974.

Bowman, K. M. The sex life of the aging individual. In M. F. De Martino (Ed.), *Sexual behavior and personality characteristics.* New York: Citadel Press, 1963.

Cath, S. H. Grief, loss and emotional disorders in the aging process. In M. A. Berezin & S. H. Cath (Eds.), *Geriatric psychiatry.* New York: International Universities Press, 1962.

Cohler, B. J. Adult developmental psychology and reconstruction in psychoanalysis. In S. I. Greenspan & G. H. Pollock (Eds.), *The course of life: Psychoanalytic contributions toward understanding personality development: Vol III. Adulthood and the aging process.* Rockville, Md.: National Institute of Mental Health, 1980.

Colarusso, C. A., & Nemiroff, R. A. Some observations and hypothesis about the psychoanalytic theory of adult development. *International Journal of Psycho-Analysis,* 1979, 60, 59–71.

Colarusso, C. A., & Nemiroff, R. A. *Adult development: A new dimension in psychodynamic theory and practice.* New York: Plenum Press, 1981.

Coltrera, J. Truth from genetic illusion: The transference and the fate of the infantile neurosis. *Journal of the American Psychoanalytic Association,* 1979, 27 (Supplement), 289–314.

Conference on Psychoanalytic Education and Research. Commission IX, *Child Analysis.* New York: American Psychoanalytic Association, 1974.

English, O. S. & Pearson, G. H. J. *Emotional problems of living.* New York: Norton, 1955.

Erikson, E. Identity and the life cycle. *Psychological issues* (Monograph 1). New York: International Universities Press, 1959.

Freeman, J. T. Sexual capacities in the aging male. *Geriatrics,* 1961, 16, 37–43.

Freud, S. Instincts and their vicissitudes. *Standard edition,* 14:109. London: Hogarth Press, 1915.

Gitelson, M. Transference reaction in a sixty-six year old woman. In M. A. Berezin & S. H. Cath (Eds.), *Geriatric psychiatry: Grief, loss, and emotional disorders in the aging process.* New York: International Universities Press, 1965.

Gould, R. L., *Transformation: Growth and change in adult life.* New York: Simon & Schuster, 1978.

Harman, S. M. Clinical aspects of aging of the male reproductive system. In E. L. Schneider (Ed.), *Aging: Vol. 4. The aging reproductive system.* New York: Raven Press, 1978.

Haiman, S. W. Male menopause? The hormones flow but sex does slow. *Medical World News,* 1979, 20, 11.

Hiatt, H. Dynamic psychotherapy with the aging patient. *American Journal of Psychotherapy,* 1971, 25, 591–600.

King, P. H. The life cycle as indicated by the nature of the transference in the psychoanalysis of the middle-aged and elderly. *International Journal of Psycho-Analysis,* 1980, 61, 153.

Kinsey, A. C. , Pomeroy, W. B., & Martin, C. E. *Sexual behavior in the human male.* Philadelphia: W. B. Saunders, 1948.

Kleegman, S. J. Frigidity in women. *Quarterly Review of Surgical Obstetrics and Gynecology,* 1959, 16, 243–248.

Kris, E. The recovery of childhood memories in psychoanalysis. *The Psychoanalytic Study of the Child,* 1956, 11, 54–88.

Levinson, D. J., Darrow, C. N., Klein, E. B., Levinson, M. H., & McKee, B. *The seasons of a man's life.* New York: Knopf, 1978.

Lifton, R. J. *The broken connection.* New York: Simon & Schuster, 1979.

Masters, W., & Johnson, V. *Human sexual response.* Boston: Little, Brown, 1966.

Myerhoff, B. *Number our days.* New York: Dutton, 1978.

Newman, G., & Nicholas, C. R. Sexual activities and attitudes in older persons. *Journal of the American Medical Association,* 1960, *173,* 33–35.

Rubin, I. *Sexual life after sixty.* New York: Basic Books, 1965.

Sachar, E. S., Halpern, F., Rosenfelt, R. S., Gallagher, T. F., & Hellman, L. Plasma and urinary testosterone levels in depressed men. *Archives of General Psychiatry,* 1973, *28,* 15.

Shane, M. A rationale for teaching analytic technique based on a developmental orientation and approach. *International Journal of Psychoanalysis,* 1977, *58,* 95–108.

Vaillant, G. E. *Adaptation to life.* Boston: Little, Brown, 1977.

Weinberg, J. Sexual expression in late life. *American Journal of Psychiatry,* 1969, *236* (5), 713–716.

Wolff, K. Definition of the geriatric patient. *Geriatrics,* 1957, *12,* 102–106.

Index